HOW *NOT* TO GET PREGNANT

Other books by Sherman J. Silber, M.D.

HOW TO GET PREGNANT
THE MALE: FROM INFANCY TO OLD AGE

HOW *NOT* TO GET PREGNANT

YOUR GUIDE TO SIMPLE, RELIABLE CONTRACEPTION

SHERMAN J. SILBER, M.D.

Illustrations by Scott Barrows

WARNER BOOKS

A Warner Communications Company

This book is not intended as a substitute for the medical advice of physicians. The reader should regularly consult a physician in matters relating to his/her health and particularly with respect to any symptoms that may require diagnosis or medical attention.

This book contains many references to actual cases the author has encountered over the years. However, names and other identifying characteristics have been changed to protect the privacy of those involved.

Warner Books Edition
Copyright © 1987 by Sherman J. Silber, M.D.
All rights reserved.
This Warner Books edition is published by arrangement with Charles Scribner's Sons, 866 Third Avenue, New York, NY 10022.

Warner Books, Inc., 666 Fifth Avenue, New York, NY 10103

W A Warner Communications Company

Printed in the United States of America
First Warner Books Printing: August 1990
10 9 8 7 6 5 4 3 2 1

Library of Congress Cataloging-in-Publication Data
Silber, Sherman J.
　How not to get pregnant / by Sherman J. Silber.
　　p.　　cm.
　ISBN 0-446-39088-7
　1. Contraception.　I. Title.
[RG136.S518　1990]
613.9′4—dc20　　　　　　　　89-29238
　　　　　　　　　　　　　　　CIP

Cover design by Anthony Russo

This book is written for:
my successful infertility patients who have had enough,
those who simply want to plan so they can cherish,
and those who do not want to ruin their chances for having
children later, even though presently it is out of the question.

This book is dedicated to:
My wife and three boys,
for whom we planned, and whom we cherish.

Acknowledgments

I want to thank my many colleagues, too numerous to name all, for their advice and consultation. In particular, I want to thank Dr. Robert Cohen, also of St. Louis, and Dr. Dan Mishell of the University of Southern California. I want to thank my office staff for the excellent typing of all the drafts. The American Fertility Society and the American Society of Andrology are to be commended for their excellent educational programs, as well as the Country Day School in St. Louis, where I have been allowed to teach reproduction to pre-adolescents, adolescents, and parents. I want to thank Bill Adler, my agent, for all his help as well. My wife deserves the greatest credit for her inspiration and guidance on this book from the moment of its conception.

Contents

Introduction

My first book, *How to Get Pregnant*, started with our six-year-old boy's view of the facts of life. "First you have to have a mommy and a daddy. . . . A little 'squirm' inside Daddy finds her egg somehow and becomes a baby." That book was my effort to help infertile couples achieve their dream of having a baby. But that six-year-old boy is now a fifteen-year-old teenager who wants to learn about sexual responsibility, and his parents are in their early forties, trying to decide how to control their family growth safely, conveniently, and even reversibly. This new book is for *everyone* of reproductive age. It should be read in schools, churches, and welfare departments; by teenagers, newlyweds, and parents—in short, everyone with sperm or ovaries.

As a physician treating the most difficult cases of infertility from around the world, I am very enthusiastic about children and family life. I love big families, I love children, and I love people who love children. I love to raise children, I love to teach children, and I love to watch how a child grows and develops. So why am I writing a book on birth control? Why is it so important for me to help people of all ages, from young teenagers to adults in their late forties, learn all about reproduction and birth control so that they can safely and conveniently avoid having children?

In 1960 the birth control pill created a revolutionary demand for simple, convenient contraception. But when the pill's side effects became publicized in 1968, many women became concerned and switched to the IUD (intrauterine device), which was even more convenient than the pill. But there are women who chose the wrong IUD and are now sterile or dead. In fact, because of subsequent lawsuits, you cannot even get an IUD in the United States now, although many varieties are quite safe.

There are many women (and girls) who go through repeated abortions, or have children they do not want, either because they cannot get an IUD, or because they are afraid of the birth control pill, even though there are new low-dose pills that are incredibly safe and reliable. In fact, these new pills even protect you from cancer of the uterus and ovary, pelvic inflammatory disease (PID), benign breast disease, acne, and even premenstrual syndrome (PMS).

Many couples who are afraid of the "dangers" of the pill and the IUD also dislike the inconvenience of condoms, contraceptive foam, and the diaphragm. So they get sterilized even though they are young and not 100 percent sure about whether they will ever want children. They do not know how to use "natural" birth control (rhythm) in a scientific way that can make it surprisingly reliable. They do not know about new techniques such as the Norplant capsule, which is implanted under the skin, GNRH nasal spray, the male "pill," or the "morning after" pill. They do not even know how sterilization can be performed in such a way as to make it easily reversible. So out of fear and ignorance, many people are either having children when they do not want them, or by using the wrong birth control method, are ruining their chances for having children in the future.

My goal is *not* zero population growth. Malthusian theory was discredited years ago. What our planet requires is that each and every child that is born (no matter how many) is truly wanted. This is the goal of birth control—not just to limit population, but to allow parents to choose to have the number of children that they can handle with love and enthusiasm. Then those children are more likely to be raised as creative, productive individuals who will open new vistas. And there will be room. Look at space, the ocean, and deserts. Our creativity can make room. The question is not how many babies should we have, but will our babies be raised well? If they are, then the numbers don't matter.

No one is "self-made." Even independent, self-assured people got that mentality because of help and assurance from someone. Too many teenage girls get pregnant because they want love, and too many teenage boys commit suicide because they didn't get it. These are kids who were born into the wrong situation at the wrong time. Every fetus has a right to be wanted, and society has a right to have it wanted—or we all pay later. Let me tell you about several patients of mine who might be like people you know.

Birth Control for Teenagers and Before Marriage

Phyllis was a lovely, thirty-year-old professional woman with her own successful business. When she was twenty years old she became pregnant (as almost 20 percent of the girls do by that age in this modern era—50 percent in some large cities), and although her boyfriend suggested abortion, she found that suggestion repulsive. Yet when at age twenty-one, young, unmarried, and immature, she had the baby, she decided that he deserved more than what she could offer. She gave him up for adoption as a one-month-old infant and has never seen the child since. Her problem was she had been fooled by TV and the movies. Her heroes and role models on the tube and screen had sold her on sex. It was just easy and beautiful. But sex is not just a holiday. It requires knowledge, forethought, and responsibility. Otherwise in a young unmarried woman it can lead to infections, permanent sterility, unwanted pregnancy, abortion, guilt, and maybe death. The promise of "carefree" sex in the 1960s was a fraud.

At age twenty-eight, Phyllis felt she desperately needed a secure method of birth control and so had her "tubes tied." She was warned that this was an "irreversible" sterilization, but all she knew about other "reversible" methods of birth control was misinformation and near-hysterical media publicity that created exciting reading but distorted the facts. So Phyllis felt her only resort was a permanent operation to prevent having children. Two years later she came to see me and my colleagues in St. Louis because she was now happily married, and she and her husband desperately wanted a family.

The sterilization procedure Phyllis had undergone just two years earlier had severely destroyed most of her Fallopian tubes, but fortunately through a very complicated microsurgical operation, we were able to restore her fertility. Phyllis's potentially tragic story had a seemingly miraculous ending, and she and her husband now have a happy family. But many women like Phyllis find out that their tubes were so damaged by sterilization that reversal is impossible. They could have used much less drastic methods of birth control with greater safety, reliability, and convenience. What neither Phyllis nor her previous doctors had realized is that even if less drastic methods of birth control were unsuitable for her, sterilization could have been performed in such a way as to make reversibility easy and reliable.

Tubal Sterilization Can Be Reversible

Although sterilization is not recommended as the first choice for reversible birth control (because to reverse it involves a major operation), nonetheless if it is the only method of birth control appropriate to the woman's situation, every woman today has the technology available to her (if she knows how to search it out) to have her sterilization performed in such a way that reversibility is just as reliable as with any other method of birth control.

Alice's story was a lot more complicated than Phyllis's. Alice was a thirty-seven-year-old professional who, at age thirty, had never been married or had children. She was afraid of the pill, and her uterus was too small to accommodate an IUD easily, so she decided to try using a diaphragm and contraceptive spermicidal foam. (She probably would not have been willing to try the foam if she had known about a very questionable lawsuit well publicized several years later that alleged that foam caused fetal abnormalities and limb defects in babies born to mothers who used it for contraception.) At first she did not mind the relatively high risk of pregnancy with this "barrier" method of contraception. But then she got pregnant at the age of thirty, had an abortion, got pregnant again at the age of thirty-one, and had another abortion. As a result, Alice went through a period of psychological misery which she had never anticipated, and decided her only resort was to have tubal sterilization.

One year later she was happily married, wanted to have children, and realized she had made a disastrous mistake. She went to a doctor who tried to perform the difficult microsurgical operation of reconnecting her tubes (which had been damaged almost as badly as Phyllis's after the sterilization procedure), but she did not get pregnant after the surgery, and subsequent X rays demonstrated that the surgery had failed. Her tubes were "hopelessly" blocked.

Alice was then told that her only hope for having children was to have a "test tube baby" through *in vitro* fertilization. Imagine, this was a woman who several years earlier had gotten pregnant easily, and had undergone abortions with the notion that someday when she was ready to have and to cherish children she would have no difficulty. Now, several years later, she was being told that she had a scant 8 percent chance of having a baby if she submitted to an arduous and complicated procedure whereby an egg would be aspirated from her ovary, placed in a laboratory dish with her husband's sperm, and the resulting embryo (if it developed) would be placed back into her uterus to see if a fetus would develop. She tried several cycles of this heroic new fertility treatment, again unsuccessfully, and she mourned the babies she now wished she had. Fortunately, my colleagues and I were able to restore her fertility microsurgically with a second operation, and she, too, now has a growing, happy family. She, too, was lucky.

Some IUDs Are Not Reversible Birth Control

Not all of the ill-conceived efforts at birth control by misinformed men and women have such dramatically happy endings. Jim and Carol were a couple in their early thirties who had been trying unsuccessfully for about a year and a half to get pregnant. After they paid a visit to my office, I discovered the wife's tragic story. At age twenty-seven, Carol decided to have an IUD inserted into her uterus for birth control with her husband. The brand of IUD that her gynecologist chose was the now infamous "Dalkon Shield." Almost all of the approved IUDs have been extremely safe (as I will discuss in more detail in Chapter 5) but the Dalkon Shield was associated with disastrous infections because the little string that trails out of the uterus into the vagina (common to all IUDs) was "braided" rather than "monofilament"—that is, like fishing line. The apparently innocent braided character of the string allowed bacteria that normally reside in the vagina to migrate up into the uterus and cause infections that could have absolutely devastating effects, including infertility and death. When physicians became aware of this complication, they stopped using the Dalkon Shield, but for Carol the damage was already done.

After delightedly using the Dalkon Shield for about seven years with no pregnancy and no infection, Carol suddenly developed severe cramping and fever. Two days later her physician removed the IUD and placed her on antibiotics. Her symptoms went away within days, and Carol thought all was well, but, in truth, the infection had destroyed her Fallopian tubes and she was sterile. If she had had the IUD removed at any time during those seven years prior to this infection, today Carol would probably have been able to have a baby. The ultimate irony in her story is that Carol was referred to me by a friend who years ago had opted for a tubal sterilization rather than an IUD, because at the time she was sure she never wanted to have children. Yet Carol's friend changed her mind, underwent microsurgery at our clinic several years ago, and now has a baby. Neither of them realized seven years ago that tubal sterilization, if performed conservatively, is a less permanent and more reversible method of birth control than the wrong kind of IUD that gets infected.

The same tragedy that befell Carol struck another couple that visited my office. Michael was a prominent religious leader who loved children dearly, and his wife, Susan, was a gifted teacher who had a deep compassion for children and a great knowledge of child development. They wanted to put off childbearing until their schooling was finished, and they were truly prepared to raise a child in a way that they knew every child has a right to be raised. But unfortunately they also chose the wrong method of birth control. Susan had a Dalkon Shield IUD, suffered a serious infection, and she, too, will never have children unless by some miracle she becomes one of the 8 percent who gets pregnant from *in vitro* fertilization, which she presently cannot afford anyway.

Why No More IUDs?

What does a couple do when they know they don't want any more children for the time being, but virtually every birth control method that they read about seems to have some kind of terrifying risk, or is unreliable, or at best is either messy (like foam) or a turn-off (like condoms)? An IUD usually is the best answer for such a couple. Take, for example, Scott and Laurie. They are both thirty-four years old, happily married, and have two children, a four-year-old and a one-year-old. The younger son has a heart problem, but the doctors feel his prognosis is good. This child, whom they love dearly, represents a great burden and takes a lot of their time and money. At this point in their lives they are certainly not ready to have another child. It would probably be disastrous not only for their marriage but also for any new child, not to mention the second one, who needs so much time, attention, and money for medical costs. They called me because they wanted a vasectomy as a last resort because there just seemed to be "nothing else."

Anyone can recognize that this is not an ideal couple for a vasectomy. But in their view, and in the view of most Americans (based on misinformation, publicity, and questionable lawsuits), what else could they believe but the common myth that they simply had no other choice but to have a vasectomy? The IUD would have been the correct choice for this couple. They knew that they did not have the time (or the self-discipline) to use "natural" or "rhythm" birth control in the scientific sort of way that would give some reliability to it. Statistically, the IUD would represent a slightly increased risk of infection if they had a variety of sexual partners, but they had a purely monogamous marriage. Therefore the correct IUD would represent no increased risk to Laurie, and would be her best choice of contraception.

But in the United States, you cannot have an IUD (except for a relatively unusual variety called the Progestasert, which has side effects that make it unpopular). Most IUDs are safe and reliable but IUDs are no longer available in the United States because the companies marketing them have had over six hundred apparently groundless lawsuits to defend. Although they have won virtually every one of those lawsuits, the expense and risk of further lawsuits became too overwhelming for a product whose profitability is not that great, and companies thus have simply stopped selling IUDs in this country. An acquaintance of mine felt so sorry for Scott and Laurie that she has decided to start a class-action lawsuit against all of the women who sued the makers of the IUD with frivolous lawsuits.

This same woman had an infertility problem herself years ago. When this was treated she became pregnant and now has two children. She was able to have a Copper 7 IUD inserted in her uterus about two weeks before it was pulled off the market. It is a relatively simple, safe, easy method of birth control—just perfect for happily married couples who do not want to take a drastic step toward sterilization and who want the simplest method possible. When this woman's Copper 7 IUD runs out of copper in about three years, she will have to have it changed. To do this she will have to go to Canada as will any other Americans for whom the IUD is the birth control method of choice. All of the women who have brought unfair lawsuits against the manufacturers of the Copper 7 IUD have, in a sense, made it impossible for this woman, or for Scott and Laurie, to have an IUD that should be available in this country and is available everywhere else in the civilized world.

Obviously the best choice for Scott and Laurie in view of their one-year-old child's precarious health is not to have a vasectomy at this stage, but rather to travel to Canada and have an IUD inserted. If they can't afford a trip to Canada, they'll have to read up more about the new low-dose birth control pills and try to choose a pill that would be appropriate for Laurie's particular age and condition, or in any case, they need to know all their other birth control options so they can make the next best decision.

Abortion May Not Be Reversible Birth Control

Betty had two abortions in the past because she really knew nothing about birth control. She later studied the subject in detail and subsequently went on birth control pills for fifteen years. Now, as a woman in her late thirties, Betty was happily married and desperately wanted children. But what she did not discover until several years after discontinuing the pills was that her entire uterus and Fallopian tubes had been massively scarred by infections that had occurred as a result of the two abortions performed during her impetuous youth. She had no chance now of ever having a child. Ironically, if she had been sterilized eighteen years ago, she would have had no trouble having her fertility restored with microsurgery.

What It's Like to Have Children When You Don't Want Them Just Because You Don't Know Anything About Birth Control

As tragic as being unable to have children is, having to raise children when they are unwanted, when your life is not happy, your mind is not settled, you are unmarried, or your marriage is unstable is more tragic. An example is a patient of mine named Bill. Bill is a brilliant man in his midforties who knows everything about children and loves them dearly. But when he was barely twenty years old he got his teen-aged girlfriend pregnant and felt an obligation to marry her. They did not love each other and had nothing in common, but he would not consider an abortion (nor would she) and he decided to do the "honorable" thing, hoping he could make the marriage work. After all, he was young and very idealistic.

He never knew, and, like most men, still does not know anything about birth control. His wife managed that, and after becoming disenchanted with the "messiness" of foam for birth control, she had an IUD inserted. After three years she decided the marriage needed another child to help "hold it together," and so she had the IUD removed. In their midtwenties they found themselves with two children and very little in common with each other. They had another child nine years later, and at this point the marriage was in shambles. These children grew up with very little self-esteem, having been brought up in a stormy marriage where each spouse was more concerned about his or her own career than with children they were not ready for and who were basically "in the way."

Now Bill is happily remarried, and he thinks he wants a vasectomy. Raising his three children has been such a tale of heartache for him, his ex-wife, and the children, that out of his ignorance about birth control comes a desperate grasp for permanent sterilization.

Bill's present wife, Rita, had a similarly unhappy story in her first marriage. She was also married at around twenty years of age to a happy-go-lucky fellow. Her life seemed exciting, and for about five years they tried to get pregnant, unsuccessfully. They were finally told there was no chance for pregnancy because her husband's sperm count was too low. By the time she was twenty-five the marriage had begun to sour because Rita had a much more responsible view of life than did her husband, and she gave up trying to get pregnant. She stopped seeing fertility doctors, and decided that a baby would not be appropriate anyway in this marriage. Still she did not use birth control at this point, because of course they figured they were infertile. At the time when they least expected it, she became pregnant. Adding to the confusion, while she was breast-feeding in her sixth month after delivery (she had no information on how to make breast-feeding an effective method of birth control), she got pregnant again without expecting it. At this point she found that her husband was sleeping around with other women and she kicked him out.

Now with five grown kids between the two of them, none of whom was born out of love, Bill and Rita are happily married but she does not want any more children. For a while they relied on condoms, but Bill, a typical male, did not really want to use them. So they relied on "natural" birth control, using a scientific variety of what is more commonly thought of as "rhythm." But they were not properly informed on how to do this, and besides, Bill was often impetuously anxious to make love at the wrong times in the cycle. With this approach Rita had had a couple of scares where she thought she might have gotten pregnant. So when I saw them they were at a stage where Rita would not let Bill get near her unless he had a vasectomy. So you can see why Bill so desperately wanted one! Yet this man loved children and admitted that he was not ready to take a permanent step against ever having them again.

Rita's doctor had told her that she could not take birth control pills because she suffered from headaches and premenstrual syndrome (PMS), and the pill was thought to exacerbate those conditions. In fact, for many women in their late thirties, the new low-dose birth control pills can actually relieve migraine headaches and PMS. (In my opinion, fear of the birth control pill, especially with the new low-dose varieties available, is mostly the result of medicolegal hysteria, and media hype.) We put her on a birth control pill designed to mimic her "natural cycle," and now in addition to having a healthy sex life with a reversible method of contraception, her PMS and her migraine headaches are gone. So what could have been a hastily performed vasectomy on a man who was not sure that his child-rearing days were over, turned into an intelligent birth control decision that immensely improved the quality of this couple's lives because they finally took the responsibility to understand their own reproductive systems better.

These were loving people who could have had the joy of raising a large, loving family together. But each of them got married too young (in one case because of *accidental* pregnancy), neither knew how to prevent pregnancy in an unhappy marriage, and the wife did not realize that even low sperm counts can result in pregnancy if you do not use birth control. Twenty years later, as mature adults, they still knew nothing about birth control, and almost ruined their lives once more.

Infertile Couples Also Need Birth Control Eventually

Birth control is not just a problem for highly fertile young couples. Most infertile couples who have struggled from the beginning to solve their infertility problems and who finally get pregnant, eventually require birth control, and some want it desperately. A typical example is John. He and his wife, Sarah, were a happy, loving couple who tried for many years to have a baby, with no luck. He was told that his sperm count was too low and that nothing could be done. So John and Sarah adopted an infant and loved this child so much, and were so happy with it, that they decided several years later to adopt another child. But this time there were no babies readily available for adoption. (This was in the late 1960s, when abortion had been legalized and the availability of babies for adoption became very limited.)

So John and Sarah knew that if they were going to have any more children, they would have to try once again to tackle the infertility problem they were told was "hopeless." The doctor was sure that the husband's sperm count was too low, but he did not have the benefit of modern studies that show that even with a low sperm count, women can get pregnant if they are extremely fertile themselves. To assuage the anxious couple, the doctor put Sarah on a fertility pill, Clomid. The next month she became pregnant and they were overjoyed to find out several months later that she would have twins!

Twin infants are a major job for any mother and father, especially when there is already a three-year-old running around the house. But John and Sarah never thought about birth control because they knew they were an infertile couple. What they did not know, and what their doctor was only vaguely aware of at that time, was that when an infertile woman has gotten pregnant on a fertility drug, very frequently she becomes fertile on her own for subsequent pregnancies. So six months after the birth of her twins, Sarah became pregnant again. Here was an "infertile" couple who suddenly found themselves with four little kids living in a joyous madhouse!

But the joy can quickly fade into the grim reality of providing adequately for that many children all at once. After years of trying condoms unhappily, being too afraid (because of adverse publicity) to use birth control pills or IUDs, and finding foam and diaphragms too difficult and messy, John and Sarah finally came into my office, desperately seeking a vasectomy. They were still a happily married couple despite a sex life that was made miserable by their ignorance about contraception. Sarah was in her late thirties, and John was in his early forties. The kids were almost grown. They definitely did not want more. Yet when I offered them a choice of permanent vasectomy, or a type of vasectomy that can be more easily reversed, I was shocked that they chose the more easily reversible approach.

Vasectomy Can Be Reversible

What John and Sarah did not know before seeing me, and what the public at large is not very familiar with, is that vasectomy can be performed in such a way as to make its microsurgical reversal much easier. In very qualified hands, there is over a 90 percent chance that a couple can bear children again if such a vasectomy is microsurgically "reversed." I originally developed this "open-ended" method of vasectomy, which is based on the principle of keeping the pressure within the vas on the testicular side of the vasectomy low (so that no damage occurs to the very delicate ducts between the testicle and the vas—see Chapter 7). John shocked me by saying, when confronted with this alternative, that he definitely wanted the more easily reversible approach because even though he and his wife were "sure" they did not want any more children, they were not 100 percent sure.

Anyone who thinks he is 100 percent sure he will never change his mind about his sterilization is not looking very deeply into his soul. Thousands of men who in years past had a vasectomy and were *sure* they would never want more children have come to me seeking microsurgical reversal, and most were well counseled when they had their vasectomy! It was the right decision for them in that particular circumstance, and they never would have predicted their lives and views would change so dramatically. A seemingly "permanent" decision to have a vasectomy can be surprisingly tenuous.

A humorous example is a prominent financial adviser, extremely happily married, with the "ideal American family," three children, a boy and two girls, a big suburban house, a successful career, good in-laws, and a peaceful, happy life. Rick and Theresa decided, quite predictably, that they had reached that stage in life (with their kids five, six, and eight years of age) where it was time to get the vasectomy that everybody else was getting. These were truly lovely people who seemed extremely stable in all their views on life and in their overall plan for the future. They definitely wanted no more children. They were happy with their three children. It was an absolutely consistent part of their game plan to stop having children after the third one. So I performed the conventional "close-ended" vasectomy (the common type that is more difficult to reverse microsurgically).

After a man undergoes a vasectomy, it is important for him to use other methods of birth control until he has had enough ejaculations (usually ten to fifteen) and enough time (usually four weeks) for all of the sperm still present on the other side of the vasectomy site to be expelled. A doctor should not give a couple the go-ahead on having "unprotected" intercourse until a semen specimen confirms that there are absolutely no sperm left. The most common lawsuit that urologists face results when a couple has a pregnancy after vasectomy, either because the vasectomy did not work and sperm continued to reach the vas from the testicles, or because the doctor failed to inform the patient that he must use some method of birth control until his sperm count goes down to zero.

So you can imagine my terror when Rick phoned me about six weeks after his vasectomy to tell me that Theresa was pregnant. My terror turned into disbelieving joy when I heard the excitement and happiness in Rick's voice. He was overjoyed with his wife's "unwanted" pregnancy. This gave me a great sense of relief for the baby, for them, and also for me. Rick explained that he and his wife realized when they walked out of my office after having the vasectomy that "it might be nice to have another child." So they used no birth control, unknown to me, during the succeeding four weeks after the vasectomy, hoping that the wife would become "accidentally" pregnant. When I suggested that perhaps he had made a mistake in having the vasectomy, Rick said, "No, definitely not. Four is all of the children that my wife and I ever wanted and planned for."

So how do you ever know for sure that you'll never want to have more children, no matter what? I don't believe that the patient or doctor ever know for sure. For that reason a major point in my chapter on vasectomy is that it is inhumane to perform a vasectomy in such a way as *not* to consider its possible reversal.

Eric was a fifty-five-year-old urban business entrepreneur. He had had seven children—a crowded apartment, to say the least. He did a beautiful job of raising them and had a beautiful family. Now they were all grown, and Eric had a vasectomy. Interestingly, after the kids were grown, Eric had found that he had more time to devote to his business, and suddenly, in his fifties, he found himself to be a rather wealthy entrepreneur. Then his life was shaken by the tragic death of his wife.

Several years later, he remarried a successful thirty-seven-year-old businesswoman who had never been married before nor had children. Despite his age and having already successfully and happily raised a family of seven children, this man found himself regretting what seemed to be a permanent sterilization procedure, and once again he wanted to raise kids. Fortunately, his story ended happily, with a successful microsurgical reversal of his vasectomy despite the fact that it had been performed in such a way as to make it very difficult to reverse.

How Many Children Is Too Many?

Eric's story and countless others demonstrate that there is no ideal size to a family unit, even in this hectic modern world. All that matters is the amount of time and energy that a happily married couple wants to devote to their children. The unhappy, mixed-up child does not usually end up that way simply because the family is "too big." It usually comes from parents who are not ready for it. If the pregnancy comes when you are not interested in having more children, then even one child is too many. But for Eric, seven turned out not to be enough. I feel very happy about the new children that this fifty-five-year-old man is going to be raising.

Frank, the farmer, is another example of someone who wants and loves a huge family. He had had four children by a previous marriage, and his wife had died. His new wife, Joanne, had five children from a previous marriage, and her husband had died. Every one of those nine children was well raised and had a purpose in life. But when Frank and Joanne got married, they decided that nine was not enough. Frank came to me seeking a reversal of his vasectomy so that he and Joanne could add to their growing family. Having that many children is an awesome responsibility because each child is a precious human being. If you cannot devote time and energy to their raising, and if you are not ready to present them with a system of stable values by which you live, then even one child can be a source of misery.

Having a child at the wrong time can also hurt a fragile marriage that might otherwise succeed if childbirth could have been planned. Over the past ten years I have interviewed close to three thousand couples who had previously been married, whose marriage had failed, and who were now remarried and who wanted to start a new family. Most of these couples began to feel the strains of marital discord around the time of the birth of their second child. It is a surprise for most people to learn that the birth of their first child may not significantly alter their life-style as much as they anticipated. The modern couples I've interviewed tend to take their first child on trips, to restaurants, and to engage them in almost adult-style conversation at an early age. They are surprised to find that not only is a child the great joy they expected it to be, but also that it is not as much of a burden as they'd feared.

Take, for example, Al and Mary. Al had been married before, had three children, had a vasectomy, was divorced, and subsequently remarried a wonderful woman with whom he was very much in love. Al loved and respected his first wife, as she did him, but around the time of the birth of their second child they seemed to grow apart. After three children, Al's communication with his wife had become hopelessly sparse. Al underwent a vasectomy in an effort to save the marriage from complete discord and with the hope that he and Mary would not get divorced. But they did.

Now Al was married to Mary, had a successful vasectomy reversal, and already had a beautiful child whom they loved very deeply. They were a mature couple who understood the stresses and strains on a marriage in modern society and understood how you had to work at communicating and settling differences amicably to keep the marriage happy and prospering. Yet with the birth of their second child, Al began to feel the same marital stress that had begun to disrupt his first marriage. Al and Mary had to change their life-style to accommodate the second child. Luckily, this time Al was prepared emotionally to deal with this change of life, and he and Mary are still a happily married couple, with two delightful children. But they have correctly decided to become knowledgeable about the use of birth control so that they do not put any more stress on a marriage and family that are so dear to them.

Should You Have Your Baby Now—While You Can?

Newlyweds without children should consider whether their fertility might deteriorate so much over the next ten years that they had better have a baby while they can. For couples in their thirties, any prolonged birth control could be an unanticipated disaster, if it ruins their chances for the future family life they planned on. For example, eighteen years ago Mary got pregnant without any difficulty as a teenager with just a single sexual episode, and gave the baby up for adoption because she would not consider an abortion. Nor would she consider raising a child that she was not mature enough to raise. Following that, she avoided sexual encounters for the next five years and had completely regular menstrual periods with no indication of any menstrual irregularity or ovulatory problem. Then she got married, and for six years used birth control pills. For the following three years her husband used condoms. Thus, for a total of nine years of marriage they used either birth control pills or condoms to avoid an unwanted pregnancy until she and her husband felt the time was right.

By the time they stopped using condoms her periods had become irregular, her flow was changeable, and she was never able to get pregnant, despite the fact that when she was a teenager she got pregnant with a single sexual encounter, and as a young woman in her twenties she had shown no sign of any infertility problem. In her thirties she simply underwent a premature loss of the ability to conceive, just at the time when she and her husband had finally decided they were ready for kids. For Mary, her careful family planning led to no family at all because she did not know that she would have a premature ovarian failure.

Birth Control Can Improve Your Health

For others, the failure to use birth control early is what leads to the eventual inability to have a family. Many men and women sow their wild oats while they are very young but eventually settle down and want a stable family life. During the wild early years they may have had multiple sexual partners, and the chance to catch infections such as gonorrhea, syphilis, chlamydia, or AIDS is extremely high when there is more than one sexual partner. In fact, it is promiscuity that allows the spread of all sexually transmitted diseases. Therefore, one method of birth control whose popularity is dramatically increasing in the past several years is the condom. This is the only method of birth control that protects you in a major way against catching one of these venereal diseases. In addition, the condom may protect women from getting cancer of the cervix, which also is commonly associated with a history of multiple sexual partners. Had Eva Perón known about this, she might not have died prematurely, at the height of her political power.

A patient of mine from outside the United States learned about this soon enough to avoid dying, but not soon enough to preserve his chance to have children. This patient was a wonderful, loving, devout man, married for nineteen years, completely faithful to his wife. Having children meant everything in their life, and they had been unable to have a baby because he had no sperm in his ejaculate. The doctors had no idea why he had this problem. They sent him to me to perform a testicle biopsy to see if anything could be done so that he could produce sperm. When I talked with him I found out that although he had been completely faithful during his marriage, he had had sex one time before marriage with a prostitute and had not used a condom. He related that several days afterward he developed a painless sore on the tip of his penis, but it went away immediately without treatment. About six weeks later he developed an itching rash all over his body, but this also went away on its own in several days.

I knew from his description of this episode that occurred over twenty years ago that he had acquired syphilis from the prostitute. I also knew that if he was not treated with antibiotics very soon, in several years he would develop the dreaded tertiary lesions of syphilis, which destroy the brain, heart, liver, and nervous system. It would be an agonizing death, and fortunately we were able to prevent this by treating him even at this late date. But his testicles had been completely destroyed, and because of this one episode of sex before marriage with a prostitute *not using a condom*, he would never be able to have children.

With the public's heightened awareness of "sexually transmitted diseases" brought on by the rapidly enlarging AIDS epidemic, sales of condoms in this country and around the world have skyrocketed. The condom business is booming. For we are now returning to the pre-antibiotic era where we have a venereal disease that truly kills and is completely untreatable. The only solution to AIDS at present is to prevent it. It is just a matter of time before it becomes as prevalent in the promiscuous heterosexual population as it is in the homosexual population.

Condoms are becoming so popular that 40 percent of their sales are to women. The condom marketers have not allowed this to escape their notice. If you go to your favorite drugstore today, you will see that most condoms are sold in the female cosmetics section and packaged in soft pastel boxes so that when a woman buys her tampons or her Kotex, she can also pick up a couple of dozen rubbers without being too obtrusive or feeling embarrassed. But condoms are not the only birth control method that can protect against infection in women with several partners.

The birth control pill, commonly despised for its allegedly dangerous side effects, has also been shown to give protection to its users (although not as completely as condoms) from certain types of venereal diseases that would otherwise cause sterility later by inflaming the Fallopian tubes. In fact, birth control pills have demonstrated many positive health benefits, such as protecting against cancer of the uterus and cancer of the ovary, reduction in blood loss and anemia caused by heavy menstruation, control of painful menstruation, prevention of benign breast disease, and even the amelioration of PMS in some women.

What Birth Control Method Should I Use?

Despite the relative safety of the seemingly huge variety of birth control methods available to men and women, often nothing seems to be quite right: Condoms and birth control pills are thought of as too much of a hassle, or unsafe; the IUD is not available in the United States; diaphragms or foams are messy; and "natural" rhythm requires too much discipline. Thus vasectomy in the male or tubal sterilization in the female seem to be the eventual options of choice. Most couples know so little about birth control and family planning that they never develop a rational family plan, and seek sterilization out of desperation because they think there is nothing else.

I will never forget Joe, a joke-cracking, affable salesman doing quite well with his company. He had always been joyful and humorous, despite many problems. I had known him and his wife, Sally, for five years as they struggled to get pregnant despite his poor sperm count and her poor ovulation. Now, after much effort, they had three children, and, ironically, it was obvious that they had not the foggiest idea of how to raise them. They were simply overwhelmed, Joe's sense of humor was gone, and he and Sally were frantic.

When they came to the office for the vasectomy consultation I was intending to be very conservative and cautious, warning them not to take too precipitous a step in view of their prior history of infertility. But when they brought in their three children, I changed my mind instantly. They nearly destroyed my office. They were complete brats. I have never seen any two parents so totally in over their heads. They did not want to talk about "open-ended" versus "conventional" vasectomy, they did not want to talk about alternatives such as birth control pills; condoms; IUDs; foam; the beauty of a natural, scientific rhythm method; Provera injections every three months for the wife; or anything else. They were incapable of any thought on the subject. Joe just wanted his vasectomy now, as an emergency measure to prevent his impending mental collapse. It is because of loving, wonderful people like Joe, who always wanted children but who was now reduced to a babbling idiot, that I decided I'd better write this book.

Why Birth Control? Why Plan?

I had the pleasure of being in the audience during a recent *Phil Donahue Show* in which the topic was a book on whether women can have a career and also raise kids. Before the show started, during the usual warm-up time, the producer came out and asked the audience (which was about 90 percent women) whether they thought they could go to work during the day; have a successful career; raise kids; clean house; have a good, happy marriage; and, simply put, be housewives as well as career women as well as mothers and do it all well. Everyone in the audience laughed and clearly indicated the answer was "no." The audience thought it just too exhausting to try to do it all. During the show itself, what came out on the air is that most women work because they have to, because most households today need a combined income, and that this country is not doing what it should be doing to give these women the support they need to be able to work and also raise their children. A successful career requires planning, and a successful family life does also.

In previous eras you did not have to think much about birth control. If you were a woman, you typically got married young, you had babies one after another, and you were given great praise (hopefully) for this feat. Your job was to raise the kids and watch the house while your husband went out and earned a living. You eventualy reached a stage of exhaustion where you could not wait for menopause. But at least there was no decisionmaking and no agonizing choices to be made.

The !Kung tribesmen of the Kalahari Desert in Africa, otherwise known as the African Bushmen, represent a hunter/gatherer family culture that is about forty thousand years old. It is about the simplest form of society, basically a family unit that is self-sufficient, has no agriculture, and simply lives by hunting and gathering whatever it can find to eat. Unlike in a farm community, where the more children the better (to do the chores), in this pre-agricultural primitive society, there was a realistic limit to the number of children the land could support. The !Kung tribesmen had a method of birth control they were not even aware of, that they did not have to think about. It was perfectly natural and protected them from having more children than they could handle. If they were overwhelmed with too many children it would not be as humorous as the case with Joe was. It would mean starvation.

Their method of birth control was that the women would breast-feed their children continuously around the clock day and night for four years, and the children would have no other food supplement. This continuous breast-feeding with no other food supplementation so completely suppressed a woman's ovulation that she rarely had babies more than once every four or five years despite regular, frequent intercourse. You see, she had a career as well as a family and a household to take care of. Although the men spent a great deal of time hunting for meat to make sure that the family had enough protein in their diet, the majority of food in most hunter/gatherer societies is provided by the women.

It is a hard life finding what you can from the earth to live by, and there was no room for unwanted children—no capacity to absorb unlimited numbers of children into the system. But the !Kung tribesmen did not have to read this book, because their society was much simpler than ours. Their food was so scarce that they could not supplement the infants' diet very easily, and so, in a sense, they were the first great family planners. Assuming you do not want to have your first child in your teen years, and from then on rely on continuous breast-feeding around the clock for the rest of your reproductive life, you will need to know something about your body so that you can decide to get pregnant when you want to get pregnant.

I still remember the gleam in the eyes of Bill and Rita when, as they watched my kids playing and interacting, I suggested to them, "Maybe when the air clears in a few years you might want the thrill of having a baby with love. You have had five kids between you and not a single one was born out of love." Rita said, "Isn't it sad how few people are born out of love?" This book is about how to make sure that your children are born out of love and not out of haste or ignorance.

It is my personal view that there is always room in the world for more children. But it should be when you want it so your child will have a fair chance. We are not even talking parents' rights here, we are talking about the child's right to be born with love and to be wanted. Nobody, not even abortion rights advocates, likes abortion. But it presently is the most popular method of birth control in many areas of the world. In this country alone, for every three babies that are born, one is aborted. But abortion probably wouldn't be popular if people understood and used other birth control options instead.

So why are Bill and Rita in their present dilemma? She cannot have an IUD unless she travels to Canada to get one. She was told not to take birth control pills because she had headaches and premenstrual syndrome, despite the fact that the birth control pills we finally put her on actually relieved her headaches and PMS symptoms. She probably received the poor advice she got because her doctor was worried about being sued. "Open-ended" vasectomy, despite the obvious benefit of reversibility, is not popular because urologists are worried about being sued for malpractice in case a woman gets pregnant. Foams and contraceptive sponges probably will be going off the market eventually because some lawsuits claiming without good evidence that a fetal abnormality was caused by foam have actually been won. "Natural" birth control really is reliable only if you can tolerate a certain failure rate or be willing to fall back on the option of abortion. Condoms are a good option for many people, but only if you use them. As this book unfolds, these apparent dilemmas will become easy for everyone to solve. It just requires a little knowledge.

More people than ever are now having babies they really do not want, and poor sex education is to blame. The Surgeon General of the United States, Dr. C. Everett Koop, a gifted pediatric surgeon and a politically conservative, religious man, has openly advocated sex education for children as well as adults. As Phil Donahue said on that show about more help for working mothers, "We really don't like our children." We are tolerant of a terrible educational system and give teachers inadequate pay, no support, and no respect. In the past, your children were your bread and butter, your social security, and the more the better. But all that has changed.

If a child comes into the world unwanted, it is a tragedy, and he or she will come back to pay you for it. It is the point of this book that a child is such a precious gift to cherish that you should not have one until you want one. If you want lots of them, that's great; if you want none, that is your choice. Learn all you can about your body and birth control so that you can avoid the tragedy of getting pregnant when you are not ready, while preserving the ability to have as large or as small a family as you want when you are ready . . . and to stop bearing children when you have had enough.

1

How You Get Pregnant

Getting pregnant is not all that easy a task. The journey which sperm must make through the female genitals to fertilize the egg, as well as the simultaneous adventure of the egg erupting from the ovary to be swallowed by the Fallopian tube, fertilized, and then hustled along into the womb to implant, constitutes an incredible odyssey fraught with excitement and peril every step of the way. Failure of the sperm or egg to make an important connection anywhere along this complicated itinerary will prevent pregnancy from occurring. Before I describe this incredible journey that sperm and egg must make for a pregnancy to occur, let me first map out the structure of the female organs in which the adventure takes place.

The Female Reproductive System: An Introduction to the Vagina, Uterus, Tubes, and Ovaries

The vagina is an elastic canal, about four to five inches long, into which the male inserts his penis during intercourse. At the end of this canal, in the deepest recess of the vagina, is a structure called the cervix, which is the entrance to the womb, or uterus. The uterus is a hard, muscular, pear-shaped structure with a narrow, triangular cavity inside, so small that it would barely hold a teaspoonful of fluid (see Figures 1–1 and 1–2). Yet this is where the fertilized egg, or ovum, must implant itself in order to grow during the next nine months into a baby. The uterus has a remarkable capacity to expand so as to allow

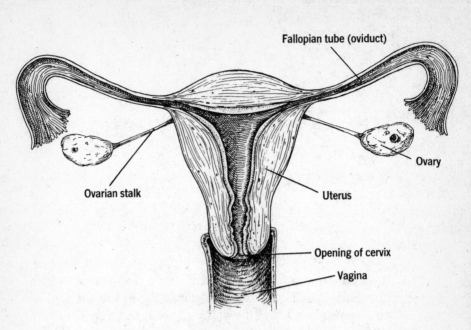

Fallopian tube (oviduct)

Ovary

Ovarian stalk

Uterus

Opening of cervix

Vagina

FIGURE 1–1. The Female Reproductive Organs.

room for this growing baby. As it expands during the nine months of pregnancy, the uterus pushes aside and squashes all the other organs of the abdomen. At the end of the nine months, its muscles contract during labor to squeeze the baby out into the world.

Far back in the corner of the uterus is a microscopic canal on each side that leads into the Fallopian tubes, through which the egg must pass. (The Fallopian tube is the structure that is cut when a woman undergoes tubal sterilization.) The microscopic canals leading from the uterus into the Fallopian tubes are only about one-seventieth to one-hundredth of an inch in diameter (the size of a pinpoint). The tubes are four inches long and hang freely in the abdomen. They widen at the end into a large, flowerlike opening near the ovaries, but they are not directly connected with them.

The ovaries are the organs that make the female's eggs and sex hormones. They sit outside of the uterus and tubes, held by stalks called the ovarian ligaments. When an egg is extruded every month from the surface of one of the ovaries, it is released freely into the abdominal cavity rather than directly into the tube. The open end of the tube, called the fimbria, comes to life like an octopus tentacle when ovulation

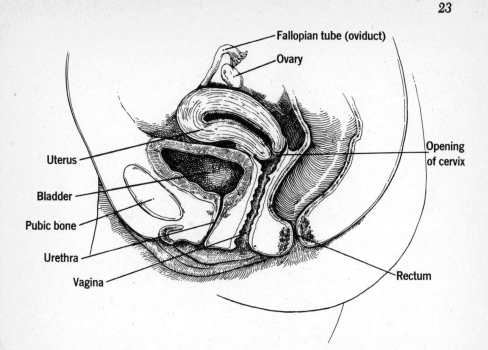

FIGURE 1–2. The Female Reproductive Organs (side view).

occurs, and actively grasps the egg after its volcanolike eruption from the surface of the ovary. The end of the tube thus reaches out for the egg and swallows it, to transport it ultimately into the uterus (see Figure 1–3).

Unlike the testicle, which is continually churning out billions of new sperm, the ovary never produces any new eggs. When a woman is born, she has within her ovaries all of the eggs she will ever have. No new eggs are formed. While the male seems wastefully to produce billions of sperm every week, the female simply matures one of her existing eggs for ovulation each month. She eventually runs out of this limited supply, and her ovaries shrivel up at the time of her menopause, usually sometime between age forty-five and fifty-five. The ovaries mature and release only about four hundred such eggs during the course of a woman's lifetime. Generally, the most fertilizable eggs are released earlier in life. Thus with advancing years, though a woman may still be able to get pregnant, she is much less fertile than she was in her youth.

The fact that the woman's eggs have already been manufactured and merely need to be extruded properly (whereas the male's sperm

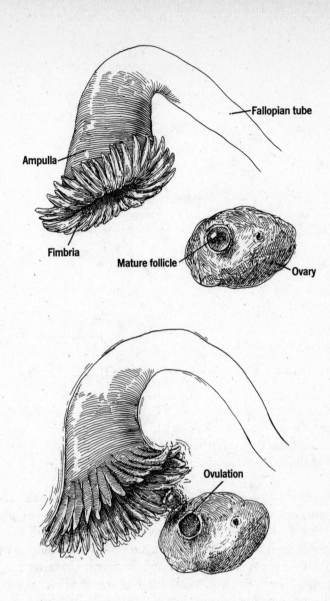

FIGURE 1–3.

must be continually manufactured by an inexorable assembly-line process) makes it much easier either to inhibit or increase the fertility of a woman than a man. When a woman's internal clockwork goes wrong and she ovulates improperly or not at all, usually it is not difficult to improve her fertility with hormone or drug therapy. The eggs are already there, and only require a little bit of guidance. Hormonal manipulations to control, or improve, the woman's fertility are much more likely to be successful than hormonal manipulations of the man. In a similar vein, when birth control is desired, it is much easier to stop ovulation in the woman, without affecting the eggs stored in the ovary, than to completely and yet reversibly "turn off" sperm production in the man.

Hormones That Control Ovulation

The process whereby a matured egg is extruded from the ovary is called ovulation. Since the majority of women who seem unable to have children owe their problems to a disturbance in ovulation, and since the birth control pill works by preventing ovulation, we need to understand how this repeatable, monthly series of changes takes place in the ovary, and unravel the hormonal events which regulate the clocklike orderliness of the menstrual cycle. All of the events taking place during the month between menstrual periods are directed at preparing the womb and the cervix for the moment of ovulation, so that the sperm and the egg have the best opportunity for joining up and resulting in a baby.

At ovulation, the egg is extruded from the surface of the ovary out of its bubblelike compartment, called the follicle. The follicle is a spherical structure that bulges up from the surface of the ovary, and which contains the egg within a mass of sticky fluid. The growth of this follicle is stimulated by the hormone FSH (follicle-stimulating hormone) produced by the pituitary gland in the early phase of the monthly cycle (see Figure 1–4). The time required for the egg to develop a proper follicle for ovulation is about fourteen days. Although FSH stimulates many eggs during the month to form follicles, one of the eggs almost always gets a head start over the others, and once it obtains that lead it never relinquishes it. The other eggs developing that month simply degenerate. Occasionally, however, two follicles successfully reach maturity, and both are ovulated. In that circumstance, if both eggs are fertilized, the woman will have fraternal, or nonidentical, twins. Indeed, some of the drugs used to stimulate ovulation in women who would not otherwise ovulate may work better than expected and cause the development of more than one follicle. Therefore, multiple births are

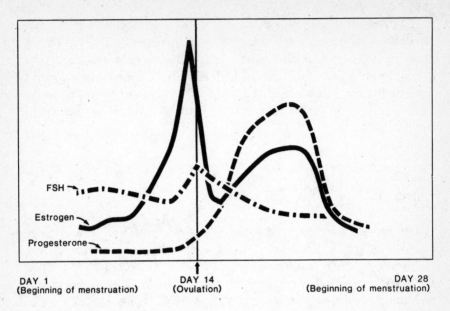

DAY 1
(Beginning of menstruation)

DAY 14
(Ovulation)

DAY 28
(Beginning of menstruation)

FIGURE 1–4. Hormone Changes Associated with Normal Ovulation.

somewhat more common in women who take so-called fertility drugs to help them ovulate.

Two or three days prior to midcycle, when the follicle has reached its maximum size, it produces an enormous amount of the hormone estrogen. This increased level of estrogen just prior to ovulation stimulates the cervix to make more of the cervical mucus that will allow sperm invasion. This dramatic increase in estrogen production also stimulates the pituitary gland to release another hormone, LH (luteinizing hormone). The sudden release of LH is what triggers ovulation (see Figure 1–5).

Under the influence of the midcycle LH surge, the wall of the follicle weakens and deteriorates, and a specific site on its surface ruptures. The bulging follicle is then extruded from the surface of the ovary through this ruptured area (see Figure 1–6). The whole event is quite dramatic. Observed under a microscope, ovulation appears similar to the eruption of a volcano. Occasionally women actually feel several hours of discomfort in their lower abdomen during ovulation (called *Mittelschmerz*). In women who require hormone treatment to stimulate ovulation, the follicle may grow so large that when ovulation occurs it is extremely violent, and they may even become sick enough on occasion

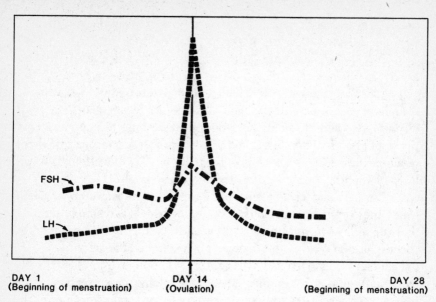

DAY 1
(Beginning of menstruation)

DAY 14
(Ovulation)

DAY 28
(Beginning of menstruation)

FIGURE 1–5. Hormone Changes Associated with Normal Ovulation.

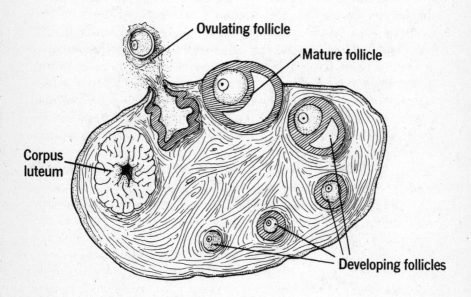

FIGURE 1–6. The Ovary.

to require several days of rest in the hospital. Ovulation is a dramatic intra-abdominal event.

The ruptured, empty follicle then undergoes a sudden change, called "luteinization." Prior to ovulation, the follicle can produce only estrogen. The rupture of the follicle at ovulation transforms it into a completely different endocrine, or hormone-producing, gland that manufactures a different female hormone, progesterone, which has an entirely different function. The production of progesterone forms the basis of all of our methods for determining the time of ovulation. It is the basis of "natural," or scientific "rhythm" birth control.

The new endocrine gland that forms from the ruptured follicle is called the corpus luteum (Latin for "yellow body") and simply signifies that the follicle turns yellow as it changes its identity. As soon as the corpus luteum begins to produce progesterone, the cervical mucus (which had become maximally receptive to sperm invasion just prior to ovulation) suddenly becomes sticky and totally impermeable to the invasion of sperm. In addition, progesterone causes the entrance of the cervix to close dramatically, even though just prior to ovulation it had been gaping in readiness for the entry of sperm.

Although estrogen stimulates the buildup of a thick, hard layer of tissue called the endometrium, which lines the uterus prior to ovulation, this lining does not become receptive to the fertilized egg until after ovulation, when the secretion of progesterone causes it to soften. The corpus luteum manufactures this progesterone over a very limited time. If no pregnancy develops, the corpus luteum ceases to produce progesterone by ten to fourteen days after ovulation. With this cessation of progesterone production by the ovary, the soft lining that was built up in the womb to prepare for the nourishment of the fertilized egg is shed and the woman menstruates. The drop in progesterone (and estrogen) production by the ovary during menstruation, stimulates a new increase in FSH. A new follicle then develops, estrogen production resumes, and the cycle begins again.

Let's examine in greater detail how all this activity coordinates with the menstrual period.

The Menstrual Periods—What Do They Mean?

SEX AND THE MONTHLY CYCLE

There are only several days in any given month when the female is very fertile—that is, when intercourse has a good chance of leading to pregnancy. This fertile period occurs just prior to ovulation. One of the most effective ways to increase the likelihood of pregnancy is to have intercourse around this fertile period of the month. Conversely, a good way to avoid getting pregnant is to delay intercourse until well *after* ovulation.

In comparing humans to the rest of the animal kingdom, there is nothing unusual about the female's being fertile only during a limited period of the month. What should be surprising is that we are the only animal that enjoys sex continuously throughout the month without any regard to whether it is likely to lead to a baby. The female of most species will accept a male for only a very brief period around the time of ovulation, when conception is most probable. This is called behavioral estrus, or "heat." When the female is not in heat, she is completely uninterested in sex, or even actively hostile toward any male that approaches her.

In the wild, the females of many species become sexually receptive only once a year, and if they fail to conceive at that proper moment in the year, sexual receptivity does not occur again until the next breeding season. In other animals, receptive cycles of heat may occur at several intervals throughout the year. The structure and activity of the reproductive tract in all female animals changes cyclically to allow maturation of the egg, and preparation of the uterus for reception of the fertilized egg.

The cycles undergone by all animals except humans are called estrus cycles. Only humans have menstrual cycles. In a menstrual cycle, the buildup of the lining of the womb is so lush, and the drop in hormone level supporting the lining is so abrupt, that at the end of the cycle the lining actually sheds and the woman bleeds for four to five days in what is commonly known as her period. In all other animals, however, this shedding does not occur, and the lush lining of the womb merely returns to the thinned-out condition that marks the beginning of the next cycle. This is important in understanding how birth control pills and Provera injections protect against cancer of the uterus in humans, but not in other animals (see chapter on birth control pill).

Since all animals except humans have no interest in sex until the time of heat, which is just prior to ovulation, they do not have to worry about when they ovulate to increase the likelihood of pregnancy. Nature has taken care of their timing for them. Animals would be completely unable to practice rhythm birth control.

There are a few animals that are exceptions, in that the female is almost always receptive to sex, such as the rabbit and the cat. However, in these cases the act of intercourse actually induces ovulation. Rabbits and cats will not ovulate except in response to the sexual act. So even the occasional rabbit with fertility problems need not worry about the timing of intercourse. In fact, rhythm birth control could never work with her either. In all animals except man, sex appears to have just one purpose, and occurs only when that purpose is likely to be fulfilled.

Therefore, the concept of sex as a truly pleasurable event that may occur at any time is uniquely human. At the same time, however, human beings uniquely find it very difficult to know, without benefit of special tests, when they have ovulated or when intercourse is most likely to lead to pregnancy.

A number of biologists speculate that one of the distinguishing features of human life is the enduring family unit, which facilitates the transmission of learning over hundreds of generations. They theorize that one reason our civilization has achieved ascendancy over other animals is the continuity of learning provided by this stable family unit. It is conceivable that the continual enjoyment of sex, unrelated to heat and the necessity for reproduction, is one factor that has held our family unit so closely together. This theory is pure speculation, but it emphasizes that we should not be disturbed by the difficulty of knowing when to have intercourse to get pregnant or not to get pregnant but rather we should be happy that an inclination toward intercourse does not specifically depend on the relatively infrequent event of ovulation.

HORMONES AND MENSTRUATION

Since most women are unaware of when they ovulate, we must try to understand the events in the menstrual cycle more fully. We will arbitrarily call the first day of the menstrual cycle "day one." Day one is the day on which bleeding commences. Menstruation normally takes place over about four to five days. Thus the fourth day of bleeding would be the fourth day of the menstrual cycle. Bleeding usually ceases by day four or five and in most cases resumes about twenty-three to twenty-five days later—namely, on day twenty-eight to day thirty of the cycle. Although the first day of menstruation represents a shedding of the lining of the uterus that has built up in the previous month's cycle, it is actually the *beginning* of the next cycle.

On the first day of menstruation (day one of the cycle), the hormone FSH is already stimulating development of a follicle that will take precedence over all other follicles trying to develop for that month (see Figure 1–4, "Hormone Changes Associated with Normal Ovulation"). (Interestingly, FSH, which in females causes the follicle to develop, is the exact same hormone that in males helps to stimulate sperm production.) As the follicle develops over the next ten to fourteen days, it produces increasing amounts of the female hormone estrogen but no progesterone. The estrogen in turn slows down pituitary production of FSH so that the FSH level begins to drop prior to ovulation. By day twelve to day fourteen of the menstrual cycle, the follicle usually is quite ripe and appears on the surface of the ovary as a fluid-filled bubble ready to burst. In the meantime, the estrogen that has been produced by the follicle during this first half of the cycle is stimulating the uterus to prepare a thick, hard lining, and the cervix to produce enormous quantities of optically clear mucus, with high water content, maximum elasticity, and the greatest receptivity to sperm penetration. Furthermore, the entrance to the cervix, which generally is closed, has begun to open between day nine and day fourteen, to the point where it is almost gaping with an abundant outflow of clear mucus just prior to ovulation. Estrogen has prepared the way.

The final effect of estrogen (in high quantities) is to trigger the release of the hormone LH from the pituitary gland. This surge of LH then causes the follicle to burst, and ovulation occurs, normally about thirty-six hours after the beginning of the LH surge.

After ovulation the ruptured follicle forms the yellow corpus luteum that produces progesterone. Over the next ten to fourteen days progesterone makes the lining of the uterus delicate and spongy so it can adequately nourish the fertilized egg. It also causes the cervical mucus to dry up and the cervix to close. If the egg is not fertilized, the corpus luteum has a very specific, limited lifetime of ten to fourteen days. At the end of that time, if the woman is not pregnant, the ovary stops producing progesterone; the uterine lining can no longer support itself and is shed on what becomes day one of the next cycle.

How Does the Egg Reach the Tube After Ovulation?

The journey of the egg through the Fallopian tube and finally into the uterus after fertilization is extraordinarily hazardous. The Fallopian tube is not simply a passive channel through which the egg is transferred. Many events must work in precise synchrony for pregnancy to occur.

The egg must first be picked up from the surface of the ovary by the fimbria at the time of ovulation and then transported into the wide, ampullary end of the tube. There are, on the surface of the fimbria, millions of microscopic hairs, called cilia, which constantly beat in one direction, toward the uterus. These microscopic hairs beat at a fantastically rapid speed and create a kind of conveyor-belt effect, moving the egg along the Fallopian tube toward the uterus. When the egg is grasped by the fimbria, it is absolutely incredible to watch it being ushered along (almost like magic) and then disappear into the tube. If you tried to pull the egg away from the fimbria as it slides rapidly into the tube, you would find that it requires a considerable amount of tug. It appears almost as though a mysterious force field is in operation. But it is simply the constant beating of these microscopic cilia that lure the egg into the tube within a matter of minutes.

The cilia must dig into the sticky gel that surrounds the egg (called the cumulus oophorus) and move the egg along by transporting the whole sticky, gooey mass, rather than by specifically moving the tiny egg itself. The egg is invisible to the naked eye, but the gel that surrounds it is easily visible. If this sticky substance were not present and the egg were just placed bare upon the surface of the fimbria, the beating of the cilia would never move the egg along. The cilia are able to dig in and transport the egg only if it is encased in this sticky, gooey material.

Because the ovary hangs freely in the abdominal cavity, it would seem remarkable that the egg ever gets into the tube. You would think that the egg would just fall off the ovary and be lost. However, the diligently maneuvering fimbria, like tentacles at the end of the tube, sweep over the surface of the ovary at the time of ovulation to swallow the egg. The numerous cilia on the surface of the fimbria beat at a rate of twelve hundred times per minute and account for the fimbria's incredible grasping power.

The process of grasping the egg and moving it into the interior of the tube requires only about fifteen to twenty seconds. Once the egg is safely within the tube, it is transported within five minutes to a narrow region halfway toward the uterus, called the isthmus. Here the egg must sit and wait for a successful sperm to challenge its way into the egg's outer membrane, making a direct hit and thereby establishing pregnancy. While the egg is held in this position by the tight resistance of the narrow region of the tube, the much tinier sperm are nonetheless able to travel in the opposite direction from the uterus.

After the egg is released from the ovary, it is only fresh (and thus capable of fertilization) for about twelve hours. If the egg is not penetrated by sperm soon after ovulation, it becomes overripe and dies. That is the whole basis for "natural" or scientific rhythm birth control (which really works if you know what you're doing). The likelihood of intercourse taking place during a specific twelve-hour interval during any month is rather slight, so Nature must provide a mechanism for delaying some of the sperm so there is a continuous flow of smaller numbers of healthy sperm over a two- or three-day period into the site of fertilization. That way, if intercourse is perhaps one or two days off the twelve-hour limit, some sperm still can arrive at the site of fertilization at the right time.

Let's now look at the male reproductive system to see how sperm are produced and what route they must take to join up with the egg in the tube for fertilization.

The Male Reproductive Tract: An Introduction to the Testicles, Epididymis, Vas Deferens, and Penis

The testicle actually has two major functions. In addition to making sperm capable of fertilizing the female's egg, it also makes the male hormone testosterone, which is responsible for male sexual characteristics and male sexual behavior. A normal male has two testicles side by side in the scrotal sac (see Figure 1–7). They are located in these exteriorized compartments because the testicles can't produce sperm at normal body temperature. By residing outside the abdominal portion of the body, the testicles are cooled to a temperature about four degrees F. lower than the 98.6 degrees F. body temperature. If your testicles were inside your abdomen, it would be too hot for them to produce any sperm.

The scrotum has a remarkably delicate temperature-regulating mechanism that keeps the temperature of the testicle at 94 degrees F.

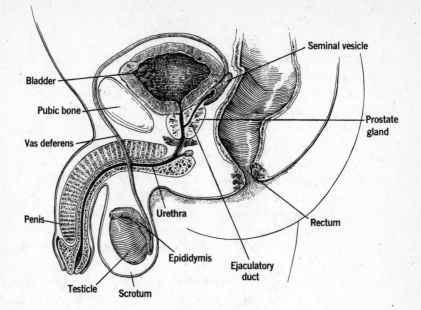

Bladder

Pubic bone

Vas deferens

Penis

Urethra

Epididymis

Testicle

Scrotum

Ejaculatory
duct

Rectum

Prostate
gland

Seminal vesicle

FIGURE 1–7.

at all times. Taking a cold shower causes the muscles of the scrotal sac to contract and pull the testicles very close to the body to conserve heat. On the other hand, when it is warm, the scrotal muscles relax, and the testicles fall farther away from the abdomen to cool off. This is an automatic reflex over which the male has no control. In addition, the scrotum works just a like a radiator, with a network of "cooling" veins carrying scrotal blood coiled around the artery that brings in the warmer abdominal blood.

The testicle consists of several hundred microscopic seminiferous tubules in which sperm are manufactured. These tubules converge and collect into an area called the rete testis, which is like a river delta near the upper part of the testicle. From here the sperm empties through a series of five to seven very small ducts out of the testicle into a delicate, coiled, twenty-foot-long microscopic tubule called the epididymis, and from there to the vas deferens, which is where a "vasectomy" is performed (see Figure 1–8). Clumps of cells called Leydig cells, which manufacture the male hormone testosterone, are sprinkled like pepper through the substance of the testicle around the sperm-producing tubules (see Figure 1–9).

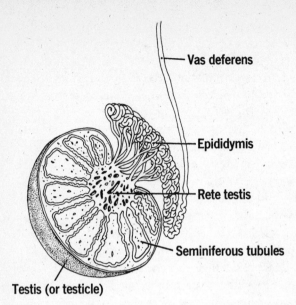

Vas deferens

Epididymis

Rete testis

Seminiferous tubules

Testis (or testicle)

FIGURE 1–8.

FIGURE 1–9.

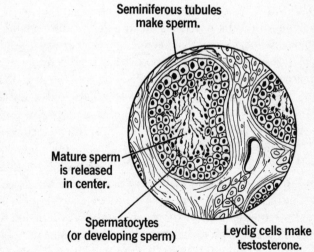

Seminiferous tubules
make sperm.

Mature sperm
is released
in center.

Spermatocytes
(or developing sperm)

Leydig cells make
testosterone.

Whereas sperm are carried out of the testicle into the vas deferens to be ejaculated at the time of orgasm, the testosterone manufactured by the Leydig cells is picked up by tiny veins coursing through the testicle and carried into the circulation. Because testosterone drains into the circulation this way, rather than via the vas deferens, a man can undergo a vasectomy (in which the vas deferens is cut for sterilization) without altering his hormone production or sexual drive.

The Leydig cells are remarkably sturdy. It is very difficult for any sort of illness or disease to interfere with an adequate production of testosterone. However, the tubules that manufacture sperm are extraordinarily delicate, and the slightest imperfection or generalized illness, such as a flu virus, can hurt sperm production. That is why so many men suffer from fertility problems and yet have no lack of virility.

Both the production of testosterone (which accounts for male sex drive, beard, pubic hair, and other sex characteristics) and the production of sperm in the testicles are stimulated by hormones produced by the pituitary gland, which sits just underneath the brain. These pituitary hormones are in turn regulated by releasing factors produced by the most primitive area of the brain, called the hypothalamus. This primitive region of the brain stimulates the pituitary gland to produce and release the two hormones FSH (follicle-stimulating hormone) and LH (luteinizing hormone). These names were given to the pituitary hormones on the basis of their function in the female. They are exactly the same hormones that stimulate the ovaries in the female. Without these hormones, either in the male or the female, the testicles and ovaries would immediately shrivel up and cease to function.

In the male, FSH helps to stimulate and maintain proper sperm production, and LH stimulates and maintains production of testosterone. When LH stimulates the testicles, the testosterone thus produced signals the brain that there is enough male hormone around, thus turning off the brain's production of the releasing hormone as well as the pituitary's production of FSH and LH. This fact is being exploited in the attempt to develop a male birth control pill. By giving a man testosterone tablets, or shots, the pituitary is signaled to stop producing FSH and LH. The testicles then will cease to make sperm. This method is similar to how female birth control pills work, except in this case the woman takes female hormones to suppress the same FSH and LH production that stimulates her ovulation.

The way in which the brain regulates production of sperm and hormones by the testicles is so important that we might dwell on an interesting example of a patient of mine who was born with *no testicles* at all and who underwent a successful testicle transplant from his identical twin brother. This patient did not undergo puberty when he went through his teens. He remained a eunuch while all of his classmates underwent the usual growth spurt and sexual development that occurs at puberty. Because of the absence of the male hormone testosterone, he had no pubic hair, no sexual drive, no voice change, and no growth spurt. However, the levels of FSH and LH production from his pituitary were extraordinarily high. Since there was no testosterone being produced (by virtue of the fact that he had no testicles), his brain responded by making excessive amounts of releasing hormone in an effort to drive the testicles that didn't exist into greater hormone and sperm production. When we successfully transplanted a testicle into him (using microsurgical techniques that will be explained in more detail in subsequent chapters), he began to produce testosterone almost immediately. At that point his FSH and LH levels came down to normal. After thirty years this patient's brain was finally being given the message that there was an adequate amount of testosterone in the circulation.

Sperm Production—the Assembly Line

The testicles normally produce huge amounts of sperm, far in excess of what is needed. Out of perhaps two hundred million sperm inseminated with one act of intercourse, only about four hundred ever reach the vicinity of the egg, and only one of those sperm has even a 15 percent chance in any given month of fertilizing the egg. Male fertility in many respects is a simple numbers game that any bookie would understand. But quality is more important than quantity, and a man who produces very small numbers of sperm can still get a woman pregnant.

All of the cells that eventually develop into normal sperm are called germ cells. The germ cells, which are lined up in an orderly array along the inside of the tubules within the testicle, are held in place and nourished by shapeless nurturing cells called "Sertoli cells." As each germ cell develops into a sperm, it sits with its head imbedded within the membrane of this maturing Sertoli cell. In the final phase of sperm production the sperm develops an oval head and a tail necessary for locomotion. As it develops, it moves toward the center of the tubule. When the product is complete, the mature sperm is released from the Sertoli cell into the tubule and swept along the tubule to make its escape, along with millions of others, from the testicle.

The developing sperm are passed along to the center of the tubule as though on an assembly line. They are passed from one stage of production to another at an absolutely unalterable speed of sixteen days for each stage. The total time it requires to produce every sperm is about seventy-two days. Neither sickness, testicular damage, nor hormonal manipulation can alter this inexorable rate. If you can imagine an automobile assembly line with a slow, steady, unstoppable movement from one stage of production to progressively more complex stages of production until the final car comes out for inspection, then you will have a pretty good understanding of how sperm are produced and, indeed, how sloppy the results often can be. In fact, one reason for the extravagant number of sperm produced by the testicles might be that only a small percentage will actually have all their nuts and bolts in the right place.

A deficiency in sperm production does not result from a slowing down of the speed at which the developing sperm proceed along the assembly line. Rather, it results from the absence of specific hormones or enzymes (like an absent worker, or a missing part) at any one of the stages of production. If there are a deficient number of early precursors, then the total number of sperm produced will be low. There is no pill or drug that can possibly increase or decrease the *speed* of sperm production. The *amount* of sperm production can be increased or decreased either by changing the availability of parts or by stopping the assembly line completely.

A simple understanding of this concept should make the reader depressingly aware of how difficult it is to improve sperm production in a man with a low sperm count, and how tricky it is to decrease sperm production to zero in a man with a high sperm count who wants reversible contraception.

How Many Sperm Do We Need?

Why do men need to produce such an enormous number of sperm simply to fertilize one egg? How could Nature be so wasteful? Why should there be so many obstacles in the female genital tract that make it mandatory for a large number of sperm to be wasted just so that one will make it? Wouldn't it be easier if Nature had provided women with a simple little test tube in which one sperm could be mixed with one egg and a baby thus formed?

There are a number of reasons for this overproduction. First, the time during which an egg in the female can be fertilized after it is ovulated is brief, about twelve hours. Therefore, it must be fertilized promptly after its release from the ovary. This requires the continuous presence of a reasonable number of fresh sperm in the Fallopian tube. Therefore, it is necessary for a much larger number of sperm to be available lower down in reservoir regions of the uterus, to be released upward continuously and slowly. Another reason that sperm must overcome so many obstacles in the female genital tract is that intercourse is not a sterile process and the female genital tract must be protected against infection. The same immune and physical barriers that allow only a few lucky sperm to gain access to the egg also protect the female against invasion by bacteria. Finally, it may be that sperm production is such a complicated biological process that there will be many defective products, again as on the automobile assembly line, and only the true "gems" are allowed access all the way to the egg. In any event, it is clear that if the quality of sperm is good, then not very many are necessary to make a man fertile.

How Sperm Reach the Ejaculate

LEAVING THE TESTICLES

After the completed spermatozoa are released into the center of the seminiferous tubule, they flow along it toward the exit point at the upper edge of the testicle. Sperm are pushed toward this exit point by contractions of very delicate muscle fibers. They do not yet move on their own. After they exit from the testicles, sperm are transferred into an amazing structure called the epididymis. The epididymis is a twenty-foot-long, coiled tube of microscopic size (one three-hundredths inch in diameter) that runs back and forth in loops like a strand of spaghetti but that actually traverses a distance of only one and one-half inches. The epididymis transfers sperm from the testicle to the larger vas deferens, the hard, muscular tube (one-eighth inch in thickness) that is severed when a man has a vasectomy.

It takes the sperm about twelve days to travel this entire twenty-foot journey through the winding length of the epididymis into the vas deferens. Sperm are propelled along this highly contorted microscopic tunnel by frequent contractions of its thin muscular wall. Most of the sperm are then stored at the end of the epididymis near where it joins the vas deferens. Here the sperm await their call to be rushed through the vas deferens and ejaculated at the time of orgasm.

WHAT HAPPENS TO SPERM IN THE EPIDIDYMIS?

The epididymal tubule is not just a bridge between the testicle and the vas. Sperm that leave the testicle still are not capable of fertilization. They must pass through the epididymis, the final tuning and inspection station of the assembly plant, before they obtain their ability to move in a straightforward direction with sufficient velocity to fertilize the female egg. If sperm were to be captured either from the testicle or from the beginning region of the epididymis, before the twenty-foot-long journey to the vas deferens, and used for artificial insemination, there would be no chance of pregnancy occurring. Only the sperm that have gone through at least part of the epididymis are capable of fertilization. During this seemingly endless journey through the winding turns of the epididymis, the sperm continue to mature, and they develop their incredible swimming ability.

Sperm motility probably is the most important determinant of the male's fertility. The sperm inside the testicle can only vibrate their tails weakly and barely wiggle around. Sperm from the beginning regions of the epididymis can swim, but only in circles. Unidirectional, straightforward swimming is achieved only by sperm that have traversed a part of the epididymis.

Sperm remain fresh and alive in the epididymis for less than a month. Old age comes quickly to a little sperm, and if it has to sit around for a month in the epididymis waiting to be ejaculated, it will be of no use. This does not mean that the man who has intercourse only once a month need not fear an unwanted pregnancy. There still are fresh sperm arriving every day that upon ejaculation will be capable of fertilizing. However, a man who has an ejaculation only once a month will have a much higher percentage of dead, ineffectual sperm in his ejaculate, despite having a higher overall number of sperm stored up.

Although this would seem to be a rather short life-span for sperm, it should be remembered that once they are deposited in a specimen jar, they are capable of living only for two to six hours. If they make it into the female genitals before that period has passed, they are capable of surviving for two to seven days.

THE FLUID THAT SQUIRTS THE SPERM OUT

Most of the fluid in the ejaculate does not come from the testicle, the epididymis, or the sperm duct. That is why vasectomy results in no change in the amount of fluid in the ejaculate. After vasectomy there is just no sperm in the fluid, but there still is plenty of fluid. During sexual intercourse, the epididymis and vas deferens muscles contract powerfully and propel sperm through the vas deferens up and out of the scrotal sac along its course through the abdomen, and finally to the ejaculatory duct, which sits just behind the opening from the bladder. The ejaculatory duct empties into the urethra, the canal inside the penis that carries the ejaculate out of the body.

Most of the ejaculate fluid comes from the seminal vesicles and the prostate gland and is expelled very forcefully behind the sperm, pushing them into the ejaculate. Thus the first squirt of the ejaculate contains most of the sperm. At this time the internal sphincter of the bladder clamps down to prevent the semen from accidentally going backward into the bladder, and simultaneously prevents urine from leaking forward out of the bladder. The external sphincter, which sits just in front of the ejaculatory duct, then opens up and allows the ejaculate to enter the holding area just near the base of the penis, called the bulbous urethra. Finally the very powerful muscles around the bulbous urethra contract and squirt the ejaculate out of the penis with remarkable force. This highly coordinated symphony of complicated muscular contractions that propel the sperm from the epididymis all the way up through the abdomen and out of the penis is what the male subjectively feels as orgasm.

The volume of ejaculate is quite variable from person to person and from species to species. The human ejaculate normally is about one teaspoonful, whereas the pig's ejaculate is close to a full pint, and it takes the pig a full half hour of orgasm to complete his ejaculation. The pig's penis has screw-like grooves which actually fit similar grooves in the female pig's cervix. He literally "screws" his penis into the cervix, locks on, and ejaculates all of this sperm directly into her uterus for over a half hour.

It is clear that many of the complicated fluids secreted by the prostate gland, the urethral glands, and the seminal vesicles are not really necessary, except to provide a vehicle for sperm to enter the vagina. In fact, dilute solutions of salt water appear to be a better vehicle for sperm than the semen in which they are naturally bathed at the time of ejaculation. The major function of the semen appears to be the provision of a very temporary environment for them during the brief moment of transition from the man's vas deferens to the woman's vagina. Within minutes the sperm that will fertilize the woman have already entered the cervical mucus and are on their way.

How Do Sperm Reach the Egg?

EJACULATION INTO THE VAGINA

Most of the spermatozoa in the ejaculate are contained in the first portion that squirts out of the penis and enters the vagina. Thus at the moment of ejaculation, the female's cervix (the opening leading into her uterus) is bathed by a high concentration of sperm. Sperm begin to invade the very thick fluid called cervical mucus, which protects this opening to the uterus, within just a few minutes after ejaculation. The sperm invade the cervix by virtue of their own swimming ability. Nothing about the sexual act will help those sperm get into the cervix. They simply have to swim in on their own, and this requires a great deal of coordinated, cooperative activity on their part.

Ejaculation is a very tense moment for the sperm, as the vagina presents a harsh, acid environment that normally would immobilize them quickly. Only the alkalinity of the semen, the fluid in which the sperm are ejaculated, allows them to survive temporarily in this antagonistic vaginal environment. However, even the semen is a potentially dangerous milieu for the sperm. Any sperm that remain in the semen for over several hours will deteriorate. To survive long enough to get to the egg and fertilize it, the sperm must gain rapid access to the cervical mucus. Most sperm that have not penetrated the cervical mucus within an hour after orgasm will not be able to do so later on, because by then they will have lost their ability to swim into the friendly environment of the cervix. The invasion must take place promptly, and any sperm left behind will never be able to catch up.

INVASION OF THE CERVICAL MUCUS

Spermatozoa can be seen invading the cervical mucus within seconds after ejaculation. But most will not make it. Of some two hundred million sperm deposited into the vagina near the cervix, only 100,000 ever get into the womb. Over 99.9 percent of the sperm never have a chance of getting beyond the vagina.

Once the sperm enter the canal of the cervix, they are capable of fertilizing the egg for as long as two to seven days. Since the egg is fertilizable for only twelve, or at most twenty-four, hours after ovulation, it is important to have a continuing flow of sperm across the tube so that whenever the egg arrives, there will be sperm available to fertilize it. The canal of the cervix thus acts as a receiving station through which platoons of spermatozoa migrate, and in which some are detained to ensure a continuous supply of smaller numbers over a more prolonged period to the Fallopian tube, where fertilization takes place.

To understand how you can use natural, or scientific rhythm birth control, you will need to understand more about the remarkable liquid that covers the opening of the womb, the cervical mucus. The cervical mucus presents a very effective barrier to bacteria and thus protects the womb against infection. It is a selective filter that favors normally active sperm and excludes bacteria and other objects (including poor-quality sperm) from access to the cervix. It doesn't even permit access to normal sperm except during a specific time at midcycle, when ovulation is imminent. Cervical mucus resembles a thick, clear liquid that can be poured (like any liquid) from one container into another. However, in a technical sense it is not a liquid, because if one wishes to pour only a portion of the cervical mucus from one tube into another, it would be impossible to do so without literally cutting it with a scissors. Thus, although it seems to behave as a thick liquid, it also has the characteristics of a very pliable, transparent plastic.

The cervical mucus is very scanty at the beginning of the cycle. It gradually becomes more and more abundant up to the middle of the cycle (when ovulation is about to occur). By this time the mucus is pouring out of the opening of the uterus. At this moment when fertilization is possible, near the time of ovulation, the mucus can be stretched out into a very thin strand without breaking. At all other times in the cycle it is sticky, and instead of stretching, it will break. All these changes in the cervical mucus that occur around midcycle are designed to help sperm gain access to the uterus. The more liquidlike character, the greater transparency, and the greater stretchability (called *Spinn-barkeit*) of the cervical mucus favor the successful invasion of an army of sperm. When the mucus is sticky and thick, not so abundant, and translucent rather than transparent, it is difficult if not impossible for any sperm to gain access. Learning to become aware of this difference helps make rhythm birth control work.

Just prior to ovulation, under the effect of the female hormone estrogen, the amount of mucus production rises tenfold and its water content increases. The otherwise dense and impenetrable microscopic fibrillar mesh gives way to a more open microscopic structure with much larger gaps between the fibrils. The molecules of the mucus then become arranged in parallel rows longitudinally along the canal of the cervix. This parallel arrangement encourages the sperm to move in one direction rather than in a haphazard motion, again aiding sperm invasion.

When the semen reaches the cervical mucus, a clear line can be seen separating the two different fluids. Soon phalanges of sperm begin to penetrate the mucus, forming branching structures that invade deeply into it. Observing the attack of the sperm on the cervical mucus under the microscope is an exciting event. Sperm at first seem to bounce against the cervical mucus without any evidence that they will ever be able to gain access. Furthermore, their movements while in the ejaculate are haphazard, and not specifically aimed toward the mucus. However, within a matter of minutes one or two spermatozoa in a given area can be seen to make an indentation in the line separating the cervical mucus from the ejaculate. Once one sperm has been able to initiate penetration of the mucus, other sperm quickly follow at exactly that point of entry. The sperm then continue to invade the cervical mucus much like a single-file line of army ants. Only one or two spermatozoa can pass at a time through this line of entrance.

Once initial penetration has occurred, more sperm are able to continue easily across this beachhead into the cervix. They swim in a straightforward direction along the parallel row of cells representing the microscopic molecular structure of the mucus. Then once this initial beachhead has been established, sperm swim through the cervical mucus at a speed of about one-eighth inch per minute. In about thirty minutes they can travel almost four inches, which is the distance required to reach the Fallopian tubes. However, pregnancy would not be likely if all the sperm got into the Fallopian tube at one time, because they would soon pass through it into the abdominal cavity. Unless they were lucky enough to pass through the Fallopian tubes at exactly the moment of ovulation, or within twelve hours of that time, they would be long gone by the time the egg arrived. Thus Nature had to invent some mechanism for allowing a continuous assault upon the site of fertilization by a smaller number of sperm at any one moment.

Some of the sperm are transported rapidly and directly into the uterus, but most of the sperm are led into crypts, or little cavities, along the inside wall of the cervix, where they are stored. There is then a slow release of the spermatozoa from these storage sites. Thus the cervix acts as a reservoir from which, over a period of time, spermatozoa are slowly released into the uterus and Fallopian tubes.

CAPACITATION OF SPERM

During the course of their odyssey toward the site of fertilization, the sperm undergo a process called capacitation, which is not fully understood. Unless sperm reside for a certain time outside the semen, for some unknown reason they are not capable of fertilization, even though in every other respect they appear normal. It used to be thought that this process of capacitation could occur only in the specific fluids of the female reproductive tract while the sperm migrate on their journey toward the egg. However, recent scientific work with test-tube fertilization has demonstrated that capacitation of sperm (until now considered one of the greatest problems in successfully achieving *in vitro* fertilization) can occur in relatively simple fluids available in any laboratory.

In fact, merely removing the sperm from the semen is all that is needed for capacitation. It is the semen itself that somehow keeps the sperm from being able to fertilize. Thus sperm seem to have a natural tendency toward developing their own capacitation for fertilization, and this simply requires a period of several hours outside the semen. The fact that sperm require time to be capacitated could represent still another reason for the delaying mechanisms the sperm encounter before gaining entrance into the tube where fertilization of the egg finally takes place.

Fertilization of the Egg in the Fallopian Tube

The goal toward which all of these processes lead is the fertilization of the egg by the sperm (see Figure 1–10). This is a beautiful and moving event to observe under the microscope, and only recently have scientists

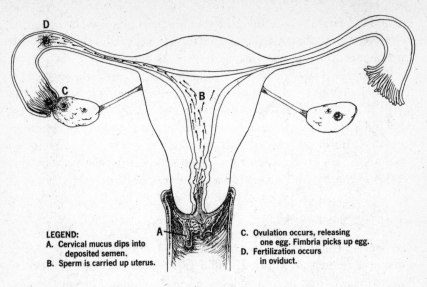

LEGEND:
A. Cervical mucus dips into deposited semen.
B. Sperm is carried up uterus.
C. Ovulation occurs, releasing one egg. Fimbria picks up egg.
D. Fertilization occurs in oviduct.

FIGURE 1–10.

come to understand fertilization well enough to duplicate it in a test tube and produce a normal baby.

Fertilization of the egg occurs in the widened region of the female's Fallopian tube called the ampulla. In most animals the egg will find sperm waiting when it arrives in the tube, because the period of sexual receptivity usually begins just before ovulation. Humans are the only animals in which there is no fixed relation between sexual intercourse and ovulation, and therefore the eggs may very well have to wait in vain in the ampulla for the arrival of spermatozoa. The egg is capable of being fertilized for a period of only twelve hours after ovulation. If it has to wait too long for sperm to arrive, it will deteriorate.

For a sperm to enter and fertilize the egg, it must first dig its way through several layers of protective shields. All of these outside walls protecting the inner confines of the egg represent an impressive barrier to sperm penetration, and a sperm cannot break its way through these protective membranes without the aid of chemicals released from its warhead, the acrosome. The acrosome surrounds the front portion of the sperm, much like a battering ram. Chemicals released by the acrosome first dissolve the jellylike cumulus oophorus, enabling the sperm to pass through it and reach the zona pellucida, the very tough inner membrane that represents perhaps the most formidable obstacle to sperm. To penetrate this barrier, the sperm cannot just haphazardly liberate chemicals, or the egg might be damaged. The attacking chemicals must remain closely bound to the surface of the sperm and cut an extraordinarily narrow slit in the membrane that allows only a single sperm to enter.

When this first sperm has successfully invaded the egg, a remarkable event takes place. The genes within the egg fuse with the genes within the sperm as these two microscopic entities initiate the development of a new human being. At this moment the membrane surrounding the egg becomes transformed into a rigid barrier so impenetrable that other sperm, despite all the chemicals in their acrosomes, cannot possibly enter. Often many sperm can be seen attempting to enter the egg in competition with the one that made it first, but their efforts are totally in vain.

Humans are relatively wasteful in the management of their sperm and eggs. If pregnancy does not occur in one month, it may occur in another. It's just that haphazard. However, in other animals the process is much more precise. In the domestic hen, for example, sperm are capable of living for four weeks after they've been deposited in the female, and large numbers of eggs are fertilized as they pass through the hen during the next month. In bats, sexual intercourse takes place only in the autumn, and the animals then hibernate for the winter. Three or four months later, when they wake up, the females finally ovulate, and the sperm are quite capable of fertilization despite their long period of dormancy in the female. The honeybee is perhaps the most careful utilizer of sperm in the animal kingdom. After one nuptial flight with a male, the queen bee has a sufficient supply of sperm to last for several years. She rations out one or two sperm for each egg that is to be fertilized and thus can produce millions of offspring over a period of years with the sperm received from one episode of intercourse. In certain spiders, the male deposits fewer than ten sperm in the female at the time of intercourse, but each of these carefully rationed sperm is a jewel. The female may save them for up to a year to fertilize her eggs. The reproductive act seems to be efficient and precise in almost all members of the animal kingdom other than humans. The human reproductive mechanism is clearly developed in such a way that fertilization of the egg is not its only purpose.

EARLY DEVELOPMENT OF THE FERTILIZED EGG

Over the next three days the fertilized egg first divides into two cells, then four cells, then eight. The fertilized egg, or embryo, does not pass into the uterus for implantation until it is two or three days old. Thus all of us have spent the first few days of our embryonic life in our mother's tube before being allowed into the uterus. If the embryo is transferred into the uterus too soon, it will not be ready to implant and will die. If the transfer of the egg into the uterus is delayed too long, a tubal, or ectopic, pregnancy occurs (i.e., the fertilized egg implants in the tube rather than the uterus). This eventually destroys the tube and requires surgery. Because the journey of the egg from the ovary to the site of fertilization, its nourishment in the tube, and the continuation of its journey into the uterus are so intricate, problems with this transportation process are frequently responsible for female infertility.

After about seven days, when the pregnancy has been established in the uterus, the embryo itself begins to make a hormone called HCG (human chorionic gonadotropin), which stimulates the corpus luteum of the ovary to keep making progesterone for the next three months to suppress menstruation and loss of the pregnancy. After three months, the fetus makes its own progesterone, and the ovaries are no longer needed for production of the hormone. After nine months, the baby is ready to be pushed out of the uterus by the mother during labor.

The presence of HCG signifies an established pregnancy and thus is the basis for almost all of the routine pregnancy tests. When the doctor samples the patient's urine or blood and checks for pregnancy, he or she really is checking for the presence of HCG. If it is present, then the pregnancy test is positive. Since previous methods of analyzing this hormone were not very sensitive, the diagnosis of pregnancy could not be made with certainty until about four weeks after the missed period. However, with sophisticated modern methods pregnancy can be diagnosed with a simple test that the woman can perform herself in her home on the very first day she has missed her period.

2

Natural Family Planning

(ALSO CALLED SCIENTIFIC RHYTHM, OVULATION DETECTION METHOD, OR PERIODIC ABSTINENCE)

Introduction

For many of you who are afraid of the potential dangers (real or imagined) of birth control methods, the end of this chapter may be where you decide to stop. You see, there is an almost foolproof method of birth control that requires no "birth control." This is an approach that practicing Catholics, Moslems, Orthodox Jews, Fundamentalist Christians, or anyone with an aversion to interfering with the natural process of conception can follow. I'm referring to "natural" family planning, or scientific rhythm. Please note that I distinguish this scientific approach from the classic method of rhythm birth control recommended in the old days by the Catholic Church and others. With the old rhythm method, you just went by the calendar and hoped you were hitting it at the right time. So many women hit it at the wrong time, and got pregnant when they didn't want to, that this method of birth control became ridiculed and humorously referred to as "Vatican roulette." I would not want to recommend a method of birth control that was so unreliable and nerve-racking.

But there is a scientific approach to rhythm that costs nothing, requires no medical intervention, no manipulation of any kind, and is quite effective in protecting you from getting pregnant. You don't need surgery, you don't need to take the time to put on a condom or a diaphragm while in the midst of your sexual desire, and you don't have to do anything to interrupt your body's normal chemistry. You simply have to read this chapter and learn how to recognize precisely when during your monthly cycle you are safe from getting pregnant and when you are not safe from getting pregnant.

If that is your inclination, you may never need go beyond this chapter. For others who find that this natural method of birth control requires too much discipline, recordkeeping, and willpower to avoid sex during sometimes lengthy fertile portions of your cycle, you will want to go on to the rest of this book to learn about your many "simpler" options. As you read through the rest of the book, you will find out how relatively safe most methods of birth control can be if you choose wisely and understand how to use them. The disadvantage of these other methods is that they are not "natural," and you may have the emotional fear of unexpected side effects such as women in the 1960s and 1970s experienced when they suddenly found out that the birth control pills and IUDs that catapulted us into the sexual revolution were not always safe (even though we know that the newer low-dose pills are safe for the right woman).

To follow this extremely appealing natural method of birth control, you must understand your reproductive cycle and, in a sense, know your body. Many people have been given the wrong advice because their advisers weren't sufficiently knowledgeable. You will hear a lot of rumors and inaccurate tales about how to recognize the fertile and infertile times in your cycle. What I want to do in this chapter is give you an authoritative guide you can rely on rather than guess with.

Before the publication of my previous book *How to Get Pregnant*, a large number of infertile couples had been incorrectly told that to maximize their chances of getting pregnant, they should wait until the wife's morning temperature went up, indicating ovulation. They were to abstain from sex to save up all of the husband's sperm until that magic moment. What these couples and their ill-informed advisers did not realize is that they were in fact practicing a relatively crude form of rhythm birth control. Once her temperature goes up, the wife has *already* ovulated, and the chances for pregnancy are much less rather than greater. I cannot tell you how many thousands of infertile couples achieved pregnancy after reading this little clarification advising them to have sex *before* the temperature goes up rather than *after*.

In the same fashion, I want this chapter to clarify how you can reliably know when it is "safe" to have sex without the fear of pregnancy.* This will not be a loose, casual piece of advice but a total effort to get you to understand yourself enough so that you have confidence in this method of birth control should you choose it.

In the Old Testament, there is a fascinating reference to "periodic abstinence" that has incredible scientific merit today and yet has been neglected in most of the popular literature. Because of this biblical commandment, Orthodox Jews cannot have sexual relations with their wives until seven days after menstrual bleeding has stopped. This is called the *mikva*, and is described in great detail in Leviticus. This first use of rhythm for timing of sex has potentially profound effects that are only now in the 1980s becoming apparent.

The average woman experiences about five days total of menstrual flow. The first day of menstruation is day one of her cycle. The most fertile women are those who have predictable, regular, twenty-eight-day cycles, with ovulation on day fourteen. For this extremely fertile type of woman, the most fertile day of her cycle would be day twelve or thirteen—that is, just prior to ovulation, when her cervical mucus is abundant and her cervix is widely dilated. If the couple have intercourse at that time, the sperm will remain in her reproductive tract ready to fertilize her egg over the next forty-eight to seventy-two hours. Thus, if the man happens to have a low sperm count, the biblical commandment of *mikva* assures that he will be saving up all his sperm for a minimum of twelve days and will release it into his wife at exactly the most fertile time of her cycle.

But there is another, more subtle, birth control benefit to this biblical timing of sex. As women approach their late thirties, the risk of becoming pregnant with a mentally retarded Down's syndrome ("Mongoloid") child rises significantly. For women in their twenties the risk is less than one in two thousand. Over the age of forty the risk rises to as high as one in twenty-five. The birth of a Down's syndrome child is so devastating that most women who get pregnant over the age of thirty-five have an amniocentesis, a procedure whereby a little bit of fluid is taken out of the uterus and examined for any genetic or chromosomal abnormalities in the fetus. If they had avoided having sex

---

* By "safe" I do not mean that a given method is 100 percent safe. I only mean that the chance of becoming pregnant while using that method is extremely low. No method of birth control (save total abstinence) is 100 percent safe. But if natural birth control is followed carefully and scientifically, it is certainly as safe as most popular methods of birth control. "Safe" is a relative term.

until day twelve, this problem would be less likely to have occurred.

The reason is that as women approach their early forties, their ovaries begin to run out of eggs and therefore the pituitary gland produces more of the hormone FSH (which superstimulates the few remaining follicles that are left). Thus middle-aged women tend to ovulate early in the month, on days nine, ten, or eleven rather than on day fourteen, as they did in their youth. Thus middle-aged Orthodox Jewish couples who follow the ancient biblical proscription against sex until seven days after menstruation ceases will usually be having intercourse after the wife has ovulated and thus when she is very unlikely to get pregnant. So at an age when the woman has the greatest likelihood of having a genetically abnormal child, pregnancy is very unlikely to occur. In a sense, this turns out to be rhythm birth control for older couples.

At one of my son's games last fall a parent who knew of my work came up to me and said she would like to have a tubal sterilization. She was almost forty years old, an energetic lady full of vim and vigor, who was having terrible headaches on the birth control pill. Her doctor had been prescribing for many years a brand of pill (Ovral) that contained very high levels of hormones and was therefore probably not safe for her. I suggested that she try a different, low-dose (low-hormone), triphasic pill that would mimic a normal cycle more "naturally" (see Chapter 4). But she was understandably terrified about the pill, and yet afraid to stop taking it because she didn't want to get pregnant. So she seemed like a good candidate for a tubal sterilization.

The problem was that her husband was against sterilization and she, too, was somewhat fearful of "going under the knife." They didn't want to use condoms or diaphragms, and she did not realize (nor did it ever enter her doctor's mind) that like the Orthodox Jewish woman who can't have sex until seven days after menstruation ceases, she could use rhythm birth control and be safe. No more pills, no operation to worry about, no potential irreversibility to worry about, no messy foam, and no having to stop, go to the drawer, and pull out a condom or a diaphragm while in the heat of passion.

Another couple that came from the other side of the country had a similar problem. The husband desperately wanted a vasectomy and wanted me to perform it on him before he left town. Yet it was clear that he was hoping that someday they could have more children, and she also had not ruled the idea out. But he was desperate because IUDs were no longer available in this country (they didn't know you could travel to Canada or another foreign country to get one), and she was afraid at her age (over thirty-five) to take birth control pills. She had gotten pregnant four months earlier, at a time when they could not afford a child and desperately did not want one. She found herself feeling guilty about being relieved at having had a miscarriage two months later. They were now living in total abstinence. Like most married men, he was not interested in using a condom, and she was so concerned about getting pregnant again that she would not let him go near her.

They, too, were perfect candidates for natural birth control methods. They were clearly able to endure periods of abstinence of longer than one or two weeks. Both were nature-loving, ecologically minded people who hated the notion of any chemical or mechanical interference. They watched their diet carefully; ate no red meat or fatty foods; lived strictly on vegetables, fruit, and fish; and ate no food with preservatives in it. They were amazed to find out that rhythm, which had been so ridiculed over the previous twenty-five years of their postpubertal life, actually works. They left St. Louis with no operation and no pills.

But the drawback is, scientific rhythm is not easy. You are going to have to read and understand thoroughly everything in this chapter and may even want to get some further guidance from some of the natural family planning centers in just about every major city in the United States and in most of the countries around the world.

Natural birth control isn't the right option for an undisciplined young girl who is just beginning to experiment with sex. The teenage pregnancy rate in this country is incredible and outscores that of every other civilized country in the world. It staggers the imagination to think that 20 percent of American teenage girls get pregnant. In large cities the figure is closer to 50 percent. When I visited one of the largest birth control clinics in the country I met a thirteen-year-old girl who already had one child. She goes to high school and takes the child with her because the high school has a day-care program for teenage mothers. She quite reasonably decided she didn't want any more children for a while and requested an IUD. The clinic doctors decided not to put in the usual Copper 7 model, which loses its potency about every three years and needs replacement, but rather to insert an older (but still relatively safe) Lippes loop model, which requires no replacement. The reason for this choice is that neither she nor the doctors felt that she would have enough discipline to come back in three years to have the Copper 7 replaced. Someone at this immature stage of life is in no position to undertake the discipline and planning that natural birth control requires.

Natural birth control is an ideal method of birth control for mature couples who are able to discipline and organize their lives. It is perfect for those couples whose religion opposes birth control, because virtually all religions favor this method, including the Roman Catholic Church. It is the ideal birth control method for "back to nature" people who do not want to "poison" their body. It is ideal for mature women who feel bad about avoiding having children but know the advantages about delaying and spacing a family. With increasing health consciousness, not to mention the rise of religion in the 1980s, natural birth control is appealing to an increasing number of Americans. It is birth control without the stigma of birth control. It is basically "pronatal" and is perfect for couples whose concept is to "choose rather than control conception," doing nothing at all to interfere with future fertility. In fact, although it involves abstaining from sex during the fertile phase of the month, the principles of scientific rhythm can be applied exactly in reverse to make it much easier for you to get pregnant when you want to have a child. Even after you have had all the children you want, if you're a woman in your late thirties this is an ideal method because in addition to being more mature and disciplined, you are less fertile than you were fifteen years ago anyway, and why should you have to go through the risk of IUDs, birth control pills, hormonal manipulation, or a surgical operation for sterilization?

When I first appeared on *The Phil Donahue Show* in 1980, I talked about how sperm are only able to get into the uterus at just the right time of the month prior to ovulation, and that at all other times the cervix is a closed, sticky barrier to sperm penetration. The whole audience joined me in my focus of helping infertile couples learn how to get pregnant. But at the end of the show, when we hardly had time for a thoughtful answer, one woman asked why we couldn't use this knowledge to avoid pregnancy without the need of birth control pills, IUDs, and all their problems. So in a sense this chapter is a belated answer to that question.

Natural or scientific rhythm is a very highly effective method of birth control, but I can't emphasize enough that it works only if you are disciplined, motivated, and prepared to spend a great deal of time learning how to do it. For it to work effectively you must understand your body. Furthermore, it may require abstinence for at least eight, possibly eleven days of the month, and if you don't want to have sex during menstruation, possibly as many as sixteen days. So don't go into this chapter thinking it is a panacea. This approach has been used by women throughout the world with success and enthusiasm. But because it requires understanding and discipline, about two thirds of those who begin this method eventually choose the "easier" path of birth control pills, IUD, condoms, diaphragm, or sterilization. The one third who continue using "natural" birth control, such as "back to nature" enthusiasts, the health-conscious, and practicing Catholics, simply can't imagine why anyone would ever use any other method of birth control. We will begin with a review of the normal menstrual cycle and go from there into how you can use this knowledge to keep from getting pregnant.

Review of the Normal Menstrual Cycle

In almost all animals except rabbits and cats, there are only a few days (just prior to ovulation) in which sex can lead to pregnancy. With rabbits and cats sex causes ovulation. Natural birth control would be impossible for them. In all other animals (except humans), sex isn't even desired except just before ovulation, when it is likely to lead to pregnancy. Thus cows and rats theoretically could use natural birth control, but they would never buy the idea, because their sexual desire is triggered chemically by a rise in estrogen level that occurs just prior to ovulation, and at no other time. In animals this is commonly referred to as being "in heat." Humans are the only animals who have the privilege of enjoying sex or wanting sex at any time of the month or year.

With humans, sex clearly has another function other than reproduction. Many anthropologists and philosophers, as well as religious leaders, believe that the sexual bond helps cement a marriage and creates the kind of stable family unit necessary for children to learn from their parents the lessons of the previous forty thousand years. But despite the fact that humans can enjoy sex at any time of the month, they get pregnant only during the fertile period just prior to ovulation.

The reason for this noncyclic female sexual desire in the human is that humans are the only animals in which the female's libido (sexual desire) is stimulated by the male hormone testosterone. Testosterone is continually secreted by the testicle in males in large amounts, and in human females by the ovary and adrenal glands in smaller amounts. In all other animals the female develops an interest in sex and goes into heat as a pure chemical response to rising estrogen levels just prior to ovulation, and she is not aroused at all by her low, constant, unchanging level of testosterone. This rising estrogen level prepares the cervix and uterus for entry of sperm and fertilization of the egg. But in humans the estrogen level does not stimulate sexual arousal or receptivity. In human females sexual arousal is simply stimulated by testosterone, whose level is fairly even throughout the monthly cycle. In other words, the level of your sexual desire is no indication of when it is "safe" to have sex.

There are four basic signs that reliably tell you where you are in your monthly cycle. You can easily determine these for yourself without the need for medical testing. They are the basal body (morning) temperature, production of cervical mucus, opening and closing of the cervix, and the calendar day of the cycle in relation to your first day of menstruation. Let's see how these four elements fit into the monthly cycle.

The first day of menstruation is day one of the cycle. Beginning on day one your pituitary gland releases the hormone FSH, which stimulates the ovary to grow follicles. As the follicle gets bigger and bigger during the first fourteen days of the cycle, the egg inside it matures and the follicle begins to make the female hormone estrogen. This production of estrogen by the follicle controls the entire cycle.

As the level of estrogen increases, it stimulates the cervix to make more and more cervical mucus. In addition, your cervix, which normally has a tiny little opening leading into the uterus, begins to enlarge. Just prior to ovulation, estrogen levels are at their highest, the cervix is wide open, and a large amount of mucus is present that is no longer sticky and thick but rather transparent, watery, and elastic. Nature's purpose here is to allow the sperm, just prior to ovulation, to enter into the mucus and thereby gain access to the uterus with maximum ease.

Once the estrogen level gets this high (usually around day thirteen in a twenty-eight-day cycle), it stimulates the pituitary gland to release luteinizing hormone, or LH. LH is the trigger that stimulates ovulation about twenty-four hours later. Once you ovulate, that same follicle that before produced only estrogen, suddenly begins to produce a new hormone called progesterone. Progesterone is produced only after ovulation, never before.

Progesterone causes the cervical mucus to dry up and the opening to the cervix to close. In addition, it causes your basal body morning temperature (your body's temperature upon waking) to rise about 0.4 to 0.8 degree F. Although we can understand how rising estrogen levels in the first half of your cycle stimulate your cervix to open and make copious amounts of mucus necessary for allowing sperm invasion, and how after ovulation progesterone causes the cervical mucus to dry up and the cervical mucus to close and no longer permit sperm invasion, we have no understanding of what benefit the rise in basal body temperature caused by progesterone could possibly be other than to make natural family planning possible.

What confounds my mind is how few women understand or are aware of these incredibly synchronized and exciting events taking place every month. The female reproductive apparatus is not just a pleasure receptacle but an incredibly complex, beautifully tuned mechanism. You can use that self-knowledge not only to have the baby that you dream about, but also to avoid having a child when you don't want it.

To know when you can and cannot safely have sex, we need to determine not only when you ovulate, but also how long after ovulation the egg is able to be fertilized, and how long prior to ovulation the sperm remain capable of fertilizing. It is clear that eggs are capable of being fertilized only for a very brief period after ovulation, somewhere between twelve and twenty-four hours. Thus if you could pinpoint ovulation precisely, forty-eight hours later you should be very secure about having intercourse without getting pregnant. For that reason there is no difficulty in deciding when to start having sex in the second half of the cycle. It is not so easy, however, to determine when it is no longer safe to have sex prior to ovulation. When in the first half of the cycle do you need to stop having sex? How long after intercourse are sperm in the cervical mucus still capable of getting you pregnant? It could possibly be as long as seven days, so if you have intercourse several days before ovulation, you may become pregnant.

There is another problem. Although humans are interested in sex at any time of the cycle, as opposed to animals, who are interested in sex only just prior to ovulation, even in humans there is a very slight increase in female sexual interest around the time of ovulation. The reason for this is that there is a slight but definite increase in testosterone level in all women around the time of ovulation just after the estrogen rise. Thus although sex occurs with almost equal interest throughout any time of the cycle, a woman's greatest interest in initiating sex is likely to be somewhat greater just around the time when she needs to be saying "No."

How to Figure Out When in the Month You Can and Cannot Get Pregnant

THE CALENDAR METHOD

The calendar method is the classic rhythm method first advocated in the 1930s. You need to understand this approach, and where it failed, to be able to use the newer, safe approaches. The calendar method of rhythm birth control is based upon the established fact that most normal fertile women ovulate fourteen days before they begin to menstruate in the next cycle. When they have varying cycle lengths—for example, a twenty-five-day cycle one month and a forty-day cycle the next month— the only thing that varies is the number of days from day one to the time of ovulation. The time from ovulation until next menstruation always is going to be about fourteen days. For example, in a twenty- five-day cycle you would have ovulated on day eleven, in a thirty-five- day cycle you would have ovulated on day twenty-one, and in a forty-day cycle you would have ovulated on day twenty-six.

The first half of the cycle—the time from day one of menstruation until ovulation—is called the follicular phase because it is during that time that the follicle is growing, developing, and preparing for ovulation as it begins to make more and more estrogen. The second half of the cycle—the time from ovulation until the first day of menstruation of the next cycle—is called the "luteal phase," when the hormone pro- gesterone is secreted by the ruptured follicle. The follicular phase may vary, but the luteal phase, at least according to this theory, always is fourteen days. That is the basis of the classic calendar method of rhythm birth control.

Forty years ago, before the advent of the pill and the IUD, rhythm was one of the more common methods of birth control used in the world. Pregnancy rates of about 40 percent per year for couples using this method were too high to be legitimately called contraception, but the rates were still considerably lower than the normal pregnancy rate per year of 80 percent for a noncontracepting couple. That means that instead of an 80 percent chance of getting pregnant in a year, couples using old-fashion rhythm had a 40 percent chance. So there was some merit to this old-fashioned method of calendar rhythm, and we'll study it a little bit more before going on, because it forms a foundation for the modern approach to rhythm that now can give you protection against pregnancy equivalent to other modern methods of birth control.

The calendar method assumes that if you abstain from sex for five days before ovulation, and for three days after ovulation, you will not get pregnant. This assumption is often quite valid. The only problem is in determining when you ovulate. Ironically, the most fertile women are those least likely to get pregnant using the calendar method of rhythm. The most fertile women tend to ovulate on day fourteen in a predictable twenty-eight-day cycle. So if they simply abstain from sex beginning on day nine of their cycle and resume having sex after day seventeen of their cycle, these highly fertile women who predictably ovulate on day fourteen are very unlikely to get pregnant using this method of birth control.

In an effort to translate this reliability to the majority of women with less regular cycles, some formulas were developed that lengthened the period of required abstinence, still attempting to prevent intercourse for five days before ovulation and three days after ovulation. The most popular formula is as follows: (1) To determine the first day of the "unsafe" portion of your cycle, subtract eighteen days from the length of your shortest cycle. For example, if your shortest cycle is twenty-five days, then your *first* "unsafe" day—the day on which you begin sexual abstinence—would be day seven of your cycle. If your shortest cycle was thirty days, then your first "unsafe" day would be day twelve. (2) To figure the *last* unsafe day of your cycle (the day after which you can again have sex), subtract eleven from the number of days of your longest cycle. For example, if your longest cycle was forty days, you would not be able to resume intercourse until after day twenty-nine. If your longest cycle was thirty days, you would be able to resume intercourse after day nineteen.

What if your cycles varied anywhere from twenty-five days some months to thirty-three days in other months? You would subtract eighteen from twenty-five and determine that day seven was the beginning of your "unsafe" period. You would subtract eleven from thirty-three and determine that day twenty-two was the end of your "unsafe" period. In like manner, if your cycles varied from twenty-three to thirty-one days, you should have no sex from day five to day twenty. (You can see that using this old-fashioned calendar method, women with irregular cycles would require a lot of abstinence.)

If you have trouble remembering this formula, simply refer to the predictable, normal regular cycle of twenty-eight days and remember that it is only "safe" to have sex earlier than five days *before* ovulation and later than three days *after* ovulation. Thus in a twenty-eight-day cycle with ovulation on day fourteen, it would be safe to have sex up to day nine, and it would be safe to resume sex after day seventeen. The calendar is easy to remember for the normal, regular twenty-eight-day cycle with day fourteen ovulation. From this you can always remember the formula that you subtract eighteen days from your shortest cycle length to determine the first day of the "unsafe" period, and eleven days from the longest cycle length to determine the end of the "unsafe" period.

In yet another effort to make the calendar guesswork method of rhythm birth control work, many experts simply recommend that instead of subtracting eighteen days from your shortest cycle to determine the beginning of the "unsafe" period, subtract twenty-one days. This extra three days of abstinence in the early follicular phase in truth gives you a tremendous margin of safety but creates a very prolonged period of abstinence. For example, if you had a regular twenty-eight-day cycle every month, you would not be able to have sex between day seven and day seventeen. If your menstruation is five days, from day one to day five, and you are not interested in having sex while you menstruate, that would leave only two days in the entire follicular phase when you could have sex! The situation is even worse if you have slightly irregular cycles and some of them turn out to be twenty-five or twenty-six days long. Subtracting twenty-one, that would mean that you could not have sex beyond day four or day five of your cycle. That means if you don't care to have sex during menstruation, you must basically abstain for the entire follicular phase.

This formula would thus seem at first glance to be a foolproof way of making calendar rhythm very effective even for women with irregular cycles, but in fact there are two other problems. First, our assumption that the sperm are capable of fertilizing only up to five days prior to ovulation is true in the majority of cases, but probably not always. There are virtually no cases of women getting pregnant who have had intercourse after ovulation, but there are occasional cases of women getting pregnant from intercourse even before the so-called five-day preovulatory fertile time. Intercourse during the follicular phase seems to be the basis for all the trouble with natural birth control, and thus you need to learn a more precise method of determining when in the follicular phase you should stop having sex, or whether indeed you can safely have sex at all in the follicular phase.

The second problem is that the luteal phase is not always fourteen days. With an eleven-day luteal phase, applying the extended formula does not guarantee that you are going to be having sex *after* ovulation. For example, even in a regular twenty-eight-day cycle, you might ovulate on day nineteen instead of day fourteen (that would mean a nine-day rather than fourteen-day luteal phase). If you resume sex (as the formula tells you to) on day seventeen, you would be unwittingly having intercourse prior to ovulation and could easily get pregnant. That is why the calendar method of rhythm that was developed in the 1930s and enthusiastically endorsed by the Catholic Church has been so ridiculed.

But with the simple new approaches outlined in the rest of this chapter, you can securely determine your fertile period without guesswork. Even the Church endorses this new method over the old rhythm to the extent that any Catholic hospital in the country now offers courses on it.

THE TEMPERATURE METHOD

By determining when your basal body temperature goes up, you can very effectively determine when you have ovulated, and therefore when it is "safe" to resume sex. The problem with the temperature method is that it does not tell you when you should stop having sex in the *first* half of the cycle because it does not predict when you are going to ovulate. It tells you only when you have ovulated, and therefore when you can resume sex in the *second* half of the cycle. We will worry about the first half of the cycle later in the chapter. Right now let's learn how you can know for sure that you have already ovulated and that you are beyond the fertile time in your cycle.

This temperature method of natural birth control dates back to the 1950s, is very reliable, and when used properly can protect against pregnancy as effectively as condoms, IUDs, or even birth control pills. But like birth control pills, it requires discipline. Your "basal body temperature" rises about 0.4 to 0.8 degree F. after you ovulate, and if you remember to take your temperature every morning in the proper fashion, you are very unlikely to be misled.

The basal body temperature is your temperature *immediately* upon waking up in the morning, before getting out of bed or having any activity whatsoever. This temperature always will be lower before ovulation than after ovulation. The production of progesterone (which can occur only after ovulation) raises the body's basal temperature 0.4 to 0.8 degree F. By taking your morning temperature, you are actually measuring production of progesterone. Charts for recording these monthly temperatures are available at almost any pharmacy, or from your doctor (or make your own following the examples in this chapter). It is easier to read the temperature with a special Ovulindex thermometer (again, available at any pharmacy) than with a standard thermometer. The new digital thermometers are even easier to read.

The only pitfall with this otherwise superb and inexpensive way of determining your ovulation is that if you do not take your temperature first thing in the morning, before you even move to get out of bed, it may give a falsely elevated reading and be difficult to interpret. Every evening before going to bed you must place the thermometer by your nightstand within easy reach. If you forget to do this, you will have to get out of bed in the morning to get to your thermometer. Even this slight degree of activity can raise your temperature above the basal level and make that day's temperature reading ambiguous. Upon awaking in the morning you simply grasp the thermometer before doing anything else, put it in your mouth under the tongue for three minutes, and lie still. After you have finished taking and recording your temperature in the morning, you can go about your daily activities. Every evening make sure that before you go to sleep, you shake down your thermometer and put it on your nightstand so that it will be within easy reach the next morning.

When you have taken your temperature, you then record it on a chart according to the date and the day of the cycle. Remember, the day on which menstrual bleeding begins, even if only lightly, is considered day one of the menstrual cycle. Mark your temperature on each day with an X or a dot. On the top line of the chart record the day of the cycle (day one through twenty-eight or higher), and on the next line you can put the date. At the end of the cycle, when the first day of the next menstruation begins, you begin charting your temperature for another month.

Remember that the temperature can be affected by such things as colds, flu viruses, keeping late hours, or having a poor night's sleep. Make sure to note such events on the chart so that if there are a few atypical readings that don't go along with the rest of the temperature pattern, you will be able to discount them. Remember that the basal body temperature refers to the body temperature after a period of normal, restful sleep. The body temperature normally reaches its lowest level after all mental and muscular activity has ceased for several hours. That is why the best time to record this basal temperature is just upon awakening. Your temperature during the rest of the day is affected by your daily activities and will not be an accurate reflection of whether or not you are making progesterone, and consequently of whether or not you have ovulated.

The basal body temperature of a fertile woman follows a very characteristic pattern during each menstrual cycle (see Figure 2–1). A low temperature range spans the first fourteen days beginning from the first day of menstruation. This low range is generally in the area of 97.2 to 97.6 degrees F. Around day fourteen there is a sudden increase in the basal body temperature of as much as 0.8 degree F. which is maintained daily until menstruation begins and the temperature drops abruptly again. If instead of menstruating you become pregnant, the temperature will remain elevated, because progesterone continues to be produced, and progesterone is what increases your basal body temperature.

If the temperature does not go up, you have not ovulated. If the temperature goes up after day seventeen or eighteen in the cycle, rather than on day fourteen or fifteen, this indicates late ovulation. Keep in mind always that you have no way of telling directly whether you have ovulated. All of our methods of measurement are indirect, based upon progesterone production.

One potential problem with the temperature method is that there will be some small variation in temperature from day to day, and for that reason you cannot consider yourself "safe" simply on the basis of one day's temperature elevation. Likewise, illness or lack of sleep can affect your temperature. But there is a relatively simple system for dealing with that problem. It is called the "3-2-6 rule." You are "safe" to have sex on the day that you have recorded three consecutive basal body temperatures at least 0.2 degree F. higher than the *highest* of the six low consecutive temperatures recorded just before the temperature rise begins. This rule may sound too complicated, but don't run away. It is actually very simple once it is explained. Just keep in mind the simple guideline "3-2-6," and the explanation will be easy to follow.

Basically what I am saying is that on the third day after your temperature rise you are safely "infertile." On the first or second day after your temperature rise, I don't feel comfortable in assuring you that you are "safe" to have sex, because of the possibility of temperature variation that I mentioned earlier.

The day on which the temperature begins to rise is identified as soon as you observe one temperature higher than the preceding six.

64

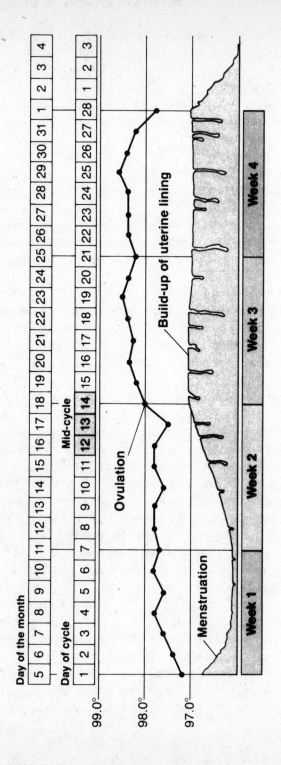

FIGURE 2–1. Basal Body Temperature.

Once this rise begins, you must look at your preceding six temperatures and find the *highest* one. To be sure that you are "safe," you must have a temperature 0.2 degree F. higher than the highest temperature of the preceding six days, for three days in a row. If you have a normal fourteen-day luteal phase, this will leave you about ten or eleven days to have "safe," comfortable, unanxious sex until you begin to menstruate.

When you can have sex during the first half of the cycle is very difficult to know using the temperature method alone. If you care to have sex during menstruation, you may comfortably do so until day five of the next cycle. If you wish to follow the calendar method guidelines, you may continue to have "safe" sex in the follicular phase of the next cycle only up until the day determined by subtracting twenty-one from the number of days of your shortest cycle; this means that in most cases you will not be able to have sex with assurance of safety beyond day five or seven. This is the major problem with using the temperature method alone, and that is why there are other signs I will teach you to watch for later in the chapter.

Although most of the time the temperature method works reliably for the second half of the cycle, there are times when it can be confusing. You should have little fear of getting pregnant, however, as long as you treat the confusing cycles as potentially fertile. With the few hints that follow, you will be able to prevent most of this potential confusion. But remember that the only bad consequence of having a confusing cycle is that you will have to abstain from sex that month or use some other method of birth control, such as a condom. You should not get pregnant simply because you have one confusing cycle, so long as you follow the rule that you are potentially fertile unless proven otherwise. You can "safely" follow this method only when the cycle is not confusing.

You can expect irregular temperature readings if you had a poor night's sleep, if you were awakened several times during the night, if you use an electric blanket, if you have a temperature elevation from a cold or the flu, or if you got up and went to the bathroom and walked around before taking your temperature upon awakening. Nobody is perfect, and these things are going to happen to you. These should not interfere in most cases with determining your "safe" period so long as you make a note on your chart next to that day's temperature reminding you that it may be in error. You then simply discount that day's temperature reading in applying your "3-2-6" rule. Just pretend that that day didn't exist, and the rule still will effectively safeguard you. Let's give a few examples.

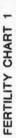

FERTILITY CHART 1

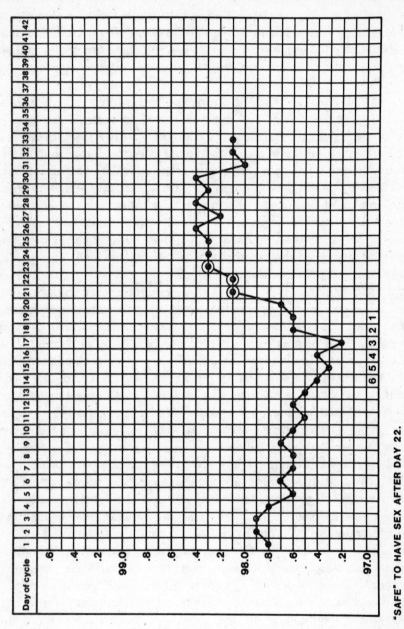

"SAFE" TO HAVE SEX AFTER DAY 22.

FIGURE 2-2.

In Chart 1 (Figure 2–2), the temperature first begins to rise higher than the preceding six temperatures to 97.7 degrees F. on day twenty of the cycle, but this temperature elevation is only 0.1 degree F. higher than the highest of the preceding six. For it to count as a true temperature elevation, following the rule of "3-2-6," the temperature must be at least 0.2 degree F. higher than the highest of the preceding six days. This happens on day twenty-one of her cycle, where the temperature climbs to 98.1 degrees F., a full 0.4 degree F. higher than that of the previous six-day period. She then has an elevated temperature on day twenty-one, the same temperature on day twenty-two, and even a higher temperature on day twenty-three. Day twenty-three thus is the fourth day of an elevated temperature, but the third day of a temperature that is at least 0.2 degree F. higher than the highest of the six temperatures preceding the rise. Therefore, it is "safe" to have sex on the evening of the twenty-third day of her cycle and thereafter.

What about when there are erratic temperature elevations caused by a poor night's sleep or when having the flu? Chart 2 (Figure 2–3) gives a simple example of how little difficulty this should cause. The important thing in this case is just to disregard the erratic temperature reading and skip over that day as though it didn't exist. For example, the woman in Chart 2 had an erratic temperature elevation of 98.3 degrees F. on day thirteen of the cycle. She simply made a note that she had a flu with fever and chills and was not feeling well that day. She then knows to discount that temperature in figuring her "safe" period. The temperature goes down again to what it should be on days fourteen, fifteen, sixteen, and seventeen. On day eighteen she notices her first legitimate temperature rise, to 97.9 degrees F. Counting backward six days, she simply disregards the temperature of day thirteen and figures that her highest temperature of the preceding six days is 97.8 degrees F. It isn't until day twenty-one that she has a temperature elevation 0.2 degree F. higher than the highest of the previous six. Undoubtedly day twenty-three would normally have been an elevated temperature also and should have been a "safe" day for sex, but because she had a poor night's sleep, the temperature went erratically too high again, and to be completely "safe," she disregarded that day's temperature and found that on day twenty-four the temperature still was over 0.2 degree F. elevated. Therefore, this was the beginning of the "safe" period of her cycle.

When the temperature rises abruptly over one or two days, the "safe" period after ovulation is easier to determine than when the tem-

68

FERTILITY CHART 2

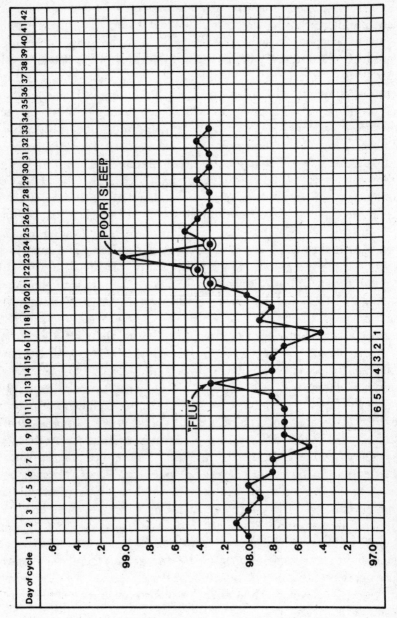

FIGURE 2-3.

"SAFE" TO HAVE SEX AFTER DAY 23.

FERTILITY CHART 3

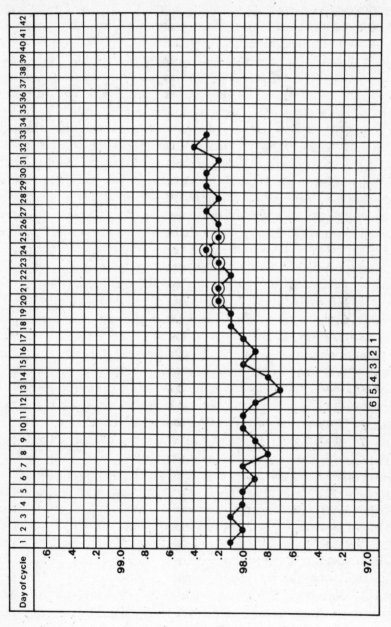

FIGURE 2–4.

"SAFE" TO HAVE SEX AFTER DAY 24.

perature rises gradually or in a stepwise fashion. For example, in Chart 3 (Figure 2–4), the temperature first begins to rise on day eighteen to 98.1 degrees F., but it rises only 0.1 degree F. from the previous day. The temperature stays the same on day nineteen. Finally, on day twenty the temperature has risen to 98.2 degrees F., 0.2 degrees F. higher than the highest reading of the six days preceding the initial temperature rise. This lasts for two days in a row, but dips down again 0.1 degree F. on day twenty-two. This means that when the temperature once again rises on day twenty-three to 0.2 degree F. above the highest reading of the six days preceding the temperature rise, we have to begin the countdown to "safe days" all over again. The temperature then stays up for two more days in a row and, therefore, only on the evening of day twenty-five of the cycle can this woman feel she is "safe." Viewing this cycle in retrospect, it becomes fairly clear that this woman would have been "safe" as early as day twenty-one, but she could not know that at the time, and if this method is going to be reliable, you must follow the rules of three consecutive temperatures that are 0.2 degree F. above the highest reading of the six preceding temperatures before the rise. This way you will be taking very little chance.

The preceding three examples were meant to be difficult to see if I could scare you away. The following examples are really more typical of what most women encounter during most of their cycles. Chart 4 (Figure 2–5) shows a cycle in which ovulation probably occurred on day thirteen, and the temperature began to rise abruptly one day following ovulation. The third consecutive day of elevated temperatures was on the sixteenth day of the cycle, and therefore from this day on sex was "safe" until the end of the cycle. It is easy to tell in retrospect that this woman ovulated on day thirteen, but she still must follow the rule of three consecutive days of elevated temperature. What if the temperature had gone right back down again on day fifteen of the cycle instead of going up to 98.2 degrees F.? It could have simply been a spontaneous variation. The rule of "3-2-6" protects you against these spontaneous variations leading to ill-advised sex before ovulation.

Chart 5 (Figure 2–6) demonstrates how the temperature method protects you against the risk of pregnancy inherent in the old-fashioned calendar approach to rhythm birth control. This woman has an otherwise normal-looking twenty-nine-day cycle. In retrospect she clearly ovulated on day twenty or day twenty-one. She then had three consecutive temperature elevations on day twenty-two, twenty-three, and twenty-four that were 0.2 degree F. above the preceding six days. Thus the

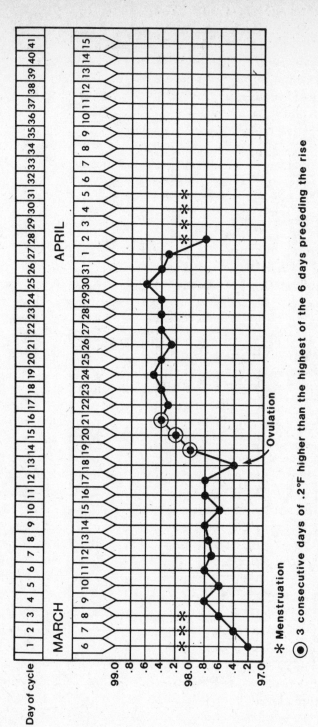

FIGURE 2–5.

72

CHART 5

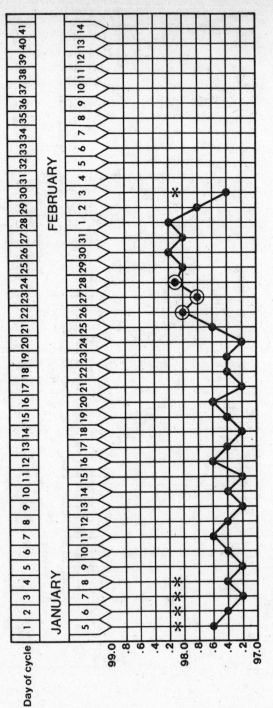

* Menstruation

⊙ 3 consecutive days .2°F higher than the highest of the 6 days preceding the rise

"SAFE" TO HAVE SEX AFTER DAY 23.

FIGURE 2–6.

first day that she could "safely" have sex would be day twenty-four of the cycle. If she had followed the calendar method of rhythm, subtracting eleven days from twenty-nine, she would have concluded that it was "safe" to have sex after day eighteen. Calendar rhythm method relies on the assumption that there will be a fourteen-day luteal phase. This lady clearly would have been having sex in the most fertile time of her cycle had she followed the old-fashioned calendar method. Simple use of the thermometer every morning can protect you against this disaster.

The biggest problem, and one that really has no solution, is for women who are relatively infertile and who do not ovulate every month. This is an incredible irony. Natural methods of birth control are unreliable only in women who often do not ovulate! Since these women might ovulate in some months, they still need birth control, but they cannot rely on the natural approach. Chart 6 (Figure 2–7) shows why. This is the chart of an infertile woman who required medical treatment eventually to get pregnant. She never ovulated on the cycle shown. Nowhere is there a consistent three-day temperature rise that fits the rule of "3-2-6." To practice reliable natural birth control, this couple would have to abstain for the entire month, and if she never ovulated for the whole year, they would have to abstain for the whole year! Even if she were a very late ovulator and did undergo a temperature rise perhaps as late as day thirty-six of the cycle, they still would have had to abstain from sex for over a month. For this reason, infertile women cannot rely on natural birth control.

But as will be explained in the chapter on birth control pills, there is another reason these women should not rely on natural methods, because nonovulators are in great danger of developing cancer of the uterus later in life if they are not hormonally treated when they are young. Thus no matter what their religious or natural health inclinations are, it is medically advisable for these women to undergo hormone treatment whether or not they wish to get pregnant. Furthermore, the Catholic Church does not disapprove of the birth control pill being used for such women because it is required to protect them from the severe risk of developing cancer of the uterus later. You will read more about that in the subsequent chapter on birth control pills, but suffice it to say now that natural birth control is not applicable to these infertile women, but this is in no way a criticism or a failing of this method. It is just one category of women who will have to forget about that approach to family planning.

74

CHART 6

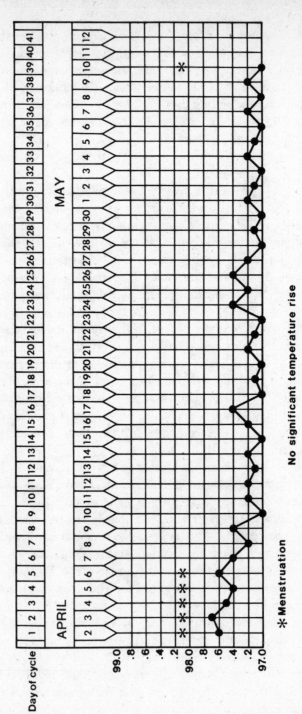

FIGURE 2-7.

By now I hope you have an understanding of how the temperature method of documenting your "safe" period works. The major deficiency in this method is that it requires that you abstain from sex during the first half of your cycle even though there may be a period during the first half of the cycle in which you would be "safe" from getting pregnant. To solve this deficiency we will now go on to other equally simple methods.

CERVICAL MUCUS (BILLINGS) METHOD

In the 1970s Drs. John and Evelyn Billings from Australia showed women how to examine their own cervical mucus daily to determine when their fertile period begins and ends. The advantage of adding cervical mucus self-checks to the temperature method is that it allows you to have sex during the first half of the cycle. With the temperature method alone, you have good protection from getting pregnant, but you can have no sex in the first half of the cycle (unless you use a calendar calculation, which is unreliable and still allows very little if any sex during the first half of your cycle). However, by examining your cervical mucus you may be able to have more sex during the first half of your cycle as well. This will also help you in the second half of the cycle, when your temperature chart may be ambiguous and you need to be certain that you have passed the potentially fertile time and are ready for sex again. You are more secure when you have two markers to go by instead of one.

The cervical mucus method alone is somewhat risky in terms of birth control but adds immensely to the reliability as well as the amount of sex that is possible with the temperature technique. Although the basal body temperature chart is the best *single* method of determining when ovulation occurs, examination of the cervical mucus is a simple way to double-check. Before going into the details of how you examine your cervical mucus to determine when you enter and when you leave the fertile phase of your cycle, we will review again how and why cervical mucus is produced in the normal cycle.

During the earliest phase of the cycle, the cervix is closed, and very little cervical mucus is produced. However, beginning around day nine or ten, under the influence of estrogen produced by the developing follicle, the production of cervical mucus begins to increase and the cervix begins to open slightly. When follicular production of estrogen has reached its maximum, usually around day thirteen or fourteen in

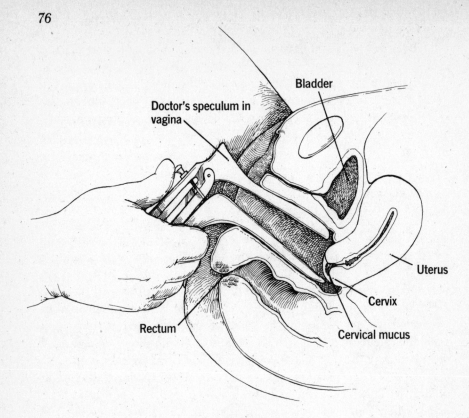

Doctor's speculum in vagina

Bladder

Uterus

Cervix

Rectum

Cervical mucus

FIGURE 2–8.

a normal cycle, the cervix is gaping open and an examining physician can actually see into it because of the optically clear, copious, watery cervical mucus flowing out (see Figures 2–8 and 2–9). At this time, one or two days prior to ovulation, the cervical mucus is most receptive to invasion by sperm, and the cervix is wide open in anticipation of their entrance. The physician can actually grasp a sample of this cervical mucus with a small clamp and spread it out several inches. It will not break. It has the perfect, clear, watery, copious, elastic consistency required for sperm to launch a successful invasion (see Figure 2–10).

Then, when a woman ovulates, and progesterone is produced, the entrance to the cervix will dramatically close and the production of the cervical mucus will stop. What mucus is left will be sticky and tacky and will have lost its optical clarity. At this point sperm would have no chance of invading the mucus (see Figure 2–11). Finally the mucus disappears. If the physician sees a "preovulatory" cervix (with a gaping opening and optically clear, abundant mucus) on day fourteen, if the

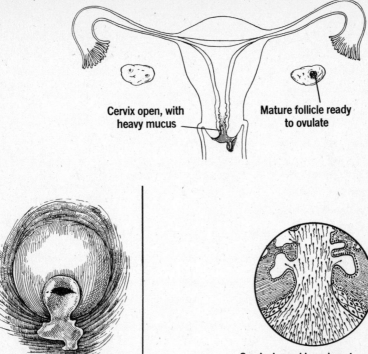

Cervix open, with heavy mucus

Mature follicle ready to ovulate

Clear, abundant cervical mucus oozing out of widened cervical opening

Cervical canal broadened, so that sperm invade cervical mucus easily

FIGURE 2–9.

temperature goes up the next morning, and if the cervical opening then closes abruptly, he or she can be fairly certain the woman has ovulated (see Figure 2–12). If, however, her temperature never rises and the cervical opening never closes until after menstruation, this indicates she is not ovulating. When the temperature goes up, there is a simultaneous closing of the cervical opening with a cessation of cervical mucus production. If the cervical opening is gaping with abundant mucus on day twenty, but then the temperature goes up on day twenty-one and the cervical opening closes, ovulation occurred late in the cycle, on day twenty or twenty-one.

Occasionally one sees the temperature begin to rise slowly but not reach its proper "luteal" level until about four days later. Slow rises in temperature may sometimes confuse the actual day of ovulation, but then the cervical opening and drying up of the mucus will clarify that

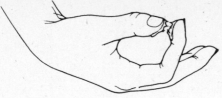

A. Early cycle—sticky, does not stretch too far

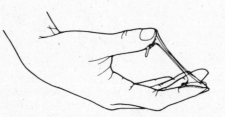

B. Closer to ovulation—spreads a little more before breaking

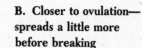

C. Just prior to ovulation—very thin, watery, and stretchable

FIGURE 2–10.

ovulation has occurred. Occasionally the temperature may appear to rise, indicating ovulation, but the cervical opening does not close at the same time. The cervical opening may continue to appear gaping with abundant and copious mucus for several days after the temperature has supposedly risen. This is the reason to double-check the cervical mucus against the basal body temperature charts. If they don't match, assume you are not "safe" until they do.

These simple self-tests can make you incredibly aware of your own body's cycle, whether you want to avoid pregnancy, or whether you want to get pregnant. The only other way to learn as much about your cycle is to do daily blood hormone tests and ultrasound exams for several cycles, which tend to be extremely expensive (over several thousand dollars). Otherwise you simply cannot gain any more information about your ovulation from complicated medical tests as you can by taking your temperature and checking your cervical mucus.

Now I will describe how you can check your cervical mucus. If

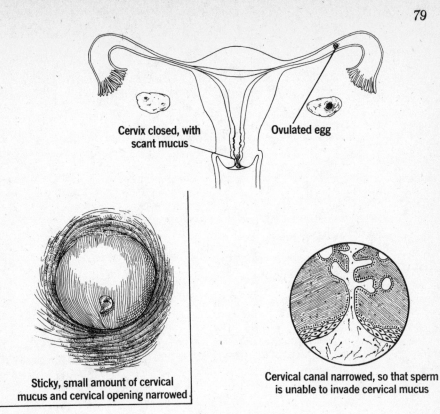

Cervix closed, with scant mucus

Ovulated egg

Sticky, small amount of cervical mucus and cervical opening narrowed

Cervical canal narrowed, so that sperm is unable to invade cervical mucus

FIGURE 2–11.

you have any confusion about this, you should have no difficulty getting personalized assistance and instruction from a qualified physician or a nurse at a family planning program, or at any Catholic hospital in the United States.

Every day you must check the opening to your vagina called the introitus. Early in the cycle, your cervix will be closed and dry. It is "safe" to have sex until mucus production begins. With early mucus production you will feel a moistness at the introitus that you didn't feel before. As mucus production continues, this moistness will progress to a feeling of wetness. When you feel the early mucus with your fingers, it will be thick, tacky, sticky, pastelike, opaque, and clearly inpenetrable to any but the most hardy sperm. As soon as you feel this early mucus it is time to stop having intercourse. Sometimes you cannot see the mucus easily in your fingers, and then you must go by the sensation of slipperiness, or lubrication.

As your cycle progresses toward ovulation, the mucus will become

80

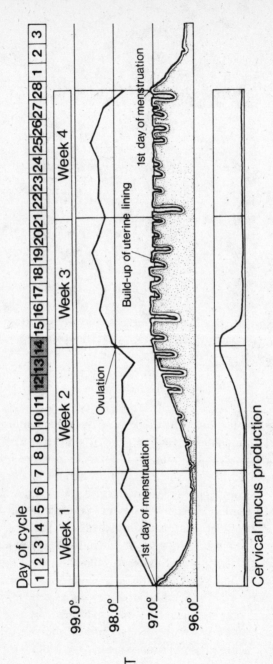

FIGURE 2–12.

more profuse, watery, slippery, stretchy, transparent, and elastic. When you get a small bit of it between your fingers you will find that you can stretch it for more than two or three inches in a string that will not break. Before this peak phase of mucus production, you wouldn't be able to spread the mucus between your fingers more than two inches. It would be tacky and break and would have no stretchability. This stretchability is called *Spinnbarkeit* and indicates that you are getting near the time of ovulation.

At this point you will certainly have a sensation of slipperiness and lubricativeness at the introitus and should not have a difficult time getting a sample of mucus that you can examine between your fingers. Nonetheless, if you have any difficulty being certain of when your mucus production begins and when it peaks, feel free to seek out instruction readily available in virtually every major city in the country, usually at Catholic hospitals. Once you feel comfortable that you can identify the mucus correctly, you can feel safe in having sex beyond calendar day five or seven until you feel the mucus in the vagina just begin to become wet. You must then continue to check your mucus every day, because by following its increase in amount, elasticity, slipperiness, and wateriness, and then its decline, you will be able to know when it is once again "safe" to have sex.

You won't have to look very hard to find the mucus. Usually it is readily detectable right at the opening of your vagina. The very earliest mucus means you are beginning to enter the fertile phase, even though you are not as fertile as you will become when the mucus is more abundant. The early mucus is sticky, tacky, and pasty. When you try to spread it between your fingers it will break and not stretch. For women trying to get pregnant, this mucus is very difficult for sperm to penetrate. I advise these women to wait until the mucus becomes abundant and watery, because then the sperm will have an easier time penetrating and it will be closer to ovulation. But for those who do not want to get pregnant, the presence of any mucus, even this pastelike early mucus, is an indication that you are at some risk, however small.

Every day prior to ovulation your mucus will begin to become more abundant, thinner, and more watery. It is readily detectable right at the entrance to the vagina and feels wet rather than moist and pasty. You are getting more and more likely to get pregnant if you have sex.

Just prior to ovulation, when your estrogen level is the very highest (and, of course, no progesterone has been secreted yet because you have not yet ovulated), your mucus will be clear, like raw egg white, more abundant in amount, and you can stretch it between your two fingers several inches (sometimes even as far as nine or ten inches) just like a long, transparent thread. Once your mucus becomes this abundant and this elastic, you are in what is called the peak of your mucus production. This is the most fertile day of your cycle.

Although you are now getting ready to ovulate, it is impossible to know yet exactly when that is going to occur. After you ovulate, the follicle turns into a corpus luteum and begins to make progesterone. The progesterone will oppose the effects of estrogen, cause your cervix to close, and cause your mucus to become sticky again, dry up, and eventually disappear. If you are using the mucus method alone for birth control, you must have three complete, dry days after the peak mucus is observed before you are "safe." In other words, on the fourth "dry" day you are "safe" to have intercourse. You may be "safe" before then, but there is no way to be sure. Although you may have ovulated several days earlier, it is hard to be certain, and that is why we bracket the period of time around which you can feel "safe."

COMBINED TEMPERATURE AND CERVICAL MUCUS METHOD ("SYMPTOTHERMAL")

It should be apparent now that the cervical mucus method is best used for determining when in the first half of the cycle you need to stop having sex, and the basal body temperature is best used for determining when in the second half of the cycle you can begin having sex again. The greatest security comes when the two are not in conflict. But there are a lot of problems with the cervical mucus method when used alone.

During the first half of the cycle, when you are relying on the cervical mucus method, you cannot have sex more frequently than every other day. The reason for this is that semen deposited during intercourse might be confused with mucus up to about thirty-six hours later. Douching after intercourse to wash out the semen will not help. Therefore, if you have sex every other day rather than every day, cervical mucus testing should be reliable. If there is any doubt and you try to convince yourself that there is no mucus but that the wetness you feel is just semen, you may be making a big mistake. You must consider yourself able to get pregnant as long as there is any sensation of mucus.

If any aspect of the cervical mucus determination confuses you, remember you can always go safely by the temperature charts, avoiding sex altogether during the first half of the cycle. Without being able to determine your cervical mucus, you will not be able to have sex in the first half of the cycle other than by subtracting twenty-one from the number of days of your shortest cycle. The calendar determination using the rule of twenty-one is very safe and effective, but for all practical purposes means only a few days of intercourse are allowed after menstruation even in women who never have cycles shorter than twenty-eight days.

Remember that the temperature method alone is an extremely effective and "safe" method of contraception after ovulation. The combined temperature, calendar, and cervical mucus method allows sex before ovulation as well, but at the potential expense of effectiveness. In one study women who used the temperature method alone and who had sex only after ovulation, had only a 2 percent yearly failure rate. This is not much different from the effectiveness of the intrauterine device (or even the birth control pill when you take into account that many women forget to take their pills). On the other hand, in a different study, with sex before ovulation until appearance of mucus, there was a 12 percent failure rate. A way to lower the failure rate further and still allow some sex in the first half of the cycle is to use the calendar (rule of 21) method also to estimate the onset of the fertile period, going by whichever comes earlier. The mucus and basal body temperature can be used together to estimate the end of the fertile period by whichever comes later. With this approach some enthusiasts for natural birth control claim an effectiveness rate of 98 percent, still allowing some sex (but not a lot) in the first half of the cycle.

Let's review: From day one of your cycle, you may have "safe" sex either until you first begin to notice mucus, however sticky and however early, or until the calendar calculation (the number of days of your shortest cycle minus twenty-one) approaches, whichever comes first. Thereafter you can have no sex until either the fourth day after peak mucus occurs, or the third evening after the basal body temperature rises, whichever comes last.

THE LH AND PROGESTERONE DIPSTICK

One more new marker on the horizon that could make this entire natural birth control as easy as child's play is the "LH dipstick." As you may recall, the hormone FSH is released by the pituitary during the first half of the cycle and stimulates an ovarian follicle to grow around the egg that is destined to be ovulated that month. As the follicle grows, it produces estrogen. Once the estrogen level reaches peak levels, it stimulates the pituitary to release luteinizing hormone, or LH, which is the trigger that causes ovulation. Ovulation occurs predictably within thirty-six hours after the LH surge. This LH surge can now be measured very easily by you in your home with a simple urine test, using a kit that is available in almost every drugstore in America. A similar kit allows you to determine progesterone.

The only problem is that the cost still is high (about forty dollars per monthly kit), and each test takes about thirty minutes of your time. I'm sure it will be even cheaper and quicker in the next five years. If you wish to use this method at the present time, you could test your urine daily, and whenever the LH surge occurs, you can be quite confident that within thirty-six hours you will have ovulated. Similarly, your progesterone will then begin to surge. If you wait another forty-eight hours after that, there will be little chance of getting pregnant. Three or four days after the LH surge, you should be safe.

Thus we now have simple, reliable methods with which you can check yourself for determining when it is "safe" to have sex without the fear of pregnancy, and these tests will be getting better and cheaper every year.

What Is the Chance of Natural Birth Control Not Working?

When figuring the success rate of any contraceptive, you must distinguish between "method failure" and "use failure." The method may be extremely safe and effective, but if it is difficult to *use*, the failure rate could be high. For example, if you have a sterilization there is no effort whatsoever involved, and the "method failure" would be no different from the "use failure" rate. But for birth control pills, if you forget to take them for a few days, you may get pregnant. It is not the fault of the birth control pill itself. The method is effective, but its usefulness depends upon your remembering to take the pills. Similarly, condoms could be an extremely effective method of contraception, except for the fact that so frequently people who rely on them forget to use them in the heat of the moment. Similarly, natural birth control, or scientific rhythm, is an extremely effective, safe method of birth control. But it can have a very high failure rate when used by people incorrectly. Many enthusiasts for this method of birth control report only the "method effectiveness rate," but I shall try to give you, from most of the studies performed around the world, not only "method effectiveness" but also "use effectiveness," under the assumption that many of the readers will want to take a realistic view of what their chances are for utilizing this extremely effective method of birth control correctly and consistently.

These are wide and overlapping ranges of failure rates for natural birth control among different groups of women, depending on the quality of teaching as well as the motivation, maturity, and self-discipline of those attempting it. The maximum effectiveness occurs when all the different fertility signals (basal body temperature, mucus changes, calendar calculations, and even LH or progesterone dipstick determination) are used. For example, when the Billings (cervical mucus) method alone has been studied in comparison to confirmed temperature plus the cervical mucus method, in a small group in the United States the combined method yielded a 0 percent method failure rate, and the Billings method alone yielded a 5.7 percent method failure rate. In Australia the combined method yielded a 2.9 percent method failure rate and the Billings method alone a 12 percent failure rate. In Colombia the combined method yielded a 5 percent method failure rate and the Billings method alone yielded a 25 percent method failure rate. Thus, no matter how you look at it, using the cervical mucus parameter alone is more likely to lead to failure than using cervical mucus plus basal body temperature.

All of the studies on the calendar method alone (pure rhythm) show a failure rate of 14 to 47 percent per year, but most of the studies are closer to 47 percent. The basal body temperature method alone had a failure rate from as low as 0.3 percent to a high of 6.6 percent per year depending on the motivation of the couple. Thus the basal body temperature method of natural birth control alone is extremely effective and reliable. The problem is that it requires abstinence for the first half of the cycle.

In a World Health Organization (WHO) study of natural birth control, all methods were most effective when sex occurred only after ovulation and never before ovulation. Most accidental pregnancies result from efforts to have sex prior to ovulation in the first half of the cycle. The next major cause for failure was that the couple did not abstain from intercourse when they knew they should have. If you have the discipline to follow the method properly, it is extremely effective.

When temperature plus calendar plus mucus were used together, couples could have sex in the first half of the cycle, but still at the expense of decreased effectiveness. With this approach, the average failure rate was 15 percent per year, although with motivated couples it was as low as 5 percent per year. With mucus alone (the Billings method), the average pregnancy rate was about 25 percent per year. As I discussed earlier, the ironic thing is that the temperature method was least effective with relatively infertile couples whose ovulation was unpredictable. If a woman didn't ovulate at all, the couple could never have "safe" intercourse because the woman's temperature would never go up. But for regularly cyclic women in a happy marriage with a willing male partner, who are highly motivated and well disciplined (particularly if they are willing to minimize sex during the first half of the cycle), natural birth control surely works, it doesn't interfere with any of your body's natural processes, and it costs nothing.

A WHO study found that a high percentage of couples discontinued this method of birth control within the first year. For example, in the United States two thirds of couples found it too troublesome to continue. But the third who did continue with it were extremely happy with their choice. The disconcerting aspect of this WHO study is that of 35 percent of women in developing countries who discontinued this method of birth control in one year's time, 19 percent discontinued because of pregnancy.

How "Natural" Is It?

The advantages of natural birth control to family planning are clear. It would appear to be the cheapest method, with the least risk to health. It is acceptable to Catholics and other religious groups. It is quite effective if very strictly followed in a disciplined fashion. It is an "acceptable" method to teach teenagers in high school sex education courses. But there are many disadvantages as well, and the rising zeal for natural approaches to health matters should not be allowed to interfere with a realistic appraisal. This method of birth control requires a very high level of motivation, complete cooperation of the male partner, lots of training time to learn how to do it, and accurate recordkeeping (some people can never get it). Any minor deviation can lead to a high failure rate. (The latter complaint, however, is no different than with the birth control pill or condom, of course.) One of the major objections with natural birth control is that since the fertile period is either not that short, or at least not that easy to pinpoint exactly, all methods require a fair period of abstinence. Furthermore, particularly for teenagers or for adults leading a promiscuous life-style, it does not protect against sexually transmitted diseases or infection, as do the condom or the birth control pill.

The other question is: How "natural" is it? It is "natural" for women to be slightly more interested in sex with the midcycle surge of testosterone, which occurs right around the time of ovulation. While it is true that human females, unlike any other animal, are interested in sex at any time of the month, nonetheless they are more likely to initiate sex just prior to ovulation, because of the slight increase in testosterone that always occurs at that time. So is it "natural" to abstain from intercourse at this one time of the month when the woman feels her greatest inclination to have it?

Finally, it is clearly not "natural" for a woman to have incessant ovulation during thirty years of her reproductive life-span. Let me clarify this point because it is very important. In the "natural" state, women become pregnant for the first time at a rather young age, then breast-feed until they get pregnant again, which hopefully is about four or five years later. Then after they deliver the next child they breast-feed it until they get pregnant again. This goes on for at least twenty years during the most fertile time of a woman's life. During this entire reproductive life-span, the woman in a "natural" state (like the !Kung tribeswomen) ovulate only occasionally (at which point they get pregnant). All of the rest of the time they are breast-feeding, and ovulation is inhibited. So the notion of avoiding pregnancy despite monthly ovulation, the key to natural birth control, really is a very unnatural phenomenon. In a truly natural setting, a woman has very few ovulations in her lifetime.

This "natural" condition of very few ovulations would be more closely matched by going on birth control pills, which inhibit ovulation. In fact, women who use birth control pills have an extremely low risk of cancer of the ovary compared to women who have not used birth control pills (see Chapter 4). In the truly "natural" state, such as the !Kung tribeswomen live, cancer of the ovary is very rare, just as it is in women who go on birth control pills for a very prolonged period. It is the incessant monthly ovulation of modern women that seems to predispose them to this deadly cancer. I bring up this point only to demonstrate that life is a risk in whatever direction you turn. Sometimes in an effort to avoid all risks by returning to a nonmodern life-style, we fool ourselves. There are a wide variety of methods of birth control available to modern women, and if they understand their reproductive system and understand these methods of birth control, they can choose an approach that is extraordinarily safe for them. Natural birth control is extraordinarily safe, but you should not infer from this chapter, and from my enthusiasm for it, that it is really any safer than other modern medical methods from which you can choose.

To give you an example in reverse, some have suggested that women who use natural birth control are more likely to have fetal abnormalities. Follow-up studies in large areas have demonstrated that this notion is clearly absurd. There is no way that natural birth control by delaying intercourse until after ovulation is going to lead to any greater likelihood of fetal abnormalities. But the absurdity of that fear can underscore how easy it is to incorrectly blame fetal abnormalities on other methods of contraception such as the birth control pill, or spermicidal foam.

ABSTINENCE

One method of natural birth control available to teenagers, and which seems to gain no commentary in most books such as this, is abstinence. There are other things in life for a teenager to do than fornicate. But it does no good for moralizing parents to pontificate or prescribe abstinence for their children. Our society is too democratic, even at the teenage level, for any such prescription to be effective. In the world we live in, teenagers must decide and will decide for themselves what they are going to do with their bodies. It is up to all postpubertal human beings to decide for themselves when, with whom, and how often they will and won't engage in sex. We all (including teenagers) need to be aware of the consequences of sexual exploration, to be responsible, and to save ourselves from misery that comes from not being responsible. If contraception is too complicated and troublesome, abstinence until one is a little more mature might be a very wise, stress-relieving decision.

When Robert Redford or James Bond make love to a woman on the screen, it all seems so easy, so joyful, and so utterly free of any responsibility. Bond does not have to interrupt his foreplay to go to the hotel room dresser to get out a condom, nor does his partner for the evening have to check her basal body temperature chart to see if it is safe. Nor is she seen in the morning remembering to take her birth control pill. Bond is not seen showing up at the urology clinic with pus dripping out of his penis from a sexually transmitted disease, nor is the female companion for that evening shown eight years later undergoing a complicated microsurgical operation to try to open up tubes that were blocked from an infection she got because she failed to make her strange lover wear a condom, or was using the wrong IUD. All around us our society is hyping up sex and making it seem like we are truly free from any need of forethought or contraceptive planning.

Against this incredibly sophisticated selling of sex all around us, the notion of abstinence as a method of natural birth control may seem naïve. But I have never been thought of as naïve, and abstinence must be a birth control option for young people.

3

Breast-feeding
as Birth Control

One of the points of this book is that without proper family planning, the future of the civilized world is at great risk. Children need to have the complete attention of their parents for several years at the beginning of their lives before the parents become distracted with the management of another infant who also needs their full attention. For forty thousand years, nature has provided humans with a natural method of birth control for child spacing, and it is only recently that we have abandoned it. We are genetically the same as our hunter/gatherer forebears from forty thousand years ago who relied upon a strong family unit and the proper upbringing of children. These ancestors of forty thousand years ago did not need to go to a modern birth control clinic, welfare department, or local gynecologist to get birth control pills, condoms, or have a diaphragm fitted after having a child in order to prevent getting pregnant again too soon. They just breast-fed their child, and never needed to worry about getting pregnant again until they stopped breast-feeding.

You may be shocked to hear that. Everything you have heard tells you that breast-feeding is not a reliable method of avoiding pregnancy, and that you must use some birth control method before resuming intercourse after having had a child unless you want to get pregnant again in short order. If that were true, how is it that the primitive !Kung Bushmen of the Kalahari Desert in Africa breast-feed their children exclusively, use no other birth control, and have an average of only 4.7 pregnancies per family, with children spaced at least four years apart? They live a life-style very much like our ancestors did forty thousand years ago, with a simple family unit. They own nothing, have no agriculture, no town system or community, and live as natural, untechnological humans. Yet the importance of delayed puberty and child spacing in the development of social morals, a value system, mental acuity, and skills is as critical to their survival as it is to ours. Without this child spacing, human beings could never have developed to the sophisticated level of modern man. A child has so much to learn that he or she must get a good start, and essential in this is child spacing. This is not a modern, zero-population piece of propaganda. It is simply the fact of how human beings were designed to be nurtured, and it requires no interventional birth control method other than the normal feeding of your child exclusively with breast milk.

The word "exclusively" is the critical factor in making breast-feeding a secure method of birth control. Unless you are *fully* breast-feeding, you must use some other modern method of birth control, of course. If you are breast-feeding just for the experience of breast-feeding, but give your child supplementary bottles, or put him or her on solids fairly soon, then you are not exclusively breast-feeding, and you are liable to become pregnant. That is why the popular belief has arisen that breast-feeding is an unreliable method of birth control. But this popular belief is wrong, and if you are interested in fully breast-feeding your infant, you need not worry about contraception to space your children. The contraceptive protection afforded when fully breast-feeding your child is as good as any other modern contraceptive.

But it may not be right for you. The !Kung women carry their children everywhere, and give their baby access to the breast whenever he or she wants it throughout the day or night. There is no feeding schedule, and no other food or drink is given to the child. These women may suckle their child as often as four times an hour for brief periods whenever the child wants it. The child sleeps with the mother in the evening, and although he suckles less frequently in the evening, he still is able to have the breast whenever he desires.

This characteristic of human breast-feeding is different from other animals. In most other animals, including cows, milk is thick and creamy, and its high fat content sustains the infant for a longer period of time between feedings. Human milk, on the other hand, has to be given more frequently if the child is to have a continuing sense of being adequately nourished. (The only other animals that suckle the child as frequently as the human are the chimpanzee and the gorilla, whose milk is quite similar to human milk and quite different from that of cows, sheep, goats, deer, rabbits, or other animals.) That means that giving your child a "relief" bottle with cow milk (which is what most infant formula consists of) is likely to sustain him for much longer than giving him a period of suckling at your breast. Thus everything in our modern life-style tends to lean away from the continual suckling required for full breast-feeding and thus complete protection against pregnancy during breast-feeding.

The chimpanzee and the gorilla suckle their young several times an hour day and night, secreting a milk quite similar to that of humans. They sleep with the infant at their breast at night. They obviously use no artificial methods of birth control, and they have sex freely during the time they are raising their infant. Yet they, too, like "natural" humans, have a birth interval of about five years between offspring. In fact, many anthropologists maintain that it is this natural spacing of our children related to the contraceptive effect of breast-feeding, beginning with the great apes and then the human race, that has allowed us, along with our tremendously flexible, large brain capacity, to transcend all other animals. It has given us the time required to teach our infant what he needs to know to use his tremendous brain capacity for forging a better way of life.

The continual suckling of the infant by the !Kung women in no way interferes with their sexual activity. The family unit remains strong and the husband doesn't go wandering around looking for sex elsewhere because he is not getting it at home. Yet, without any understanding of modern reproductive physiology, the !Kung woman knows that she need not fear the difficulty of having to raise another infant close on the heels of the one to whom she is presently devoting all her energy. Modern psychologists tell us that giving the child a good solid four or five years of extensive attention and nurturing is all he needs to carry with him for the rest of his life. Four or five more siblings can follow and take up all of the mother's and father's time, but it won't matter because the child has had the four or five years that he needed to become a secure, relatively autonomous, self-sufficient human being capable of dealing with the perplexities of growing up.

The !Kung are not the only rural or ancient people who practice this method of full breast-feeding with no schedule. For example, in Rwanda, mothers carry their babies everywhere, getting adequate nutrition for themselves from the food they gather and their men hunt, giving only breast milk to the infant. The human species has spent more than 90 percent of its existence leading this type of nomadic hunter/

gatherer life, and "civilization" with its pressures is too recent to have had any appreciable impact on our genetic makeup. When we look in Africa, Australia, New Guinea, and South America, we see that it is natural and critically important for human families to space their children, and for this necessity, Nature provides.

When I visited a well-known family planning clinic that helps minority groups, an institution where over 2 percent of the nation's births occur, I was impressed by the attention and devotion to trying to help economically underprivileged with their family spacing. But these costly efforts seemed an ironic by-product of the warping effect our modern society has produced. These women are given a large supply of condoms and spermicidal vaginal foam to use until four weeks after delivery, and then they start on birth control pills. If they are breast-feeding they use the progesterone-only birth control pill, and if they are bottle-feeding they use the regular birth control pills, which dry up the breast milk. If they forget to pick up their refills on time many will become pregnant again within a year. The reason they don't use breast-feeding for birth control is that they have the infant on a schedule so that they can either rush off to work during the day, or do their shopping. Meanwhile, because of the tendency to forget to take the pill in the midst of all these other duties, as well as the perhaps unfounded fear that the pill could be potentially harmful, doctors are busily trying to develop "simple" approaches that require less effort (such as the IUD, which is now off the market in the United States, or hormone implants under the skin to release constantly a low level of progesterone to suppress ovulation without the requirement of remembering to take the pill). But somehow we are failing, and these women are having their children too fast, with too little spacing, and with too little time to give them the early start they need to become secure, autonomous, productive human beings.

I have a very sophisticated patient from out of town who was initially infertile and required treatment with our office's full armamentarium of modern techniques to help her get pregnant. She breast-fed her child, did not have to go to work, and was very knowledgeable on the issue of child spacing. She asked me whether breast-feeding alone would prevent her from getting pregnant again too rapidly, because she believed in having at least two years with this first child before going on to the next. In fact she felt she had no alternative because she did not believe in any other method of contraception for philosophical as well as medical reasons. I told her that yes, breast-feeding would prevent her from getting pregnant, but only if she did it fully, did not schedule the child, and did not give him any other source of supplementary food. Probably because of her prior infertility problem, she did not take this precaution seriously, and just assumed it would be difficult for her to get pregnant again. But at six months, as soon as she started giving the child supplementary food, she became pregnant again. Even women who are infertile most frequently find that after their first pregnancy—which may have taken years to come by—the next ones will follow rapidly in succession if some method of birth control is not used.

There are certainly other advantages to breast-feeding aside from contraception. Breast-feeding is simpler than preparing a bottle. Breast milk has all the nourishment the infant needs, but more importantly, it protects against so many of the illnesses that are most likely to kill the child (particularly in developing countries) during the first year of life. Breast-fed babies have four times fewer respiratory infections, twenty times fewer episodes of diarrhea, and substantially less asthma, hay fever, and stomach feeding problems than bottle-fed children.

When I worked in Alaska with the Eskimos twenty years ago as a young doctor, the infants there had a disastrous epidemic of what is called "pathogenic *E. coli* diarrhea." The pediatricians had their hands full day and night with this severe, potentially life-threatening diarrhea problem among native people who had never experienced such a problem before. It is only now, years later, after studying reproduction for the past twenty years, that I have a better understanding of how this happened. Before the coming of the white man's influence, Eskimo women of course breast-fed their children. With the introduction of bottle feeding and supplementary foods, breast milk became less important in the feeding of the infant. Yet in the primitive conditions they lived in, which many in a modern setting would have to call poverty (although others would consider it their natural environment), the potential for infection and contamination of food was great. With breast-feeding, the infant did not have to worry about that contamination. But now it was getting its food from bottle milk formula mixed with the local water supply and naturally was susceptible to the most deadly diarrheal infections.

It is fascinating that when the World Health Organization recognized this problem, they passed a code against all marketing of bottle formulas in the developing world. But the United States, where most bottle milk formulas are manufactured, was the only country that refused to endorse this code. Health authorities around the world could barely believe that we were so tied into our own popularity of bottle feeding in the United States (a developed country where the consequences of bottle feeding are not at all so disastrous) that we did not recognize what a health hazard we were creating for infants around the world in poorer areas. Their only protection against the frequent bouts of diarrhea and infections that threatened their lives is breast milk. Not only is the breast milk already sterile, but also it contains antibodies passed on from the mother to the infant for virtually every disease the mother is already protected against from her prior experience. The interesting phenomenon about child spacing is that in developed countries where there is very little breast-feeding, and where modern methods of contraception are used, the time between infants is no greater than in developing countries where the mothers breast-feed until they get pregnant without using any contraception.

Prevention of ovulation in breast-feeding women is caused by one of two events. Medical science is not certain exactly which is more important. First, suckling of the infant on the breast creates a reflex reaction that directly inhibits the brain from releasing the hormone that allows the pituitary to make LH. Thus ovulation is directly inhibited. The other mechanism is that the suckling of the infant on the breast stimulates the pituitary gland to release the hormone prolactin, which is the hormone that stimulates the breast to make milk. You can measure the levels of prolactin in breast-feeding women. Women who only partially breast-feed their child have lower levels of prolactin than women who breast-feed their children for most of their nourishment. The highest level of prolactin is in women who breast-feed their infants entirely, on no set schedule other than demand, and with *no supplemental feedings whatsoever* (including water). It is this very high level of prolactin that inhibits the pituitary's release of the hormone LH, which is necessary to trigger ovulation.

It is the sucking stimulus itself, not milk production, that inhibits ovulation. Levels of prolactin are directly related to the number and duration of suckling episodes. These levels are not quite as high in women who try to set up a schedule, even though their child might be feeding exclusively at the breast. Thus the frequency of suckling is more important than the total amount of milk given the child. It is the introduction of supplementary food, or scheduling the breast-feeding rather than allowing it to occur on demand, that allows the prolactin level to become low enough that ovulation can occur.

Breast-feeding is getting to be more common in America as more women are becoming aware of its benefits. But the majority of women in the developed world are not going to want to feed their child constantly on demand, as the !Kung tribeswomen do. It simply doesn't fit into the modern life-style, however regrettable that may be. So why do I seriously bring it up as a method of natural contraception for spacing of children? The reason is that even if you decide to breast-feed fully only for the first three months (a reasonable proposition for many women even in our modern society), it will be reassuring to know that you are at no risk of becoming pregnant and have plenty of time to decide upon another method of contraception until such time as you begin either to supplement your infant's food with the relief bottle, solid food, or begin to schedule his feedings.

The second issue you need to be aware of in case you have a strong zeal to follow the ways of the "hunter/gatherer" women of the Kalahari Desert is that most World Health Organization studies show that infants who are solely breast-fed for the first six months have the same growth curve as infants who are bottle-fed or given supplemental feedings. But many studies seem to show that sometime between six months and one year, infants who receive all of their nutrition from breast milk without any supplemental foods have a slower growth rate. Some enthusiasts for exclusive breast-feeding would dispute these figures, but the only responsible thing I can do is bring them to your attention. For this and reasons of convenience, you most likely will decide that no matter how long you wish to breast-feed your infant, you probably will want to add supplemental food or at least schedule his feeding pattern sometime before one year is up. But just think of the benefits of knowing that you have that much time before having to embark upon more conventional methods!

4

Birth Control Pills

It may surprise you to hear that not only are today's birth control pills very safe, but they also have far-reaching health benefits that actually make not taking them more risky than taking them. An ironic twist is that over the past twenty-six years there has been such well-publicized concern over speculated risks and dangers of the pill that there seems to be little media interest now in the fact that the birth control pill is safe and virtually free of the symptoms that made some women turn against it in the 1960s and 1970s. The birth control pill is the most thoroughly researched drug of the twentieth century. There is not a single pill, drug, or medication, including aspirin, that has been studied as carefully, scientifically, and reliably as the birth control pill. So for those of you who have given up on natural birth control, which I am obviously very enthusiastic about, you need not despair. The pill is reliable, easy to take, and if you make sure to take the right pill with the right dose, it is safe. There are over thirty different formulations presently on the market, with different hormone ingredients and different dosages. This chapter will help you simplify this seemingly confusing mass of available products into a simple understanding so that you can make sure you are prescribed a truly safe low-dose pill.

I feel uncomfortable in reporting this extremely good news about the pill because of my personal enthusiasm for more natural approaches in medicine, avoiding any drug you don't have to take. There is in all of us an immediate reflex fear of the pill for that very reason. But unless we are living out in the Kalahari Desert walking around with loincloths and no permanent shelter, living truly "natural," digging up wild plants and gathering whatever food we can in the forest, it shouldn't matter whether our method of contraception is "natural" so much as whether it is safe. The new birth control pill formulations you will learn about in this chapter are not only safe but also give you significant protection against diseases that otherwise, as a modern woman, you would be extremely prone to develop. The birth control pill protects you against cancer of the uterus and cancer of the ovary. It usually corrects painful periods, prevents anemia from too much menstrual blood loss, combats acne, prevents benign breast disease as well as benign ovarian cysts, and even protects you somewhat against pelvic inflammatory disease that would otherwise result from various venereal infections. It even mitigates the symptoms of PMS (premenstrual syndrome).

Most of these are diseases of modern life, and the pill, a modern invention, protects against them. Even rhythm birth control is not completely natural. The "natural" human condition for women is either to be pregnant or breast-feeding. This means that in the natural state women have very few ovulations during their lifetimes. But women who use rhythm birth control ovulate every single month without getting pregnant. This incessant ovulation creates a strong risk for cancer of the ovary, which women of a previous era did not have to worry about. Yet the birth control pill prevents this incessant ovulation and thus helps minimize the risk of this otherwise prevalent cancer. As soon as we started to cook our food, we stopped being "natural." Our goal shouldn't necessarily be to be natural, but simply to be healthy.

About fifty million women in the world today use birth control pills, but its use has declined from the 1960s because of unwarranted fears about its "dangers." Between 1970 and 1976 about 36 percent of married women in the United States used the pill. But in 1975 articles began to emerge about the risk of heart attacks or cancer, grossly exaggerated by the lay press, and the use of birth control pills declined dramatically. Today only about 17 percent of married women in the United States use birth control pills. Many gynecologists would much rather perform a sterilization procedure than prescribe pills. In the first place, they might get sued if you develop any one of the many illnesses that have been incorrectly ascribed to the pill, and second they get paid a lot more for performing a sterilization, which most women view as safer than the pill.

Since 1960, when the pill first became available to the public, there has been a dramatic reduction in dosage of the pill. In 1960 women were getting almost tenfold the hormone dose necessary to prevent ovulation and conception. This produced unpleasant symptoms, such as nausea, breast swelling, weight gain, bloating, headaches, and sometimes acne or nervousness. The original birth control pill in 1960, Enovid, contained 150 micrograms of estrogen compared to 35 micrograms of estrogen in present-day pills. The original birth control pills had 10 milligrams of progestin (a synthetic form of progesterone), compared to 1 milligram today. The early pills, even with this high dosage, were moderately safe. But in the 1960s advanced epidemiological studies showed that certain diseases that carried a low risk of about one in thirty thousand in a normal population, such as pulmonary embolism or stroke, had three to five times that frequency in women who were using birth control pills. This still meant that women on the pill had only about a one in five thousand chance at most of developing these complications, but that was certainly enough to scare off many otherwise healthy users.

In fact, the newer formulations of birth control pill have reduced the dosage so dramatically (while still maintaining efficacy) that the aggravating side effects are very uncommon, and the life-threatening ones have been eliminated for most users. As you read through this chapter you will be able to learn just how this remarkable refinement in the safety of the pill occurred, determine whether the pill is now safe for you, and determine which pills are the right ones for you to take.

There are three major areas of concern for any woman about to take the birth control pill: (1) Is there assurance of fertility after discontinuing the pill? (2) Is there a risk of cancer, heart disease, and other life-threatening side effects? and (3) Can you expect aggravating symptoms such as weight gain, breast swelling, nausea, etc.? Before we deal with these questions, we must review how hormones are produced in a normal cycle and how the pill affects them.

Review of Normal Hormone Production in Women

The key hormones are FSH and LH (released by the pituitary gland), and estrogen and progesterone (released by the ovary), along with (to a lesser degree) testosterone, the male hormone. Figures 1–4 and 1–5 on pages 26 and 27 summarize how all these hormones stimulate and inhibit each other during the month. On day one of menstruation, the level of FSH goes up and stimulates the follicle to produce estrogen.

As estrogen is produced by the follicle, it depresses the pituitary's production of FSH. Thus during the first two weeks of the cycle, as the estrogen level goes up, the FSH level goes down. The rising estrogen level begins to crescendo by day twelve and stimulates the pituitary gland to release a huge and sudden burst of the hormone LH. This sudden burst of LH by the pituitary is what causes ovulation. The ruptured follicle then becomes the corpus luteum and begins to manufacture progesterone for fourteen days after ovulation. The ideal complete cycle takes twenty-eight days.

During the first two weeks of the cycle, the ovary produces only estrogen. During the second two weeks of the cycle (assuming ovulation has taken place), the ovary produces progesterone and estrogen. The addition of progesterone converts the lining of the uterus from a relatively thick, hard, "proliferative" surface to a more soft, spongy, "secretory" surface.

The corpus luteum (the ruptured follicle that makes the hormone progesterone) normally has a life-span of about fourteen days. The only thing that can prolong its function is a pregnancy. In the absence of a pregnancy, the corpus luteum ceases dramatically to make hormones by fourteen days. When the hormone levels drop to near zero, the lining of the uterus is shed. This is the first day of menstruation. Because menstruation reflects a reduction of hormone production by the ovaries to near zero, the FSH level then jumps again abruptly to high levels and the cycle starts once more. The initial rise of FSH on day one is essential. Without this initial rise in FSH to stimulate follicle development, none of the other events of the cycle will occur in proper sequence. Although ovulation is actually triggered by a rapid rise in the circulating levels of estrogen on days twelve to fourteen, causing the pituitary to release LH, the initial condition required for a normal cycle is a high level of FSH during menstruation.

Lack of ovulation is a true disease and should not be regarded simply as a problem with becoming pregnant. Even if a woman does not want to become pregnant, she should be concerned about this condition because the hormonal imbalance resulting from or causing poor ovulation leads to heavy buildup of a hard uterine lining that does not shed properly like the soft lining of an ovulatory woman. Not only can this lead to irregular bleeding and occasionally a painful ovarian enlargement (which may even necessitate surgery), but also over many years it can lead to the development of cancer of the lining of the uterus. So an infertile, nonovulating woman is deficient in progesterone and at high risk of developing cancer of the uterus. One way or another, she needs treatment. She either needs to have her ovulation stimulated to shed her uterine lining or to get pregnant, *or* she must be on birth control pills to help *prevent* cancer. But more on that later in the chapter.

How Does the Pill Work?

The birth control pill consists of estrogen and progestin (synthetic progesterone) given daily for three weeks out of every four, with menstruation occurring during the off week. Its major effect is to prevent ovulation by inhibiting the midcycle surge of LH release from the pituitary gland. In addition, the progestin in the pill alters the cervical mucus, making it thick, pasty, and scanty, thus preventing sperm penetration. Third, it decreases the thickness of the lining of the uterus, again because of the predominant progestin effect. So the pill does three things: It prevents ovulation, it prevents sperm penetration of cervical mucus, and it decreases the receptiveness of the lining of the uterus to sperm or egg.

Why does the pill have to have both an estrogen and a progestin? Estrogen normally inhibits the pituitary's release of FSH, and progestin inhibits the pituitary's release of LH. If the pill had estrogen only, FSH would be inhibited and the follicle should never develop. If the pill had progestin only, follicles should develop, but they could never ovulate because of the inhibition of LH release at midcycle. It was discovered in the late 1950s and early 1960s that this nice theoretical thinking was erroneous. In pills that contained only estrogen during the first half of the cycle and then progestin and estrogen in the second half of the cycle (the so-called sequentials that are no longer on the market), it was quickly discovered that the FSH was not inhibited enough by estrogen alone, and some of these women got pregnant. Furthermore, these pills did not have a predominant progestin effect and therefore did not have the health benefits of the modern pill.

There are birth control pills that contain only a progestin with *no* estrogen, but these also do not reliably prevent ovulation. The progestin provides only reasonable contraception by thickening the cervical mucus so as to prevent sperm penetration and inhibiting ovulation perhaps 20 percent of the time. But ovulation is consistently prevented only by taking a combination of estrogen and progestin. The estrogen prevents

FSH release by the pituitary and thus minimizes follicle development, and the progestin plus the estrogen inhibit the LH surge. A pill containing only progestin has a pregnancy rate of about 2 to 3 percent, or even higher if not taken exactly at the same time of the day every day.

The combination of estrogen and progestin in the pill is also necessary for regular, predictable periods. The estrogen in the pill serves to stabilize the uterine lining (endometrium) so that irregular shedding and breakthrough bleeding can be avoided. Progestin alone would lead to a small, thinned-out, irregular uterine lining with inconsistent, unpredictable bleeding. The estrogen in the pill helps to build up the lining enough so that despite the progestin dominance, there is enough stability to allow a nice, clean, predictable menstrual period. Furthermore, because the estrogen works in combination with the progestin to inhibit ovulation, the presence of both of these ingredients allows both of their dosages to be reduced dramatically to very safe levels.

One last word on how the pill works must be mentioned so that you can understand why we still do not have a reliable "male pill." The birth control pill is not able to suppress completely the pituitary's release of FSH and LH, which stimulate the ovary's production of hormone. The amount of estrogen production by the ovary in women taking the pill is about the same as that of those not taking the pill in the early phase of a normal cycle. This means that although there is enough suppression of the pituitary by the pill to prevent the woman from ovulating, you can't turn the ovary off 100 percent.

This same phenomenon occurs in the efforts to make a "male pill." If you give a normal amount of testosterone to a man, you can inhibit his FSH and LH production dramatically, just as you can in a woman by giving her progestin and estrogen. Indeed, you can decrease his sperm count to very low levels, but you can't reliably reduce his sperm count to zero. The system is "too vigorous" to turn off completely, at least with the present methods, and it takes just a few sperm to fertilize a fertile woman. With a woman you don't have to turn the system off completely; you just have to prevent ovulation. But with a man you would have to turn the system off completely to get the sperm count to zero.

Is Future Fertility Going to Be Impaired by Taking the Pill Now?

Since the pill works by inhibiting ovulation by means of hormones that the ovary would normally be producing on its own in response to stimulation from the pituitary gland, the biggest question on women's minds is whether ovulation will resume when the pills are discontinued. Take, for example, Nancy. She became pregnant in 1975 and subsequently went on birth control pills. Prior to that time she had completely normal twenty-eight-day cycles with normal menstrual periods. Three years later she went off her birth control pills and never menstruated again after that and never got pregnant. We finally were able to get her menstruating again by stimulating her with Clomid, but her periods varied between twenty-eight and thirty-five days, she finally gave up treatment, and as far as I know she has never had another child.

Robin is a thirty-four-year-old woman who has married at age twenty-two and who went on birth control pills for the first two and a half years of her marriage. She was menstruating regularly prior to taking the pills, with predictable twenty-eight-day cycles. Yet when she discontinued the pills two and a half years later, she never menstruated again and for ten years had been trying unsuccessfully to get pregnant. We now have her periods going again with what is called a "GNRH pump" in an effort to stimulate her ovaries, which have failed to receive any FSH or LH stimulation over the past ten years since she stopped taking the pill.

These women clearly blame birth control pills for their present infertility. But I have seen just as many women who never took birth control pills undergo just as sudden a change in their periods (or total loss of menstruation) simply because they got older. So how do we know whether the infertility in these women, which became apparent only after discontinuing birth control pills, was caused by the pills or would have occurred anyway? The menstrual irregularity and inferility of some women is actually improved by birth control pills. Take, for example, Sheila. She had irregular, painful periods before getting married and going on birth control pills. On the pills her cycles were painless and obviously regular. Once she discontinued the pills she noted that her cycles were now normal.

Jan had three children, and used no birth control pills after the birth of the third one. Yet her periods became irregular and she stopped ovulating without any clear reason other than just the passage of time. Bobbi never had children, and used only condoms and barrier methods for birth control. She had perfectly regular twenty-eight-day cycles and was ovulatory and perfectly fertile until around age thirty-five, when her periods suddenly began to become irregular. Unfortunately, this was just around the time that she decided she wanted to have children. If she had taken the pill all of those years, she might have concluded that her subsequent infertility was caused by the pill rather than just the passage of time. Joy is a thirty-five-year-old woman who became pregnant five years ago, had a wonderful little boy, and has been unable to get pregnant since that time. She went on birth control pills for one year after she had the boy. After going off the birth control pills her previously regular twenty-eight-day cycles had become variable and irregular, between twenty and twenty-six days, with poor ovulation.

The only way to know whether taking the birth control pill affects subsequent fertility is to compare a large group of women who are on the pill and discontinue it, to an equally large group of women who used some other method of contraception (such as the condom or an IUD) and discontinued it. We know that a certain percentage of women in any population are going to be infertile. Over a given period of time of trying to get pregnant, about 20 percent of women will fail to conceive after the first year, and 10 percent will fail to conceive after two years. This has nothing to do with prior use of birth control pills, or in fact any birth control whatsoever. Elizabeth is a good example of why individual reports of women who could not get pregnant after discontinuing the pill tell you nothing about whether the pill was at fault. At age twenty she got married and went on birth control pills. When she discontinued the pills, her periods did not return. When her life stabilized and her stress level was reduced, her periods returned to normal. Then three years later her periods once again stopped, only this time she had not taken birth control pills.

Fortunately, detailed studies from highly respected scientists have exonerated the pill in 99 percent of the cases from having any deleterious effect on subsequent fertility. Data from several sources in North America and England indicate that in a normal population about 25 percent of women will conceive within one month of unprotected intercourse, 60 percent within six months, 80 percent within twelve months, and 90 percent within two years. Thus a substantial portion of the population will experience a delay before conceiving. In a study from Oxford of seventeen thousand women discontinuing one method or other of contraception, comparison of the monthly and cumulative pregnancy rates was made between those women who had been on the pill and those who had used the diaphragm, the condom, or the intrauterine device. This study showed that women who stopped birth control pills on average required several months to begin ovulating. Thus these women took longer to get pregnant compared to women who had stopped other methods of contraception.

However, as time passed there was no longer an appreciable difference in fertility between women who had discontinued birth control pills and women who had discontinued other methods of contraception. Thirty-six months after stopping contraception, the percentage of women who had not gotten pregnant was no different among those who had used birth control pills than among those who had used the condom, IUD, or diaphragm. After forty-two months among women of proven previous fertility, who had previously had children and who had thereafter used contraception, 3.5 percent of former birth control pill users still had not gotten pregnant, and 3.4 percent of former diaphragm users still had not gotten pregnant. In women who had never had children before, forty-two months after discontinuing contraception, 10.7 percent of former pill users had not gotten pregnant, and 9.2 percent of women who had used other methods of birth control had not gotten pregnant.

Although there was no difference in conception rate among these women after three years, and therefore no long-term effect of the birth control pill on fertility, there was a short-term effect. Six months after discontinuing birth control pills, about 32 percent of women still hadn't conceived among those women who had had children in the past, whereas only 20 percent of such women who had discontinued other methods of birth control had not conceived. Thus among women who had previously had children, the pregnancy rate was considerably lower at six months for those who were discontinuing birth control pills than for those who were discontinuing other methods of contraception.

For women who had never had children before, six months after discontinuing birth control pills only 45 percent had gotten pregnant, and of those stopping other methods of birth control, 65 percent had gotten pregnant. The pregnancy rates became equal sometime after three years. By four years after stopping the pill, about 10 percent of women remained infertile, but this was the same no matter what method (if any) of contraception they had used previously. Thus it would appear that the pill leads to a transient but not permanent delay in return of fertility.

Yet there is a tiny percentage (less than 1 percent) of women who fail to menstruate after discontinuing the birth control pill, a condition called postpill amenorrhea, and who create a nagging controversy over whether in their specific case the pill might have turned off their hypothalamic and pituitary stimulating center irreversibly. It does seem that in this tiny percentage of women the pill might have some deleterious effect on subsequent ovulation. This deleterious effect is most likely to occur in women who had menstrual irregularity or poor ovulation before going on the pill. The good news is that with proper treatment normal fertility can be achieved in these rare patients with postpill amenorrhea. Within eighteen months the pregnancy rate for women treated for amenorrhea not related to the pill, as well as for women with amenorrhea related to having taken the pill, is 90 percent.

Weighed against this rare phenomenon of postpill amenorrhea, in which the woman stops ovulating and stops menstruating after having taken the pill, is the tremendous protection afforded to women taking the pill from permanent sterility that can be caused by pelvic inflammatory disease. Even in the presence of demonstrated gonorrhea and chlamydia infections, women who take the pill are remarkably protected against tubal disease caused by such infection invading the uterus or tubes and resulting in subsequent sterility. The reason for this protection is that the progestin (progesteronelike hormone) in the pill causes the cervical mucus to become sticky and prevent the invasion of sperm as well as any infectious organism. The progestin component of the pill inhibits colonization of the tube by bacteria that otherwise might easily find their way inside.

There is another unusual way in which the birth control pill can hurt future fertility, but it is rarely mentioned. Janice is a forty-one-year-old woman who already had three children, and was clearly quite fertile when she was young. After age thirty-six her periods (which previously had been like clockwork) became irregular and she began to develop PMS symptoms. Because she and her husband still had not given up the possibility of having a fourth child, they avoided sterilization. The IUD was making her periods heavy and uncomfortable, and so when it was removed at age forty she went on the low-dose birth control pills. She had dramatic relief from PMS, her periods became normal again, and she was happily protected from build-up of the uterine lining that occurs when you don't ovulate properly. What she didn't realize was that she was sealing her future reproductive destiny.

A year later she turned up in her gynecologist's office thinking she might be pregnant, but instead the physician discovered a huge benign fibroid tumor, which had obliterated the rest of the uterus. Two weeks later she had a hysterectomy. Her mother, who had never taken the pill, had the same exact size tumor on her uterus, and had also undergone a hysterectomy at age forty-one. Still, we know the pill in older women can cause these fibroid tumors to grow, and this can cause infertility just as readily as inhibition of ovulation.

To summarize, for 99 percent of women who have taken the pill, there is an eventual complete return of prior fertility when they stop the pill. But there is a slight delay compared to women using other contraceptives. However, about 1 percent of women stop menstruating when they go off of the pill, and about half of those had a prior history of menstrual irregularity. Thus 0.5 percent of women have suffered a permanent inhibition of ovulation related to the pill. Fortunately, when those women are treated, fertility returns in 90 percent of the cases. Weighed against this tiny risk of permanent inhibition of ovulation is the tremendous protection the pill gives against tubal disease, an extremely common cause of infertility, which is far more difficult to treat than anovulation (lack of ovulation).

Symptoms Caused by High-Dose Birth Control Pills

In the 1960s, when the introduction of the birth control pill heralded the "sexual revolution," women had to tolerate some of the aggravating symptoms that came to be assumed as an inevitable part of taking the pill. These included breast swelling, weight gain, nausea, increased appetite, and headaches. Women who had been on the pill for several years often felt tremendous relief when they discontinued them to get pregnant. With the new low-dose pills available today, women should not have to put up with any of these symptoms, and actually should have more comfortable periods, fewer headaches, and less swelling than they might possibly experience in a natural cycle without taking the pill. If you are having uncomfortable symptoms on the pill, it may mean you are on the wrong pill and probably are getting too large a dose of hormone.

You need not be bewildered or confused by the over thirty different formulations and brands of birth control pills presently on the market. All of these different brands and formulations contain basically just two ingredients: an estrogen and a progestin. Remember, estrogen is the hormone that your ovary normally produces in the first half of your cycle as the follicle is growing and preparing for ovulation. Estrogen increases your cervical mucus, keeps your bones strong, and builds up the lining of the womb. Progestin is similar to the hormone progesterone, which the ovary secretes *after ovulation* for the next 14 days. The ovary does not stop making estrogen during the second half of the cycle; it just starts making progesterone in addition. Progesterone makes the cervical mucus dry up, and softens the lining of the uterus that previously had been built up by estrogen. This softening to the lining of the uterus is critical. Unless progesterone is secreted, the lining of the uterus does not soften up, and when the time comes to menstruate, instead of a clean bleed, the lining will just flake off incompletely and you will have a continuing buildup of tissue. Without progesterone you will have irregular menstrual bleeding, and cumulative tissue buildup in the lining of the uterus.

HIGH DOSE OF ESTROGEN

Birth control pills contain an estrogen and a progestin. You take them three weeks out of four, and during the fourth week (when you don't take the pills) you menstruate. It is the estrogen component of the pill, in too-high doses, that causes your symptoms of nausea, breast tenderness, and fluid retention (which you notice as swelling around the fingers or ankles). Otherwise flat-chested females who took the birth control pill in the 1960s and 1970s suddenly became big-breasted. To some this was a benefit; to others, a nuisance. The reason for these uncomfortable symptoms was that you were getting five times the amount of estrogen, in those early pills, that you needed to suppress ovulation.

Some of the side effects of the estrogen in birth control pills, which include increased blood pressure, headaches, and the increased coagulability of the blood, are caused because it is not a natural but rather a synthetic estrogen. The synthetic estrogen in the pill comes into your body orally, and has to be digested in your gastrointestinal tract and absorbed through your liver. On the way through your liver, this high dose of estrogen stimulates the liver to produce an increased amount of some of its products called globulins. Some of these globulins, such as angiotensin, normally are used by the body to constrict its blood vessels, and other globulins help the body's blood clotting process. Thus it is not only the increased level of estrogen in your blood that is causing symptoms, but the fact that the estrogen has to go through the liver.

The estrogen component of the pill can even produce mood changes if the dose is too high. This is also caused by the metabolic effects of estrogen being absorbed through the liver. All of these aggravating symptoms, both of estrogen overdose, and of estrogen absorption through the liver, are very infrequent now because you now have available effective birth control pills with one fifth the amount of estrogen that was in all the formulations available in the 1960s and 1970s. If you are having any of these symptoms, such as nausea, breast swelling, bloating, increased blood pressure, or mood changes, your solution is not a complicated one. You simply need to find out how much estrogen is in the pill you are taking and make sure to switch to a pill that has less estrogen. An ideal pill is one that has the least possible amount of estrogen in it. If you look at Chart 2, which lists all the available birth control pills, you can easily determine which ones have the lowest amount of estrogen and ask your doctor to put you on one of those pills.

HIGH DOSE OF PROGESTIN

Symptoms of acne, nervousness, headaches, premenstrual tension, and weight gain usually are caused by the progestin component of the pill and once again should not occur in pills where the progestin content is low. You need to understand why the progesterone can produce all of these symptoms when given in the pill in high doses, but generally doesn't produce them in the natural cycle.

Natural progesterone cannot be absorbed in pill form. To make a pill form of progestin, it was necessary to create a synthetic progestin that could be absorbed orally. This was accomplished in 1951, and that is what made the birth control pill possible. We knew how to make estrogens in pill form as early as 1948, but it wasn't until progesterone could be made in pill form that oral contraception could become a reality. To make the pill form of progesterone, the male hormone testosterone had to be used as a starting point. Modification of the chemical structure of the male hormone is what led to the synthesis of the "female" progestin hormones in a form that could be absorbed by the stomach. Thus in the progesterone component (the progestin) of any birth control pill there is a tiny degree of male hormone (or "androgenic") effect. Chemically, the synthetic progesterones just don't look like progesterone. They look more like testosterone.

There is nothing wrong with having a male hormonelike effect in the progestin of the pill. Women who are not on the pill normally make a small amount of male hormone (testosterone), which is important for them to have a normal libido. The problem comes when the progestin dose is so high that the testosteronelike effects are too great. These effects include increasing oiliness of the skin, which leads to acne, nervousness, and irritability, possibly headaches, and certainly the increased appetite that all women in the 1960s reported when going on the pill.

Testosterone is the classic "anabolic steroid." This is the drug that you hear about athletes taking to increase their muscle mass and make them grow stronger. Obviously it is more effective in female athletes than male athletes because the levels of testosterone in females are normally so much lower than those of males. Any female athlete who is placed on an anabolic steroid like testosterone is likely to improve her performance dramatically. For that reason many female athletes have used these steroids to further their athletic careers. But they can also tell of the aggravating side effects such as acne, irritability, and interruption of normal menstrual cycles. They don't mind the increased appetite and weight gain, because with all the exercise they get it is associated with an increase in muscle mass and strength rather than fat.

But too much testosterone is, to say the least, aggravating, and potentially dangerous for any woman. Take, for example, Chris. She had completely normal twenty-eight-day cycles until she got married fourteen years ago and then went on birth control pills for two years. Her pills had a high dose of progestin, and before she knew it she had gained 15 pounds, and continued to gain weight during the rest of her marriage to the point where she is now 50 pounds overweight. She presently weighs 170 pounds and is only 5 feet, 6 inches tall. After going off the pill she found it difficult to lose weight again, and this increased body fat (not muscle), caused by her prodigiously increased appetite on the pill, played havoc with her ovulation because fat cells store estrogen. We could not treat her infertility until she was able to lose those 50 pounds and get back to a normal weight.

In a similar vein, it's ridiculous to have to endure such side effects as increased oiliness of the skin and acne on the pill. If anything, the female hormones estrogen and progesterone should improve the skin, which accounts for the remarkable "glow" of a woman's face when she becomes pregnant. With the development of the modern low-dose birth control pill, physicians even prescribe it as a treatment for acne. The new low-dose birth control pills have such a low progestin content that there is virtually no male hormone effect other than what you have in a natural cycle, and in fact your skin should look better rather than worse. The female hormones of the pill counteract the effects of your own testosterone production, and suppress your ovaries over production of testosterone.

The early pills contained as much as ten milligrams of the progestin called norethindrone, the most common and popular of the birth control pill progestins. Modern birth control pills contain one tenth that amount of progestin, and in fact the "triphasic" (which we will get into later) formulations give you even less than that. So if you are experiencing symptoms of weight gain, nervousness, acne, mood changes, or head-aches prior to menstruation on the pill, it means you are probably taking too high a progestin dose or too potent a progestin. Again, look at Chart 2 and consult your physician to make sure you switch to a pill that contains the lowest possible dose of progestin.

One note of caution: Because some of the progestins (as opposed to the estrogens) have different potencies, the amount of progestin alone is not as important as the amount of a specific progestin with a known potency. To make your life easier I would suggest that when you look at this table you consider only the progestin norethindrone. That is because it is the most commonly used, the least potent, and if you limit yourself to comparing the levels of that progestin it will be much easier for you to make sure you are taking a low dose. If you look at it in this simple low-dose fashion, you should be on a pill that contains only thirty-five micrograms of estrogen and one milligram of norethindrone. Furthermore, the triphasics (Ortho-Novum 7–7, Tri-Norinyl, and Tri-phasil), which give you varying amounts of progestin during the cycle, add up to considerably less progestin throughout the month than even the one-milligram formulations we have considered to be free of pro-gestin-related side effects. Thus in these new low-dose pills the pro-gestin component no longer has a clinically significant level of male hormonelike, or androgenic, effects.

The Risk of Dangerous Complications Such as Cancer and Heart Disease

BIRTH CONTROL PILLS AND CANCER

The biggest fear most women have of birth control pills is that they will cause cancer. The number one fear has been cancer of the breast. I have a friend on the East Coast who has seen one right after another of her friends develop cancer of the breast, and they all had been on birth control pills when they were younger. This friend of mine, a very sophisticated and knowledgeable woman, is convinced that birth control pills caused the cancer of the breast in all her friends simply because they all had been on the pill at one time or another. But this does not necessarily mean the pill had anything at all to do with their breast cancer. The only way to find that out would be to perform a large-scale study of hundreds of thousands of women, some of whom had taken the pill and others of whom had not, to determine twenty-five or thirty years later who got breast cancer and who did not. Since statistically 11 percent of all women are going to get breast cancer eventually, if a study reveals that 11 percent of women who had been on the pill develop breast cancer, then you can't conclude that the pill has anything to do with breast cancer.

In fact, the real risk factors for breast cancer among this woman's friends are more likely the fact that they put off childbearing until later years, and exclusively bottle-fed their children once they had them. We have known for fifty years that these factors dramatically increase the risk of breast cancer.

The fear that cancer of the breast would be caused by birth control pills relates to an article in a British journal in 1983. An epidemiologist named Pike from England attempted to show that women who had used oral contraceptives high in progestin before twenty-five years of age had an increased risk of developing breast cancer before age thirty-seven. This surprised many people, because if anything the fear was that estrogen might lead to increased risk of cancer of the breast, and that progestin would protect against it. Once a scare like this gets started, fueled by the clear awareness of women who took the pill in the 1960s that the high estrogen content did result in breast swelling and breast tenderness, it is difficult for any amount of scientific, rational study to dispel the fears. But one objective, unbiased study after another, which were very carefully and scientifically controlled, found no effect whatsoever of prior birth control pill use on the risk of developing breast cancer. Long-term oral contraceptive use for more than twenty years, even in the high-dose variety with all of its other attendant side effects and risks, did not increase the risk of breast cancer. The safety of the birth control pill with regard to breast cancer was true even in women who had a family history of breast cancer or previous benign breast disease, all predisposing factors.

It is interesting that detailed studies between 1977 and 1982 with a huge number of patients had already appeared to settle the question and rule out any risk that birth control pills increase the chance of developing breast cancer. But in science, when faced with speculation to the contrary of medical consensus, it is our burden to restudy the issue because there may be merit in any new idea or proposal no matter how farfetched it may sound. For that reason, between 1983 and 1986 an incredible amount of federal money was spent to research this issue completely. In August 1986 the results of this new far-reaching study, involving thousands of women and sponsored by the National Centers for Disease Control and the National Institute of Child Health and Human Development, reported in the *New England Journal of Medicine* once again that the birth control pill, even the high-dose variety popular in the 1960s and 1970s, created no increased risk for developing cancer of the breast.

Furthermore, all of the thirty different formulations of birth control pills on the American market were tested and there was no difference in the results no matter what brand or formulation of birth control pill was used.

What is even more exciting than the fact that birth control pills do not cause cancer is that indeed they appear to *prevent* cancer of the uterus and cancer of the ovary, which are the next most common forms of cancer in women second to cancer of the breast. When this protective effect of the pill against cancer of the uterus and cancer of the ovary was discovered, it was very ironic. In the 1970s it was popular to put women on estrogen after they went through the menopause because it helped make their bones stronger, kept their vagina soft and receptive to intercourse instead of drying up the way it normally would, and prevented hot flashes. But at that time none of these women who were placed on estrogen was given progesterone also. Without progesterone, "unopposed" estrogen leads to a continual overabundance and buildup of tissue on the inside of the womb, and over a long period of many years this will eventually cause cancer. Thus in 1970 women who were given postmenopausal estrogen alone were discovered to have a higher risk of endometrial cancer of the uterus. When these women were carefully studied for past medical history, the researchers were aghast to find that although women with cancer of the uterus were much more likely to have been on postmenopausal estrogen than women who did not get cancer of the uterus, very few of them compared to the normal population had ever taken birth control pills. This led to detailed prospective studies (studies which follow a population into the future for many years) that verified the remarkable protection that prior birth control pill use conveys against later development of cancer of the uterus.

Why should this be so? The reason is that virtually all the hundreds of oral contraceptives that have been marketed over the past quarter of a century or more have had more of a progesterone effect than an estrogen effect. It is a basic rule of female endocrinology that when estrogens and progesterones are given together, the progesterone effect always dominates. Even in the high-dose pills of yesteryear, with all that we didn't know, the progesterone effect of the oral contraceptive always overrode whatever estrogen effect there was, and this probably is why it afforded such remarkable protection against cancer of the uterus.

That was not the only area where the progesterone dominance was helpful. It is now clear that although the birth control pill does not prevent cancer of the breast, it dramatically prevents or minimizes benign breast disease. Benign breast disease can be a very frightening condition that is difficult to manage. Women with this disease form lumps and cysts in their breasts that feel just like cancer. The lumps and cysts have to be biopsied or needled or aspirated or examined very carefully through mammograms or surgical testing. A woman may experience ongoing anxiety over this benign disease even when her physician does test after test to tell her that her condition looks benign. By virtue of its progesterone dominance, the birth control pill remarkably minimizes the risk of a woman developing this benign cystic breast disease.

Probably the most terrifying cancer in women is cancer of the ovary, because it is a death sentence in over 80 percent of women in whom it is diagnosed. Eighteen thousand women develop it in the United States every year, and it is a major cancer killer among women. Birth control pills also appear to protect against developing this cancer. But they afford this protection in a manner quite different from how they protect against cancer of the uterus and benign breast disease. The risk for cancer of the ovary seems to be related to "incessant ovulation." Throughout human history women have either been pregnant or lactating for most of their life, and in any event not ovulating. Modern life has changed that, and this has increased the incidence of cancer of the ovary.

It is virtually impossible to detect cancer of the ovary before it has already spread. The survival rate is low, and among gynecological cancers in women (cervix, uterus, and ovary) it is certainly the number one killer. It is the number four overall cancer killer among women in this country, taking a backseat only to cancer of the breast, colon, and lung. The fact that taking birth control pills protects against this deadly cancer should make you think carefully before turning pills down as a method of contraception. This does not mean you need to be on birth control pills to avoid this cancer. You can also avoid this cancer by having a lot of children. Pregnancies protect against getting this cancer just as much as the birth control pills do. But if you are going to put off getting pregnant, particularly if you are going to put it off for a long time, the pill may be of great benefit.

One of the most common cancers in women is cancer of the cervix. The cervix is the opening to your uterus, its portal to the outside world that opens up and secretes cervical mucus at midcycle to allow entry of the sperm. Nowadays cancer of the cervix has a very high cure rate and is not a major killer among women in the developed world only because most women now know to get a yearly Pap smear. This almost religious routine of going to the gynecologist once a year to get your Pap smear means that if you do develop this cancer you will most certainly have it diagnosed early enough to have it cured. This was not the case fifty years ago, when cancer of the cervix was a major killer of women.

Cancer of the cervix is not protected against by the pill, nor is its risk increased by taking the pill. But if you take just a few minutes to read about what really causes cancer of the cervix, and if you fit into the category of women who are susceptible to this disease, then perhaps you ought to think about a different contraceptive that will give you protection against cancer of the cervix.

Nuns and women who have only *one* sexual partner in their life-time virtually never get cancer of the cervix. The risk of cancer of the cervix increases with the number of sexual partners and with early age of onset of sexual activity. The greater the variety of sexual partners you have, the more likely you are to develop cancer of the cervix. This may not concern you because in our modern era with yearly Pap smears, cancer of the cervix is diagnosed early, and the cure rate is very high. But if it does bother you, you need either to reconsider your life-style, or use a different contraceptive.

Cancer of the cervix, as you might have already concluded by now, is basically a "slow" venereal disease. The infectious organism has not yet been identified, nor are we certain that it isn't just a response to a general variety of sexually transmitted infections that women who have a variety of sexual partners are more likely to have. If that is your situation, you need to insist that your male partner use condoms, or that you use the diaphragm. Of those two choices, condoms offer some-what more protection against cervical cancer.

Young women with multiple partners are more likely to be on the pill because of its convenience. In fact, at one time it was thought that birth control pills might increase the risk for developing cancer of the cervix, only because so many young women with an early onset of sexual activity and a wide variety of sexual partners in their young life chose the pill as their method of contraception. Cancer of the cervix occurs equally in women using and not using birth control pills. But the real risk factors have to do with sexual activity, age at first intercourse, and the number of partners. The only problem with the pill is that it doesn't protect against this particular cancer. Therefore every woman who is sexually active should be especially careful to have an annual Pap smear whether she is or is not on birth control pills.

After more than a quarter of a century of use, with most of those years involving dosages that were way too high, we can safely say that not only does the pill not cause cancer, but in fact it prevents thousands of deaths from cancer every year.

THE PILL AND THROMBOEMBOLISM OF THE VEINS

Too much estrogen can cause increased coagulability of the blood, leading to clots in the veins and to potentially disastrous migration of one of those clots to the lungs. Too much synthetic progestin (which you'll remember is derived from the male hormone testosterone rather than from progesterone) can cause fat deposition in the blood vessels, arteriosclerosis, and therefore heart disease and stroke. The early high-dose pills created a very slight but definite increase in the risk of these cardiovascular diseases. Even today with the low-dose pills, most doctors are afraid to recommend that any woman over the age of thirty-five who smokes or has other risk factors take the pill. But the major impact of huge studies performed over the past fifteen years in women on high-dose and low-dose pills and who had other risk factors (such as smoking) for arteriosclerosis and heart disease, makes one issue very clear: Women over thirty-five should not smoke, whether they take the pill or not, and women under thirty-five who do smoke have no increased risk from taking the pill. The big question is whether women from the ages of thirty-five to forty-five who do not smoke can take the pill. We had better discuss these studies in detail so you can make a proper decision.

Most of the studies of the effect of birth control pills on cardio-vascular disease were performed on women taking the pills during the 1970s, when the estrogen and progestin doses were much higher than they are today. Furthermore, the most worrisome studies came from Britain, once again when the doses of estrogen and progestin were higher than today's levels. The pharmaceutical industry has responded remarkably over the past quarter century to these findings by lowering the dosage to the point where it is now quite safe. In fact, in both the United States and Britain, death rates from heart attacks have decreased in the general population of women age twenty to forty-five during the past fifteen years, years in which the use of birth control pills increased dramatically. Since birth control pills have been used by about 35 percent of women in this age group at some time or another, we would not have expected such a decline if the pill were a major risk. But for certain women it is a risk. For that reason you must read on, even though what follows may seem to be a bit heavy and scientific.

There are four major blood vessel problems to worry about: heart disease caused by narrowing of the coronary arteries as a result of arteriosclerosis; stroke caused by narrowing of the arteries to your brain; high blood pressure caused by contraction of the muscle in the walls of the arteries; and venous thromboembolism (clots in the veins, which return blood to your heart). High blood pressure is rarely a problem with modern low-dose pills. It is caused by high levels of synthetic estrogen in the pill that have to go through the liver before reaching the bloodstream. In the process of doing this, the synthetic estrogen causes the liver to increase its production of certain globulins. One of these globulins is angiotensin, which the body normally manufactures to constrict the blood vessels in the process of directing the traffic of blood throughout the body. Too much angiotensin can cause high blood pressure. The safety of the reduced dosage of the pill is now becoming quite apparent. In the early days of high-dose pills, 5 percent of pill users developed hypertension (high blood pressure) clearly related to pill use. Recent studies show no association between birth control pills and hypertension. High blood pressure is a common enough disorder in today's fast-paced world, but the new low-dose pill does not increase your risk of developing this problem.

Venous thromboembolism was the first serious health problem documented to be an increased risk among pill users. In 1963 and later in 1967, while women were taking pills with incredibly high dosages of estrogen and progestin (five times the estrogen and ten times the progestin dose available today), it first became apparent that venous thromboembolism might be more common in pill users. The first careful study, published by the Royal College of General Practitioners in

England in 1967, reported a four- to twelvefold increase in the risk of venous clots and emboli in birth control pill users compared to nonusers.

The reason you may not be exactly familiar with what I mean by venous thromboembolism is that it is not a common problem, like heart disease. Veins are the blood vessels that carry blood back to the heart, whereas arteries are the thick-walled blood vessels that carry blood away from the heart to all parts of the body. The arteries are very prone to developing arteriosclerosis, a thickening of the walls that narrows the inner lumen, or diameter, of the artery. Veins are, for the most part, free of these problems. However, men and women will occasionally form blood clots in the veins, which quite rarely can be dangerous by getting dislodged and passing into the heart.

The risk of this occurring in a normal population of women is somewhere between one in fifteen thousand to one in thirty thousand per year. By comparison, the risk of dying from pregnancy is perhaps one in twenty-five thousand per year. In fact, one of the commonest reasons for dying from pregnancy is this very problem of venous thromboembolism. During pregnancy, the baby, as it enlarges and expands the uterus, compresses veins that return blood to the heart. This is why pregnant women frequently get varicose veins. Blood clots are more likely to form in these varicose veins, because the blood is not moving as fast as in normal veins. For that reason women who are pregnant run an increased risk of venous thromboembolism. Major surgical procedures also increase this risk for similar reasons. Early studies in 1967 and 1969 from Britain definitely demonstrated an increased risk of venous thromboembolism in women taking the high-dose pills. This risk was approximately four to twelve times higher than the risk for nonusers. Studies in 1970 and 1971, however, demonstrated that as the dosage of the estrogen in the pill went down, so did the risk of venous thromboembolism.

With doses of estrogen greater than fifty micrograms, the risk of deep vein thrombosis is about one hundred per one hundred thousand people per year. But two detailed studies that came out of Sweden and Britain in 1980 utilizing the new low-dose pills showed that when the dosage was reduced to thirty or thirty-five micrograms of estrogen (present-day dosage), the risk went down to as low as seven per one hundred thousand cases per year. Reducing the estrogen from fifty micrograms to thirty or thirty-five micrograms has so dramatically reduced the production of globulins in the liver that the increase in blood coagulability is very little, if any. The decreased dosages in modern pills (thirty to

thirty-five micrograms of estrogen) has prevented the hypercoagula-
bility of the blood and increase in blood pressure that otherwise was
part and parcel of taking the pill. In addition, as you already know,
lowering the estrogen has reduced the incidence of unpleasant side
effects such as nausea, breast tenderness, and fluid retention.

Now we will turn our attention to the more major cardiovascular
risks of heart disease and stroke, which are related to the progestin
content of the pill.

HEART DISEASE AND STROKE

You may remember reading in the newspaper about an incredible
female athlete who, in her late twenties or early thirties, suddenly
dropped dead of a heart attack. Heart attacks are very rare events in
women under the age of forty-five. The reason they are so uncommon
in women, as compared to men, is that the female hormone estrogen
protects against arteriosclerosis, and the male hormone testosterone
tends to promote arteriosclerosis. These women athletes who drop
dead unexpectedly of heart attacks have most likely been on anabolic
steroids, all of which are derivatives of the male hormone testosterone.
They are not sanctioned, but that doesn't stop some extremely ambitious
athletes from taking them. Although the effect of taking such drugs on
the male is very small because men already have a high testosterone
level, the effect on women athletes is incredible. Their muscle mass
and oxygen-carrying capacity increase dramatically under the effects of
male hormone.

But it also increases their risk of heart attacks. Any woman taking
male hormone in an effort to increase her body muscle mass and athletic
strength also puts herself in the same category as men who normally
have an increased risk of developing heart disease in comparison to
women.

The early high-dose birth control pills had a very high dose of
synthetic progestin. Since the synthetic progestin is derived from testosterone chemically, it had a very slight but definite testosteronelike
effect. This could not compare to the tremendous testosterone effect
from anabolic steroids, but nonetheless the effect was distinct and mea-
surable. These women gained weight, their appetite increased, they
developed somewhat oily skin, and they developed a small but definite
elevation in blood levels of LDL cholesterol, which is the fatty component of the blood that leads to arteriosclerosis. When the progestin

content of the pill was ten milligrams it would make sense that there might be an increased risk of heart attacks in certain women on the pill because of the testosteronelike side effects of such a high dose of progestin. Today the progestin level is down to less than one milligram, which results in very little testosterone effect.

The first study to implicate the pill as causing an increased risk of heart attacks in women came from England in 1975. In this study, women in their thirties on the pill had a 2.8 times greater risk of heart attack than women not on the pill. Women between the ages of forty and forty-five had almost a five times greater risk than if they were not taking the pill. In 1977 the Royal College of General Practitioners in England reported similar findings but noted that the majority of women who developed heart attacks, whether pill users or not pill users, were smokers. Very few women under thirty-five who are nonsmokers get heart attacks. It was clear that even at the high dosage level of the early 1970s, it was safe for all women under thirty-five to use the pill, and for all nonsmokers under forty. But for smokers over thirty-five or any woman over age forty, usage of the birth control pill seemed possibly to cause an increased risk of heart attack.

In 1981 studies began to come out that demonstrated that the lower-dose pills were associated with a lower risk of heart disease or stroke. At this point the British studies and the American studies began to differ in their findings, most likely because in the American studies very few women were taking a pill with a progestin content of greater than 1.5 milligrams, whereas in the British studies more women were taking these higher-dose pills. In fact, in the British studies most women were taking pills with more than 50 micrograms of estrogen also. American studies in 1981 demonstrated no increased risk of pulmonary embolism or venous thrombosis, as well as no increased risk of heart attack or chronic heart disease in birth control pill users. Study after study demonstrated that the risk for heart attack and stroke diminished significantly as the progestin dose dropped, first from 4 to 2.5 milligrams and then from 2.5 milligrams to 1 milligram of norethindrone.

In the most recent reports from England, women on the new low-dose pills have thus far shown no cases of arterial disease, and the American studies continue to show no increased risk of heart attack, thrombotic stroke, venous thrombosis or embolism, and no increased risk of death between users and nonusers. The increased risk of circulatory diseases were totally attributable to smoking. Only smokers thirty-five or older have a significantly increased risk of dying from circulatory diseases, and they probably should be cautioned against using the pill. But in truth their real problem is smoking, and the best advice to them is to stop that rather than the pill.

For women who smoke heavily, the risk of getting a heart attack is about seven to thirty-four times greater than for women who do not smoke. Older women who smoke have an even greater risk of heart disease. The birth control pill adds virtually no increased risk to women under thirty-five, and little if any increased risk to women between the ages of thirty-five and forty-five who do not smoke. Because the risk of heart attack in women goes up in general over age forty-five, it would be prudent at this time for women over forty-five not to go on the pill until more detailed studies come out for women in the older age brackets who use these lower-dose formulations.

The knowledge that the new low-dose pills are relatively safe even for nonsmoking women between the ages of thirty-five and forty-five becomes very important for older women who don't want to undergo a surgical procedure such as sterilization and who are having difficulty with other birth control methods. For example, Susan was forty years old, had her last baby six years earlier, and wasn't 100 percent sure that she would not want to have another child. Perhaps she was fooling herself, but the thought of having a sterilization (a "permanent"-sounding step) was not emotionally acceptable. She had an IUD for six years and was developing heavy periods; severe migraine headaches premenstrually; and a painful, uncomfortable premenstrual syndrome (PMS). We took out the IUD and put her on ultralow-dose birth control pills. Now she no longer has headaches or PMS. Her periods are no longer painful or heavy, and her heaped-up endometrial lining is now safely reduced. The pill, even at age forty, was the ideal contraceptive for her and probably will remain so for several years.

A patient age thirty-five wanted a tubal sterilization because she was getting severe headaches on Ovral, a formulation of birth control pill prescribed by her older doctor. The dosage of estrogen and progestin in this particular pill, which was introduced in the late 1960s, is enormous compared with today's modern formulations. This woman really did not want a sterilization because although she wanted no more children, her husband wasn't as convinced. Again her ideal birth control method would be the pill, but the high-dose pill she was on not only made her uncomfortable but also created unnecessary health risks. There is never any reason for any individual to be on a high- or even moderate-dose birth control pill. There is absolutely no reason why your body is any different than anybody else's. The only safe and proper prescribing practice is to go on a very low-dose modern pill with no more than thirty-five micrograms of estrogen and no more than one milligram of norethindrone.

There is in fact no reason why you shouldn't start out on the new "triphasic" pill, which gives a varying but lower dose of progestin throughout your cycle. It is an ingenious way of giving you the equivalent of only 0.75 milligram of norethindrone per day, averaged throughout your cycle, without any increased breakthrough bleeding or decreased effectiveness of contraception. In fact, we did this with Susan as well as my thirty-five-year-old friend who thought she might need a tubal sterilization.

What Susan was not aware of before we made this decision is that her ovulation had gotten worse and irregular over the past six years, as frequently happens to women in their late thirties, thus leading to a buildup of endometrial tissue lining her womb because of a lack of progesterone. She was not aware that because of this lack of ovulation a time bomb was ticking away that gave her an increased risk of developing cancer of the uterus. We performed an endometrial biopsy of her uterus at the time we took out the IUD and started her on the pill. The biopsy confirmed that there was in the uterus a huge accumulation of tissue that could have led to cancer over the next five to ten years, except for the fact that we corrected the problem by putting her on birth control pills. A tubal sterilization, the conventional "thing to do," would *not* have given her this protection.

Health Benefits of Birth Control Pills

We have already discussed how birth control pills provide remarkable protection against cancer of the uterus and cancer of the ovary. They also help prevent benign breast disease and ovarian cysts, both conditions that can be very worrisome because they must be distinguished from cancer by the physician and can lead to a great deal of patient anxiety. For all four of these conditions the longer you have taken the pill, the more protection you get. This protection is caused by the progesterone-dominant effect of virtually every combination pill. Infertile women who don't ovulate regularly, and fat women who have excess estrogen levels because their fat cells store and release estrogen, are more at risk of developing these problems than fertile women who are not overweight. So the pill not only prevents pregnancy but also is a preventive medicine breakthrough for women.

The pill also can be used to treat specific medical problems when they occur. Women with irregular periods and heavy uterine bleeding usually have irregular ovulation, with many anovulatory cycles. If such a woman wants to get pregnant, the best treatment is to stimulate her ovulation with Clomid or Pergonal. But if she does not want to get pregnant, low-dose birth control pills are a very effective treatment. The problem with these women is that they produce inadequate progesterone. They have a heavy buildup of uterine lining that flakes off from time to time with bleeding and pain. Although a biopsy is in order to confirm the diagnosis, the birth control pill is the best treatment.

Many women develop a condition called "polycystic ovaries." They produce an inordinate amount of male hormone, have excessive hair growth, oily skin, and acne, are frequently overweight, and have irregular menstruation. By putting these women on birth control pills you suppress all ovarian activity and thereby will lower the testosterone level. The pill also provides a diagnostic test for these women if the testosterone level does not go down, it indicates that it is not coming from the ovary but rather from the adrenal gland, requiring a different treatment. Teenage acne, as well as acne in older women, is caused by too much testosterone. One of the scariest things about treating acne is that the most popular drug for treating it, Accutane, has been implicated in causing severe fetal abnormalities if taken while pregnant. How much safer than Accutane would the birth control pill be for treating acne in a sexually active adolescent? As we have already seen, the birth control pill is an excellent treatment for many women with PMS symptoms (headaches, swelling, anxiety, and depression). It is also excellent for treating iron deficiency anemia caused by heavy menstrual bleeding.

The birth control pill helps prevent three million cases of pelvic inflammatory disease (PID) every year in the developing world because it makes the cervical mucus sticky and not only resistant to the invasion of sperm but also to the invasion of infectious diseases. Africa has the highest rate of pelvic inflammatory disease (and subsequent sterility) in the world. Yet Africa also has the lowest rate of birth control pill use. In some areas of Africa, 47 percent of the female population have been found to be sterile because of scarred, blocked Fallopian tubes caused by pelvic inflammatory disease. These women would have been much more likely to be fertile had they used oral contraception. If it weren't for their hesitancy to use birth control pills, perhaps for fear that it would interfere with later fertility, they might not have become sterile. Use of the pill would have protected them against many sexually transmitted diseases that are rampant in Africa. Similarly, in certain populations of young women, use of the birth control pill is an important public health measure to ensure their subsequent fertility.

Effectiveness of the Pill in Preventing Pregnancy

There can be no controversy over the fact that other than sterilization, the birth control pill is the most effective method of contraception available, but only if it is taken properly. Theoretically, if there are no mistakes in pill-taking, the pregnancy rate should be less than 0.1 percent. But the pill really is not that effective in practice because women forget to take it. Depending upon the population studied, the actual failure rate of the pill is closer to 2 percent. That is the only reason why sterilization is more effective, simply because it requires no thought, with no need to remember to take a pill every day.

But the effectiveness of other contraceptive methods also is very high if they are used correctly. For example, the failure rate with condoms is only 1 percent if used every time. The problem with the condom is that, like the pill, people forget to use it. The failure rate with periodic abstinence, or "natural" birth control, varies from 1 to 40 percent, depending purely on the skill and discipline of the person using it. The diaphragm and foam often have failure rates of 20 percent, but if they are carefully used, the failure rate can be as low as 5 percent. Most methods of birth control are relatively effective if used properly. But second to sterilization, the pill certainly is the most effective method that does not interfere with spontaneity of the sexual act. I doubt if it will reach its former heights of popularity until the stigmas of bad side effects, potential dangers, and simply fear of tampering with one's system are eased. This fear cannot be eased by blanket assurances. It can be eased only by detailed study of the facts. That is what I hope this portion of the chapter on the birth control pill has been able to accomplish.

Formulations and Dosages: Which Pill Should I Take?

There are over thirty different brands and formulations of the birth control pill now on the market (see Table 1). But don't worry. In every one of the seemingly bewildering array of possible pills to choose from, there are only two ingredients: an estrogen and a progestin. The only thing you have to know about the dosage of these estrogens and progestins is simply that you should choose the pill that has the lowest dose. If you read through this section you will be able to narrow your choice to basically two or three preparations from this whole complex-appearing (but in truth really simple) list of possibilities. "Tailor-making" of the pill to the individual patient is not a valid concept. Everyone who opts for the pill should be on a low-dose formulation. Unfortunately, by 1980, only 30 percent of women were using pills with lower than fifty micrograms of estrogen. There is simply no point in taking any pill other than a low-dose one because of a misconception that your particular system might require a higher dose. This simply is never the case.

Only two types of estrogen are present in any of the myriads of birth control pills: *ethinyl estradiol* and *mestranol*. Mestranol works only by being changed by the body into ethinyl estradiol. This makes mestranol somewhat less potent as an estrogen than ethinyl estradiol. Thus fifty micrograms of mestranol probably would be equivalent to about thirty-five micrograms of ethinyl estradiol. You need not concern yourself with this, because most modern pills you would choose today use ethinyl estradiol.

Five different progestins can be found in the various birth control pills. Four of them are roughly equivalent in potency: *norethindrone*, *norethynodrel*, *norethindrone acetate*, and *ethynodiol diacetate*. Of these four, norethindrone is the most popular and also the lowest in potency. All other progestins are measured in terms of how they compare in potency to norethindrone. So if you just remember that norethindrone is the yardstick by which to consider the other progestins, you will have an easy time of it. The fifth progestins, levonorgestrel and norgestrel, deserve special mention because they are so extremely potent. Levonorgestrel is ten to twenty times more potent than norethindrone; 0.15 milligram of levonorgestrel is equivalent to 1.5 to 3 milligrams of norethindrone. Thus if you chose a pill such as Nordette (see Table 1), it would appear that you were taking only a very low dose of progestin. But in fact, if compared to the "standard" of norethindrone, you would

TABLE 1 Composition of Oral Contraceptives Currently Marketed in the United States

Product	Type	Progestin	Estrogens	Manufacturer
Brevicon	Comb	0.5 mg norethindrone	35 μg ethinylestradiol	Syntex
Norinyl 1+ 35	Comb	1.0 mg norethindrone	35 μg ethinylestradiol	Syntex
Norinyl 1+ 50	Comb	1.0 mg norethindrone	50 μg mestranol	Syntex
Norinyl 1+ 80	Comb	1.0 mg norethindrone	80 μg mestranol	Syntex
Norinyl 2	Comb	2.0 mg norethindrone	100 μg mestranol	Syntex
Nor-QD	Prog	0.35 mg norethindrone		Syntex
Tri-Norinyl 7/	Comb-triphasic	0.5 mg norethindrone	35 μg ethinylestradiol	Syntex
9/		1.0 mg norethindrone	35 μg ethinylestradiol	
5		0.5 mg norethindrone	35 μg ethinylestradiol	
Demulen 1+ 35	Comb	1.0 mg ethynodiol diacetate	35 μg ethinylestradiol	Searle
Demulen 1+ 50	Comb	1.0 mg ethynodiol diacetate	50 μg ethinylestradiol	Searle
Ovulen	Comb	1.0 mg ethynodiol diacetate	100 μg mestranol	Searle
Enovid-E	Comb	2.5 mg norethynodrel	100 μg mestranol	Searle
Enovid 5	Comb	5.0 mg norethynodrel	75 μg mestranol	Searle
Enovid 10	Comb	9.85 mg norethynodrel	150 μg mestranol	Searle
Loestrin 1+ 20	Comb	1.0 mg norethindrone acetate	20 μg ethinylestradiol	Parke-Davis
Loestrin 1.5+ 30	Comb	1.5 mg norethindrone acetate	30 μg ethinylestradiol	Parke-Davis
Norlestrin 1+ 50	Comb	1.0 mg norethindrone acetate	50 μg ethinylestradiol	Parke-Davis

Name	Type	Progestin	Estrogen	Manufacturer
Norlestrin 2.5 + 50	Comb	2.5 mg norethindrone acetate	50 μg ethinylestradiol	Parke-Davis
Lo/Ovral	Comb	0.3 mg norgestrel	30 μg ethinylestradiol	Wyeth
Nordette	Comb	0.15 mg levonorgestrel	30 μg ethinylestradiol	Wyeth
Ovral	Comb	0.5 mg norgestrel	50 μg ethinylestradiol	Wyeth
Ovrette	Prog	75 μg norgestrel		Wyeth
Triphasil 6/	Comb-triphasic	50 μg levonorgestrel	30 μg ethinylestradiol	Wyeth
5/		75 μg levonorgestrel	40 μg ethinylestradiol	Wyeth
10		125 μg levonorgestrel	30 μg ethinylestradiol	Wyeth
Ovcon-35	Comb	0.4 mg norethindrone	35 μg ethinylestradiol	Mead Johnson
Ovcon-50	Comb	1.0 mg norethindrone	50 μg ethinylestradiol	Mead Johnson
Modicon	Comb	0.5 mg norethindrone	35 μg ethinylestradiol	Ortho
Ortho-Novum 1 + 35	Comb	1.0 mg norethindrone	35 μg ethinylestradiol	Ortho
Ortho-Novum 1 + 50	Comb	1.0 mg nonrethindrone	50 μg mestranol	Ortho
Ortho-Novum 1 + 80	Comb	1.0 mg norethindrone	80 μg mestranol	Ortho
Ortho-Novum 2	Comb	2.0 mg norethindrone	100 μg mestranol	Ortho
Ortho-Novum 10/	Comb-biphasic	0.5 mg norethindrone	35 μg ethinylestradiol	Ortho
11		1.0 mg norethindrone	35 μg ethinylestradiol	Ortho
Micronor	Prog	0.35 mg norethindrone	35 μg ethinylestradiol	Ortho
Ortho-Novum 7/	Comb-triphasic	0.5 mg norethindrone	35 μg ethinylestradiol	Ortho
7/		0.75 mg norethindrone	35 μg ethinylestradiol	Ortho
7		1.0 mg norethindrone	35 μg ethinylestradiol	Ortho

be taking up to three times the progestin dose. If you took Ovral, which contains 0.5 milligram of norgestrel, you might think you were taking an extremely low dose of progestin, but in truth you would be taking a fairly high dose.

Since none of the progestins have any advantage over norethindrone, and since norethindrone is the least potent of the progestins, it is perfectly reasonable for you to eliminate from your mind any birth control pill that contains a progestin other than norethindrone.

To simplify your decision-making, I recommend that you look only at the pills in Table 1 that contain ethinylestradiol and norethindrone, and look for the lowest dosages of those two hormones that will give you reliable contraception. Refer to this chart as you read through what follows.

The modern standard dosage of thirty-five micrograms of ethinylestradiol, and 1 milligram of norethindrone should be a safe option. This formulation is contained in Norinyl 1 + 35 and Ortho-Novum 1 + 35. Although Demulen 1 + 35 contains ethynodiol diacetate rather than norethindrone as a progestin, ethynodiol diacetate's potency is so close to that of norethindrone that these three preparations should serve as a simple standard, the choice of which wouldn't matter significantly one over another. You may wonder why I pass over Brevicon and Modicon, which contain 0.5 milligram of norethindrone, and Ovcon-35, which contains only 0.4 milligram of norethindrone. These formulations have not been popular because they result in a lot of "breakthrough bleeding" between periods because of an inadequate level of progestin to support the endometrium. The goal of lowering the progestin content to less than 1 milligram of norethindrone is a valid one. But it cannot be comfortably achieved by having a fixed dose of progestin in each and every pill. If you do this, the lining will shed intermittently, and you will bleed irregularly during the cycle.

But this goal of lowering the progestin dose to less than 1 milligram per day has now been obtained with the newest low-dose pills called the "triphasics." With this approach the progestin content is varied throughout the cycle as a method of giving a lower overall amount of progestin throughout the month, but giving just enough progestin to prevent breakthrough bleeding during those parts of the cycle when it is most likely to occur otherwise. If you look on the chart, you will see three triphasic pills: Tri-Norinyl, Triphasil, and Ortho-Novum 7/7/7. Because Triphasil utilizes levonorgestrel for its progestin, I would recommend, for the sake of simplicity, that we exclude it from discussion because of the extremely high potency of the progestin and the difficulty in correlating its dosage to the "standard" of norethindrone. For example, on the last ten days of taking Triphasil, you would be taking 0.125 milligram of levonorgestrel, which would be equivalent to somewhere around 1.25 to 2.5 milligrams of norethindrone. That would simply be too high a dose of progestin compared to what otherwise is available in pills containing norethindrone.

Thus we basically come down to a choice of a few possible pills that simply have somewhat different dosages of the same progestin and estrogen. The most popular low-dose would be Norinyl 1 + 35, Ortho-Novum 1 + 35, and Demulen 1 + 35. It doesn't really matter which of those three you use, because they all satisfy the new requirement of being the lowest dose possible that still maintains contraceptive efficacy and results in a minimum of breakthrough bleeding. Yet I advise you to consider seriously the triphasics—for example, Tri-Norinyl or Ortho-Novum 7/7/7—because they reduce the progestin content even further and thus give you an even greater margin of safety. By minimizing the dose of progestin, they cause no significant elevation of LDL cholesterol levels. Yet they minimize the aggravation of "breakthrough bleeding" that would otherwise occur by lowering the dose of norethindrone to less than one milligram.

The final consideration in deciding which pill to take is a simple one of packaging. Virtually all of these pills come in either "twenty-one-day packs" or "twenty-eight-day packs." All modern birth control pills are taken for twenty-one days out of the month, with a seven-day "rest period." During the seven-day rest period, you menstruate. At the end of those seven days you begin taking pills again, starting on day one of the next cycle. Because the manufacturers were concerned that some women may have difficulty keeping track of a three-week-on, one-week-off schedule, they decided to offer "twenty-eight-day packs," the last seven pills of which contain no active ingredients. Thus all you would have to do is follow the routine of taking one pill every day, and the last seven days' worth of pills in the twenty-eight-day cycle would be placebos. The majority of women prefer twenty-one-day packs, because they find the twenty-eight-day pack an insult to their intelligence, and they feel stupid taking a sugar pill the last seven days of their cycle.

How to Take the Pill

The pills will come in an individual packet for each monthly cycle. In most packets, the pills are lined up in three rows of seven, representing the three weeks that you will be taking them. Each row will be underneath a day of the week, just like a calendar. Thus whatever day you punch out the pill to start your cycle will mark the day of the week on which your cycle was begun. It is on that *exact* day of the week that you will start your next cycle twenty-eight days later. It does not matter whether you start taking the pills on the first day of your menstrual period, day five of your period, or on a specific day during your period. You make this decision based purely on your own convenience. The only critical thing you must do is start taking the pill sometime between day one and day seven of your cycle. If you delay starting the pills until after day seven, you run the risk of ovulating in that cycle.

Many women prefer to start the pill on the first Sunday or first Monday after their period starts. The reason for starting on Monday is that it is the beginning of the week, and all your routines, such as starting work or classes, usually begin on Monday. So why not also start a new pill cycle on Monday? Other women prefer to start the pill on the first Sunday after their menstrual period begins because that will mean that their three-week cycle of pill-taking will end on Saturday, and most likely they will start menstruating two days later, on a Monday. Most women would usually prefer to be menstruating during the week than on the weekend.

There is no single "right" way to start the pills. Your choices are:

A. Start on day one of your period.
B. Start on the first Sunday after your period begins, or the first Monday.
C. Start on the fifth day after your period starts (the old, common, classic recommendation).
D. Start today, or any day, as long as you know there is no chance that you are now pregnant.

If you use this last approach, starting any day whether it is within seven days of the beginning of your menstrual cycle or not, you *cannot be assured* of protection that first month. Therefore this is obviously not a popular approach, but it might be useful if you just want to get into the habit of taking the pill before "it really counts." But again, as with making a choice on which pill to use, the watchword is to simplify. The simplest way to do it is to decide what day of the week you want to begin on, and begin taking your pills that day, after your menstrual period begins.

If you decide at a later date that you would rather begin, say, on a Wednesday than on a Sunday, it is no problem to switch. But you must remember to restart taking the pills within seven days of when you finished your last pill. For example, if you stopped taking the pill on Saturday night and wished to switch to Wednesday as the beginning of your new pill cycle, you should start taking the pill the next Wednesday even though it is only four days later and you may still be menstruating. You must not wait until the following Wednesday, which would be eleven days later. Remember that waiting more than seven days to begin a new cycle is the commonest way that women get pregnant while taking the pill. Missing a pill or two in midcycle is not as worrisome as starting the cycle more than seven days after the previous one.

It is important to set up a regular daily routine, planning to take the pill at the same time of the day every day you take them. Most women find it convenient to leave the pill packet right by their toothbrush. Virtually everyone brushes their teeth every day immediately upon arising. If you keep your packet of pills next to your toothbrush, then most likely you will not forget to take them.

Problems with the Birth Control Pill and How to Manage Them

We just don't see the problems today that we used to see with the higher-dose pills. Not very many women today are complaining, "I just don't like what I feel the pills are doing to my system." Not many women complain about weight gain, breast swelling, finger and ankle swelling, headaches, blood pressure increase, irritability, nausea, or any of the myriad of aggravating problems that accompanied use of the birth control pill in the 1960s. The rule of thumb among doctors is that if a woman is complaining about symptoms like these on the pill, she should usually be prescribed a lower-dose pill. The better approach is just to lower the dose anyway in everyone. There is no reason to take even moderately high-dose pills anymore. But despite this greater satisfaction with modern low-dose pills, there still are some problems.

One of the advantages of the pill is that it decreases the amount of menstrual bleeding. It does this because of the progestin component overriding the estrogen. This is one of the great benefits of the birth control pill aside from preventing pregnancy. However, 1 percent of women on the pill have periods that are so reduced that they don't bleed at all and their menstruation ceases. This is called amenorrhea. It is the extreme of a good thing—namely, decreased menstrual bleeding.

Such women need not worry that they have some kind of permanent atrophy of the uterine lining. The thinned-out uterine lining will come right back to normal when they go off the pill. But the problem is that a nonmenstruating woman is going to have monthly anxiety about whether or not she may be pregnant. In other words, if you have taken the pill dutifully for twenty-one days out of the month and then fail to menstruate during your "rest" period, you don't know for sure whether the pill has caused your uterine lining to diminish so that you no longer have to worry about periods while you are taking the pill, or on the other extreme, whether you represent a "pill failure" and are pregnant. Fortunately, this happens with only 1 percent or less of women taking the pill. Because it is so anxiety-provoking a situation, most women with this problem eventually give up on the pill and try some other contraceptive method, unless the problem can be solved by switching to a different pill.

Sadly, this is what happened to Noreen. She was taking birth control pills, and her periods got significantly scantier and scantier until one month she had no period at all during the week off the pills. She mistakenly assumed she was pregnant and decided not to restart the next cycle of pills for fear that taking the pills while she was pregnant would harm the fetus. In truth she was not pregnant, but when she discontinued taking the pills, the very next month she did get pregnant and had a baby she was unfortunately not ready to have.

What she should have done rather than stopping birth control would be to get a pregnancy test. The new home pregnancy tests are cheap, reliable, and extremely sensitive. By "sensitive" I mean that they can tell you if you are pregnant as early as one to three days after your missed period. Thus if you find that during your rest period you do not menstruate, and wonder whether you should begin taking another cycle of pills, all you have to do is run down to the local drugstore prior to the seventh day of the rest period, purchase one of the early home pregnancy tests, do a simple test on your urine, and find out whether you are pregnant. In almost all cases, if you have been taking the pill reliably, you will find that you are not pregnant and you can begin the next cycle.

You are not going to want to be doing this pregnancy test every single month, and for that reason most women whose periods cease while they are on the pill will have to switch to another contraceptive. Fortunately, they represent only a tiny fraction of women using oral contraception.

In case you find out that you are pregnant and worry that having taken the pill during those first two weeks of fetal life might in some way harm the fetus, we have good news for you. The only known possible effect of the birth control pill on the fetus is a masculinization of the female fetus, which can occur only after about eight weeks of pregnancy. Countless studies of women who have gotten pregnant while on the pill have failed to show a risk to the fetus, but for medicolegal reasons your doctor is going to protect himself from any possible lawsuit by hedging. If you are inclined to want to terminate the pregnancy, he probably will say nothing to dissuade you because he is terrified that you may sue him if by some chance the baby is abnormal, even though it would almost certainly not be related to having taken the pill. On the other hand, if you are not inclined toward terminating a pregnancy, you can feel comforted in knowing that no study yet has shown any dangerous effects on the child so long as the pill was discontinued before the eighth week of fetal life. But I, too, have to be afraid of lawsuits, and all I can give you is scientific information. I, too, would take no responsibility for a fetal abnormality because I know all too well that getting pregnant under any circumstance entails a risk of having an abnormal child.

What Do You Do if You Forget to Take the Pill?

What do you do if you miss taking a pill, or worse yet, if you miss taking a pill two days in a row? The first thing you must realize is that missing one or two pills per se does not usually result in pregnancy. It is starting the pill late, after seven days in the cycle, that usually results in pregnancy. Most doctors therefore recommend the following simple approach if you forget to take a pill: As soon as you realize that you have forgotten to take the pill for today, even if it isn't until tomorrow morning, you then take today's pill and go right ahead and take the next day's pill when you are supposed to. Most of the time women do not realize that they have missed a pill until the next morning when it is time to take the next day's pill. They should then simply take two pills that day instead of one, to make up for the day they missed yesterday. It is just that simple.

If you missed two days' pills in a row, then you have several choices. We cannot absolutely guarantee that you won't get pregnant if you have missed two days, and therefore one choice is simply to wait seven days, allow yourself to menstruate, and start a brand-new cycle all over again. Remember that if you do this, it does not matter whether you menstruate or not; what matters is that within seven days of missing your last pill, you start your first pill of your next cycle, and you throw away the packet of the cycle that you messed up.

You have another choice, which is probably less appealing, if you have missed two days' pills in a row. You can take two pills on the next day and two pills once again the following day. This will get you back on schedule, but because you can't be certain that you are completely protected against becoming pregnant, you would need to use some backup method of birth control such as contraceptive foam, the sponge, condoms, or simply abstinence.

If you miss three days' pills in a row, you definitely need to discontinue the cycle, use a backup method of birth control, and seriously ask yourself the question of whether you should be on the pill. Perhaps another contraceptive that requires less attention to a daily routine would be easier for you. I will never forget meeting at a birth control clinic a twenty-three-year-old woman who already had six children, was inundated with motherhood ever since she was an early teenager, had no husband, and who was completely over her head in confusion and worry because she had relied on the birth control pill for contraception when she did not have even the foggiest hint of self-discipline anywhere in her nature. She would have been far better off with an IUD or even a sterilization rather than relying on remembering to take the pill regularly.

BREAKTHROUGH BLEEDING

What if you menstruate before you are supposed to—that is, during the three weeks on the pill rather than the week you are off the pill? This is called "breakthrough" bleeding. This irregular bleeding is most likely to occur, if it occurs at all, in the first couple of months while on the pill. You need not discontinue the pill or get at all worried or concerned because of this irregular bleeding in the first couple of months. It occurs only occasionally. But if it does occur to you, just call your doctor of course and rest assured that it will most likely cease by the third month. It is the price you have to pay for the extreme safety and otherwise pleasant lack of side effects of the low-dose pill you are taking. You should not even think about going off the pill if you have this minor side effect during the first few cycles. Most break-through bleeding occurs because there is not enough estrogen effect to "hold" the thicker endometrial lining you had before going on the pill. In a couple of months (after the endometrial lining becomes thinned down), this breakthrough bleeding will cease.

But another type of breakthrough bleeding may occur after you have been on the pill for a while. This breakthrough bleeding is not just an adjustment in the endometrial lining of the uterus that must occur when you first start on the pill. It results from the lining becoming so thinned out that it simply does not have enough support or "estrogen effect" to hold it. This is not dangerous but just aggravating, and it has a very simple solution. All you need is a very brief seven-day course of estrogen to rebuild the endometrial lining to where it once again can hold. Your physician will put you probably on either 20 micrograms of ethinyl estradiol, or 2.5 milligrams of Premarin (a form of estrogen that is not in the pill) for seven days in addition to your regular pills. The idea here is not to change your birth control pill schedule. You keep right on taking the pill, despite the breakthrough bleeding, according to your standard schedule. But you add seven days of estrogen supplement. Once you have finished this brief, one-week extra estrogen dose, you need not worry about taking any estrogen again because the problem will have been solved and you can go right on taking the pill in the usual fashion without the fear of breakthrough bleeding.

Sometimes women try to double up on their pills or increase their birth control pill dose when they have this breakthrough bleeding, but that approach is totally unadvisable. Taking more birth control pills will not really solve the problem, nor will increasing the dose of the pill solve the problem. That will only take away all the benefits of using the safe, low-dose pill. Furthermore, it is illogical, because no matter how high a dose of birth control pill you take, there always will be a progesterone dominance, and sooner or later breakthrough bleeding will again become a problem. Increasing the progestin content of the pill you take might temporarily solve the problem, but not in the best fashion. It will mean a slightly increased risk of heart disease, and it will not solve the basic problem, which is a thinned-out endometrial lining. In other words, increasing the progestin in the pill will only hold the thinned-out lining slightly better, but it won't correct the basic problem of the lining being too thin.

Another version of this breakthrough bleeding is early menstruation. By this I mean that you start to menstruate before you have completed your twenty-one-day cycle of pill-taking. Normally you should deal with early menstruation simply by continuing to take the pills as usual so you don't get off schedule. Another approach is simply to discontinue the pills and restart exactly seven days after you stop them. If this becomes a continuing problem, the solution is the same as with breakthrough bleeding: a brief seven-day burst of estrogen in addition to your regular pill-taking. Obviously these matters should be handled by your physician, but you should understand them so you can help guide him or her according to what approach is most appealing to you.

What if You Get Pregnant While on the Pill?

What if you do get pregnant because you forgot to take the pill for the first few days, and yet did take it during the rest of the cycle? Does the ingestion of the pill during early pregnancy result in an abnormality in the baby? Well, you can certainly imagine the scare and hysteria this question has generated. Whenever an occasional congenital defect occurs in a woman who had been taking the pill, the pill would naturally be blamed. But remember that congenital abnormalities are common in any population of women. Even contraceptive foam (which hundreds of studies have clearly shown over the past forty years has absolutely no damaging effect whatsoever on the fetus), "periodic" abstinence or the rhythm method of birth control (women who do get pregnant using rhythm have impregnated an "older" egg later in the cycle) have been blamed for congenital abnormalities in the baby. But careful studies have shown that neither rhythm birth control, nor contraceptive foam, nor IUDs, nor birth control pills create any increased risk of congenital abnormalities. Earlier studies claiming such deleterious effects have been refuted by numerous, better-designed, scientific protocols.

Taking the Pill After Childbirth

What about starting the pill after you have had a baby? At one time it was popular to take the pills only prior to your first child, and then to have an IUD put in after the delivery. The IUD was considered an ideal birth control method for happily married women in a monogamous relationship. But because of the high infection rate noted in women with multiple sex partners, fear of lawsuits took the IUD off the market in the United States. Thus it will be much more common now for women to restart the birth control pill after delivering a child.

You should not take the pill within two weeks of delivering the baby because of the theoretically increased risk of venous thromboembolism. Since birth and delivery itself entail an increased risk of venous thromboembolism, which is one of the major causes of death from childbirth, and since the higher-dose pill created an increased risk of venous thromboembolism also, it simply is a wise theoretical policy not to take the pill until a few weeks after the delivery. You probably will not ovulate prior to the third week after having the baby (unless you have taken Parlodel to dry up your breasts in preparation for bottle-feeding). In fact, ovulation often is delayed for one to three months after delivery. Most women would not be interested in engaging in intercourse during the first two weeks after having their baby anyway. Thus anytime after two weeks is okay to begin the birth control pill with the following proviso:

If you are breast-feeding, the combined estrogen/progestin birth control pill will decrease the quantity of milk available to your infant, and very minute amounts of hormones will be present in the milk. In all likelihood this minute amount of hormone of the breast milk will pose no problem to the infant, as none to date has been discovered. However, because of the possibility that some future effect of this minute amount of hormone might turn up in these infants at a later date, most doctors recommend that you do not take the combination estrogen/progestin pill while you are breast-feeding.

So what can women who are breast-feeding their infant and who want reliable birth control do? There are three very reasonable alternatives. One is that you could follow the approach of total breast-feeding outlined in my chapter on breast-feeding, which will give you very reliable contraception until such time as you discontinue it. The second approach is to use barrier methods such as contraceptive foam or sponge, a diaphragm, or a condom (which will be discussed in a later chapter) until such time as you discontinue all breast-feeding. The third approach is the "minidose" progestin-only birth control pill. The most popular brand of this pill is Micronor.

Micronor represents a fascinating birth control concept. It is simply a very low dose (0.35 milligram) of norethindrone that you must take daily every day of the week, every week of the month, without a "rest" period in between. It comes in a twenty-eight-day pack and must be taken every day at the same time of day. This incredibly low-dose progestin-only birth control pill does not reliably inhibit ovulation but does make the cervical mucus impenetrable to sperm penetration because of the progestin effect. It is extremely safe, and has a pregnancy failure rate of only about 2 percent, which is no different from that of the IUD. It doesn't inhibit breast milk in the slightest and is the standard contraceptive recommended for breast-feeding mothers. The only problem with Micronor is that you never know when you are going to have a period, and the periods are of varying lengths. This would make it an unpopular birth control pill for any other time in your life, but it is a reasonable alternative while you still are breast-feeding after having had your child. As soon as you have stopped breast-feeding, you can go on to the combination estrogen/progestin pills discussed in detail in the previous section. But remember that if you are "totally" breast-feeding (as explained in my chapter on breast-feeding), you need no other birth control.

There is, of course, one fourth possibility for breast-feeding mothers. Even though the IUD is not available in the United States, physicians have no objection to managing women who have an IUD in place. If you feel very strongly that the IUD is the contraceptive method you want, you can travel to Canada or another foreign country and have an IUD inserted there. You may wonder whether some U.S. Customs agent will insist on your having a pelvic exam before coming back into the United States. But have no fear: the IUD is perfectly legal in the United States and very safe for monogamous women in a "faithful" marriage or relationship.

Who Should Not Use Birth Control Pills, and Who Should Think Twice About Using Them?

The birth control pill is clearly the most popular method of contraception in the developed world for women under age thirty. It is extremely safe for women up to age thirty-five whether or not they smoke. Most physicians feel that it is also safe for women from age thirty-five to forty-five who don't smoke. It is not recommended for women over age thirty-five who do smoke, or who have other risk factors such as obesity or high blood pressure.

Most women don't go through menopause until about age fifty or fifty-two. They certainly are very unlikely to conceive over age forty or forty-two, but during those ten years, when they least expect it, some of these women are liable to turn up pregnant if they don't use some form of contraception, and they may be very unhappy about it. On the ski slopes last year I met a fifty-five-year-old woman who was skiing with her seven-year old son. She told me how she had gone through what seemed to be menopause at age forty-four, after having had five children years earlier. She never dreamed that she had to worry about birth control any longer. But at age forty-eight, when she never would have thought it was possible, she turned up pregnant.

My children were having a garage sale a few months ago, and up walks a lady who had two children (aged twenty and fifteen), was forty-two years old, and was about eight months pregnant. She had an IUD in place until about eight years ago and tried to get pregnant from about age thirty-four to age thirty-eight, but was unable to do so. At that point she just gave up, her gynecologist gave up, and they both figured there was "no chance." So they forgot about it. Yet at age forty-two there she was preparing once more to have an infant around the house.

For women in their forties, birth control may even be more important than for women in their twenties and thirties, because of the much higher risk of fetal abnormalities. I don't recommend that you have a baby in your forties unless you really want to. You have to figure whether you have the time, the energy, the finances, and the desire to raise an infant, and whether you are willing to face the consequences of a slightly increased risk of severe, heartbreaking, congenital abnormalities (as high as 4 percent) among women in their forties.

Furthermore, most women begin to go through a change in their cycles by age thirty-five or forty, in which they have more irregular bleeding, more painful periods, and a greater likelihood of premenstrual syndrome (PMS), all related to a less regular frequency of ovulation. Having a tubal sterilization, or using contraceptive foam, or condoms, or a diaphragm will do nothing to alleviate these symptoms, which usually begin more than a decade before menopause. Therefore, the birth control pill in very low doses must be considered an option for some women in their forties.

Patrice is a case in point. Her husband, Glenn, a forty-eight-year-old man, had undergone a vasectomy reversal by me about eight years earlier. As a consequence of the vasectomy reversal, Patrice and Glenn had two happy, healthy children. Now at age forty, Patrice felt she had enough. Glenn inquired about having another vasectomy. Since I was not too thrilled about undoing the very delicate microsurgical handiwork I had performed on him eight years earlier, I told Patrice to see her regular gynecologist to discuss the matter with him. Naturally, his first recommendation was a tubal sterilization. She was reluctant to do this, and was having a miserable time with her menstrual periods, for which she needed some treatment as well. She was having headaches, and severe premenstrual syndrome associated with irregular periods, and endometrial lining buildup, associated with unopposed estrogen. Her doctor put her on low-dose birth control pills. Within three months after having some more irregular "breakthrough" bleeding, Patrice was feeling great and probably was spared what was otherwise becoming a high risk for developing uterine cancer. The pill was the perfect choice for her.

Women over forty who take the pill should simply be aware that there are theoretically slightly greater risks, though much less than suggested by the early British report on high-dose pills. The pills definitely are safer than getting pregnant. Taking the pill also is safer than allowing yourself to get cancer of the uterus or cancer of the ovary if you are in a high-risk group for that problem. If you are a smoker, have high blood pressure, diabetes, obesity, or increased blood fat levels, then you should not take on the extra risk of the birth control pill. The most important thing you could do to save your life would be to lose weight and stop smoking. A famous family planning researcher, Malcolm Potts, known for his outrageous sense of humor, has been quoted as saying that cigarettes should be dispensed only by prescription, and birth control pills should be put in the cigarette vending machines.

If you have irregular periods, or scanty periods, you probably are not ovulating regularly, and going on the birth control pill gives you a slightly greater risk of having no periods (amenorrhea) when you go off the pill and try to get pregnant. Some doctors suggest, therefore, that women with irregular or scanty periods should not go on the pill because of the possibility that it would interfere with subsequent fertility. In actuality, the exact opposite is true. Any woman with irregular ovulation is at risk for developing cancer of the uterus, cancer of the ovary, and benign breast disease. She is most likely better off going on the pill until such time as she wants to have a baby. Then she may very well need treatment to stimulate her ovulation. The more worrisome case is the woman who is ovulating normally before going on the pill and who then does not resume ovulating after discontinuing the pill. Fortunately this is a rare case, and it can generally be treated very successfully with either Clomid or Pergonal.

Some other medical conditions—high blood pressure, obesity, diabetes, liver disease, heart problems, thrombophlebitis—may cause you to think twice about taking the pill. This becomes a matter of judgment and guesswork. The bottom line for this issue is that pills should not be given without a doctor's prescription. You should have a yearly physical exam, including a breast examination, possibly a mammogram, and certainly a pelvic examination with a Pap smear. You should take steps to control your diet to diminish obesity and blood fat levels, as well as high blood pressure. One of the major advantages of going on the birth control pill is that you must have a doctor's prescription, and that requires having a physical examination and some of these important tests every year. In that sense, getting a prescription for birth control pills from your doctor is truly getting a prescription for proper health care.

The pill minimizes your risk of certain common cancers and other "female" illnesses, but it also requires your having a yearly Pap smear and breast exam, not to mention screening for blood pressure, obesity, and blood fat levels. This way, taking the pill, combined with regular visits to a good doctor, are a better assurance for a healthy future than being scared by alarmist rumors and hyped-up newspaper articles.

If after this inundation with facts, which I hope has dispelled incorrect rumors about the birth control pill, you still have an emotional reluctance to go with this method and yet you find natural birth control too difficult, fear not, because you still have some good alternatives.

5

The Intrauterine Device, or IUD

You might think that the "sexual revolution" began in the United States in 1960 with the introduction of the birth control pill, but, in fact, it was already happening at the turn of the century in Germany, when the modern IUD (intrauterine device) was first invented. Actually the IUD had its origin in antiquity. For ages people have known that the presence of a foreign body in the uterus prevents pregnancy, but in 1909 the Germans used this knowledge to develop the first practical device (made out of silkworm gut) that when placed in a woman's uterus acted as a contraceptive. Later, in 1926, the famous German doctor Ernst Grafenberg developed the first IUD that was a commercial success. The model of IUD used by forty million Chinese women today is basically a copy of Dr. Grafenberg's original model.

The IUD is a wonderfully convenient, reversible method of birth control if you are the right person for it. But Elizabeth wasn't. At age twenty, four years before getting married, she had an IUD inserted. Although she was having sex with the man who eventually would become her husband, she had several other sexual partners as well. Eight months later she developed a pelvic infection, a fever, and cramps. The IUD had to be removed, and she went on antibiotics. It wasn't until fourteen years later, after ten years of an infertile marriage, that she came to see me and finally discovered what a fateful error she had made at age twenty. Her tubes were completely and irreparably scarred. Ironically, if she had had a "permanent" sterilization at age twenty, rather than having an IUD inserted, which was thought to be "reversible" birth control, she would probably have been able to have children today. We could have performed a microsurgical operation to reconnect her tubes, and she would have probably had no difficulty getting pregnant. But because of the extensive destruction wrought by sexually transmitted disease in the presence of an IUD, the birth control method she chose at age twenty was unwittingly a permanent one.

The reason that it required seventeen years from the development of the first IUD in 1909 until it could be used successfully on a wide scale is that women using early models of the IUD were plagued with infection. The key to Dr. Grafenberg's success back in 1926 was his discovery that the infections were caused by the string (or "tail") of the IUD, which protruded from the uterus into the vagina. This string, which made it easy to remove the IUD, also provided a route of entry for bacteria into the uterus. Dr. Grafenberg's IUD design, the "Grafenberg ring," eliminated the string. His innovation solved the infection problem and thus hurled the world into the "sexual revolution" of the twentieth century. If the makers of the Dalkon Shield (which was the one Elizabeth used) had followed Dr. Grafenberg's original design, they might not now be facing $600 million worth of lawsuits, and the IUD, which is for many women a safe and reliable method of contraception, might still be available in the United States.

The IUD is simply a tiny piece of inert plastic or metal designed in a shape that fits nicely into the uterine cavity, thus preventing pregnancy. Two and a half million American women, forty million Chinese women, and thirty million women in the rest of the world presently use the IUD as their method of contraception. Unfortunately, for reasons that will unfold in this chapter, American women can obtain the IUD only if they go to some other country (such as Canada) to have it inserted. The problem is not that there is any law or prohibition against the IUD, because the FDA has approved four different models for use in the United States. The problem is that manufacturers of the "safe" models have discovered that the high cost of defending themselves against lawsuits, whether frivolous or not, exceeds any possible profits. Therefore, safe IUDs that are readily available in every other country in the Western world are not available in the United States. But if after reading this chapter you feel that this method of contraception would be ideal for you, you simply have to arrange a vacation in Canada or another country, and have it inserted there. I'm sure this will meet with no objection from your physician, who probably feels as constrained by this unavailability of the IUD in the United States as you do.

The advantages of the IUD are that it is cheap, it doesn't require continual daily effort, it is easily reversible, and it is extremely effective in preventing pregnancy. Unlike the birth control pill, you don't have to remember to take it every day, and there are no hormonal effects to worry about. Unlike the condom, the sponge, or the diaphragm, you don't have to remember to put it on before having sex. Unlike natural birth control, you don't have to keep detailed records, take daily temperatures, and monitor cervical mucus quality. Unlike sterilization, you don't have to go through an operation. All you need to do when you want to have children is to have it removed in the doctor's office and you are ready to go again. But it is not exactly that simple. You'd better choose the right IUD, and the right doctor to put it in, and you'd better be the right patient to use this form of contraception.

The IUD seems to be an ideal contraceptive in many ways, but it does have problems. In most women it causes heavier menstrual bleeding, and in some women it causes more uncomfortable menstrual cramps. Anywhere from 5 to 15 percent of women spontaneously expel the IUD because their uterus simply won't tolerate it. Because of spontaneous expulsion, and unhappiness with the heavier menstrual flow and discomfort, only about 50 to 60 percent of women continue with their IUD after the first year. But those women who do continue are an extremely happy lot because they no longer have any fuss or worry about birth control. The best part about the IUD is that it is one of the most effective reversible methods of contraception, second only to the pill. In fact, the newer models of IUD are *just as* effective as the pill, and even the older models become as effective as the pill once they have been in place for more than two years. The conventional copper IUDs have an annual failure rate of 2 percent; the newer models have an annual failure rate of less than 0.3 percent.

The main reason why condoms and diaphragms with spermicidal foam have a 10 to 15 percent annual failure rate is that they need to be used consistently, and many people don't like to use them because they interfere with the spontaneity of the sexual act. Birth control pills may be easy for the young couple who have not yet had children. But by the time the first child arrives, with all of the time, effort, and potential disruption of routine that that entails, women are ready for a method of birth control that doesn't require taking a pill every single day, taking your temperature and checking your mucus every day, or bothering to have your husband put on a condom or inserting a diaphragm or injecting foam yourself prior to every episode of intercourse.

Tubal sterilization, or vasectomy, seems very appealing to such couples. But many such couples are not ready for "permanent" sterilization, and that is where the IUD enjoys its greatest popularity. But because the IUD is no longer available in the United States and will only be used by American women who travel to Canada or another foreign country for it, we are going to see a tremendous increase in the popularity of sterilization among people who should not be getting sterilized.

The Different Types of IUDs

There are two ways in which the IUD can be designed to prevent pregnancy. One design simply works by direct contact with the uterine surface. The other works by slow release of an inert substance such as copper, or a hormone such as progesterone from the IUD into the uterus. The early Grafenberg ring seemed at first to function just by direct contact with the uterine surface, but later tests have demonstrated that it was the undetected copper contamination in German silver in those days that made the device extremely effective. Nonetheless, modifications of that early German IUD containing no copper (which worked just by direct contact) were used in Japan and Israel in the 1940s and 1950s fairly successfully. These devices didn't have the protruding string design known to cause infections, but since they produced a lot of discomfort, and were difficult to remove (because they had no tail), they never became widely popular.

POLYETHYLENE IUDS

Then, in the 1950s, the Population Council was founded under the guidance of the United Nations as a scientific body designed to help Third World developing countries deal with their population crisis. The Population Council put a great deal of money and scientific effort into the improvement of the IUD, which was aided in the late 1950s by the invention of polyethylene, a biologically inert plastic that was to revolutionize every area of medicine and biology from heart surgery to breast, face, and orthopedic reconstructive surgery. Polyethylene was a plastic that the body could accept with no dangerous reaction, and it had a remarkable property called "memory." That means that though soft and pliable, it could be bent into any desired shape and then hold that shape. With the aid of polyethylene, an IUD could be developed

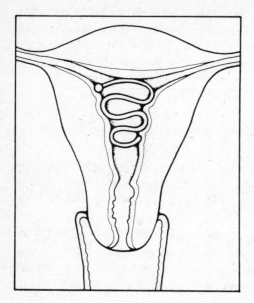

FIGURE 5-1.
Lippes Loop IUD.

that was soft, and thus not as irritating to the uterus as stainless steel or silver. It could be inserted through a narrow tube (called an inserter) in the doctor's office. Once in the uterus, with the inserter pulled out, the IUD would spring into its proper configuration.

Furthermore, a tail of *monofilament* string could now be left to protrude into the vagina for easy removal of the IUD, apparently without the risk of infection. Studies had shown that a cotton or linen braided string (which was all that was available in the days of the early German IUDs) would act as a wick and encourage harmful bacteria to migrate from the vagina into the uterus. But a monofilament string (like a fishing line), which is not braided and has an absolutely smooth surface, would not allow such bacterial migration. The Dalkon Shield did not use such a string, and many women who wore that IUD later developed serious infections and became sterile. Some even died. Three hundred thousand women have joined in a class action suit against the A. H. Robins Company, which manufactured the Dalkon Shield.

The first "safe," popular IUD, the Lippes Loop, came out in 1965 shortly after the pill (Figure 5–1). It consisted of a loop-shaped piece of polyethylene plastic with a monofilament tail. It was an instant hit.

It came in four sizes: A, B, C, and D. Sizes A and B did not effectively prevent pregnancy because they were too small and did not contact enough of the uterine surface to have a contraceptive effect. Size C was large enough to be an extremely effective contraceptive, but everyone recognized the need for an improvement because this larger size resulted in some discomfort and heavy menstrual bleeding in many women. That is when the copper IUDs hit the market in the early 1970s.

The Lippes Loop was extremely popular with many women, but the copper IUD literally set the standard for women who had had their first child and simply wanted temporary, easy contraception for a period of time before having their next child. The popularity of the IUD was enhanced also by the scare over the pill precipitated by the U.S. Senate hearings of 1971, overseen by Gaylord Nelson. In Sweden nearly every woman went off the pill and switched to the copper IUD. In Finland the use of the IUD increased ninefold (from 3 to 28 percent of all women of reproductive age). Women with heart disease, headaches, high blood pressure; smokers; and those who were afraid of the possible hormonal consequences of the pill flocked to the IUD as a safer answer to the now insatiable demand for convenient birth control. The only problem with the IUD seemed to be that it could be used only by women who had already had a child. A woman who had never been pregnant before would have a uterus too small to accept the IUD comfortably.

COPPER IUDS

The beginning of the downfall of the IUD came with the movement to extend its use to women who had never before been pregnant. The first copper IUD, called the Copper 7, was much smaller than the Lippes Loop, and its contraceptive effect relied not so much from direct contact with all areas of the uterine surface but on the release of small amounts of copper over a period of many years into the uterine cavity. This decreased the size of the IUD and made it an option even for women who had never been pregnant. Thus began the movement to put the IUD into any woman who wanted it, regardless of her sexual habits. If the development of IUDs had stopped with the Copper 7, and if its use had been limited to married women with children who were having a monogamous sex life, there probably would have been no IUD crisis today. The Dalkon Shield, which was introduced in 1970, immediately became popular for unmarried as well as married women, with younger as well as older women, and with women who had not

TABLE 2 Effectiveness of IUDs over a Two-Year Period

Device	Pregnancy Rate Per Year (percent)	Pain/Bleeding (percent)	Expulsion (percent)	Continuation of use for at least a yr. (percent)
TCU 380A	0.5	25.4	9.1	50.1
Nova T 200AG	0.7	16.0	5.7	64.7
TCU 220C	0.9	15.8	8.2	57.2
Multiload 350	1.1	N.A.	N.A.	N.A.
Lippes Loop	1.2	12.6	9.7	62.6
Multiload 250	1.4	8.9	2.5	80.5
TCU 200	1.7	13.9	7.1	61.7
TCU 300	1.7	16.7	6.1	58.3
Copper 7	2.1	11.1	17.6	54.5

had children. By 1974 over three hundred thousand women had come to regret their choice, and the Dalkon Shield finally was removed from the market. The stage was set for legal action, and twelve years later even the very safe IUDs are no longer available in the United States.

The classic Copper 7 is known to have a failure rate, or pregnancy rate, of about 2 percent per year. It has to be changed about every three years because the copper runs out. Some newer copper IUDs have been developed that last as long as ten years and that have a failure rate of less than 1 percent, making these IUDs certainly as effective as any method of birth control, including sterilization. The only reason for the continued popularity of the older Copper 7 in the United States is that despite government approval of one of the newer copper devices, no U.S. company has been willing to enter that marketplace because of the fear of litigation. But since you will now have to go to Canada or another foreign country to get an IUD if you want one, you should know about these newer models, because they have been available for years in Canada and other foreign countries.

Table 2 gives you a listing of most of the IUDs that are available. The IUDs with copper in them are smaller and therefore somewhat more easily tolerated than the plain polyethylene Lippes Loop but still allow a very low pregnancy rate. Unfortunately, they are so well tolerated that women without any children were able to have them as well. There are basically two shapes, the old Copper 7, which is literally in the shape of a number 7, and all other copper devices, which are in the shape of a "T." The copper "T" 's are less likely to be expelled by your uterus, because the two arms of the "T" help secure the device in place. More copper can be loaded onto the "T" shape, and thus these devices have incredibly low pregnancy rates (less than the birth control pill) but have the disadvantage of being somewhat more likely to cause uncomfortable menstrual bleeding than the Copper 7.

The oldest copper "T," the TCU 200, has roughly the same effectiveness as the Copper 7, but has a lower expulsion rate and is easier to insert than the Copper 7. This older "T" has never been commercially available in this country, even though it has been made available throughout the rest of the world. Given a choice between these two old standbys—the Copper 7 and the old copper TCU 200—most experts prefer the copper TCU 200 because it is easier to insert and much less likely to be expelled. The only advantage of the Copper 7 is that it is much more likely to be tolerated by women who have never had children.

There are new copper "T" devices, produced mostly in Finland but marketed by American companies in Canada and Europe, and by the Population Council throughout the rest of the world, and which you may prefer to the old TCU 200. The TCU 220C is a newer version of the TCU 200 and has a much lower pregnancy rate (less than 1 percent per year) but does not produce significantly more bleeding, pain, or risk of expulsion. The TCU 380A contains more copper and therefore has an incredibly low pregnancy rate. It is definitely the most effective of all the intrauterine devices for protecting against pregnancy. It is not significantly more likely to be expelled than the older TCU 200, but the major problem is that it is twice as likely (25 percent of users) as the TCU 200 to cause uncomfortable menstrual bleeding. Therefore many women elect to discontinue its use even though they are satisfied with its contraceptive security. Notice that the more you increase the amount of copper, and therefore the effectiveness of the IUD, the more likely you are to have uncomfortable menstrual bleeding. So there is a trade-off.

One of the best compromises in this trade-off is the Nova T 200AG. This IUD has a pregnancy rate almost as low as the TCU 380A (0.7 percent per year) and is even less likely to be expelled than the old TCU 200. It causes slightly more uncomfortable menstrual bleeding (16 percent of users) than the Copper 7 (11.1 percent) or the TCU 200 (13.9 percent) but has one of the highest satisfaction and continua-

tion rates of any of the IUDs. Because it is very unlikely to be expelled and its copper lasts for a full ten years, the Nova T 200AG
certainly is as convenient as any method of birth control now available
anywhere.

The incredibly low pregnancy rate of these newer copper "T"
IUDs—the TCU 380A, the TCU 220C, and the Nova T 200AG (all less
than 1 percent)—is extremely important for the woman's safety, because
unlike with most other contraceptive methods, pregnancy with an IUD
in place constitutes not just a contraceptive failure but a potential medical danger as well. If you get pregnant with the IUD in place, *it must
be removed.* Leaving it in would mean risking a spontaneous abortion
rate of over 50 percent, and taking it out will reduce the risk of spontaneous abortion to 20 percent (which is only a little bit greater than
the normal spontaneous abortion rate of a woman using no contraception
at all). More importantly, there is a risk with the IUD in place of a
"septic abortion," which is life-threatening, and which could lead to
permanent sterility at best. The incredibly low failure rates for these
new IUDs are not only a selling point for security from pregnancy but
also make the IUD safer for you medically.

The need for an IUD that lasts for ten years without replacement
may seem trivial to the mature thirty-year-old woman who assesses her
life situation carefully on a regular basis. But for the thirteen-year-old
girl whom I saw over a year ago at a birth control clinic, the issue of
IUD replacement wasn't so trivial. This little girl had just had a child.
She actually takes her little baby to high school with her (where they
have a day-care program for her baby and for the babies of her other
teenage classmates who have already had children). She had no intention of abstaining from sex, and certainly needed protection against
having another child before she was fifteen. She decided on the IUD
but was horrified at the thought that the device might run out of copper
by three years. Yet her only choice that was available on the American
market place was the Copper 7 and the Lippes Loop. None of the IUD
models designed to last for ten years or more (with pregnancy rates
lower than that of the pill) was available to her in the United States.
So she chose the Lippes Loop because it does not require replacement.
A month later the Lippes Loop went off the market, and less than a
year later the Copper 7 went off the market. She has no intention of
giving up her Lippes Loop until she is grown up, has her life in order,
gets married, and decides to have a regular family. This could take
twenty years, or it may never happen at all.

PROGESTERONE IUDS

There are in addition to the copper-bearing IUDs some less popular progesterone-bearing IUDs. One of them, Progestasert, is the only IUD still available on the U.S. market, yet it is probably the least desirable one. It works by releasing a small amount of progesterone into the uterine cavity, making the cervical mucus impenetrable to sperm, and reducing the uterine lining because of the intense local amount of progesterone. It runs out after about twelve to eighteen months. The pregnancy rates are equivalent to those for the Copper 7, and it results in less painful menstrual bleeding. The problem is that because Progestasert thins down the uterine lining so drastically, it results in unpredictable spotting and bleeding at any time during the menstrual cycle. Therefore, even though it is more comfortable than the copper IUDs and results in less blood loss, it is not acceptable to a lot of women because they don't like the idea of never knowing when they are going to bleed. For this reason it never became very popular despite being readily available in the United States. Possibly now that the Copper 7 is no longer available in this country and the Progestasert is the only game in town, it may begin to enjoy wider use.

A final word before we finish this section on the different types of IUDs. Most of the complications of the IUD, including pregnancy, spontaneous expulsion, painful menstruation, and even infection are related more to the skill and experience of the physician inserting it than the particular model of IUD being inserted. For example, with any given IUD studied, the pregnancy rates and complication rates vary almost as much among the different centers using that IUD as they do among different IUDs being used by the same center. So no matter what IUD you have put in, to make sure you have the safest possible contraception and the lowest possible risk of unpleasant side effects, you should go to a doctor or a clinic with a great deal of experience in using it.

How Does the IUD Work?

Most of the IUDs, whether the plain plastic varieties like the Lippes Loop, or any of the copper models, work by creating a "sterile" (no-infection) inflammatory reaction within the uterus. How that inflammatory reaction prevents pregnancy is a crucial matter, and it still is an ongoing debate among scientists. If it prevents pregnancy by keeping the sperm from reaching the egg, or by preventing the egg from being fertilized, such a mode of action would make it philosophically acceptable to most people. However, if it prevents pregnancy by not allowing the fertilized egg to implant in the wall of the uterus (as it normally must by about day six or seven after conception), it might be construed as a very early termination of pregnancy rather than as a method of birth control and be unacceptable to many people. A recent, still unpublished study from Chile makes it seem likely that the major mode of action of the IUD is to kill the sperm, or at least render them incapable of fertilizing the egg. In the Chilean study, women underwent sterilization by complete removal of their Fallopian tubes soon after ovulation. Eggs were found to have been fertilized in the tubes of about half the women not wearing IUDs but in none of the women who were wearing IUDs. It is postulated that the breakdown products of white blood cells that are released in the uterus around the IUD are toxic to sperm as they travel through the uterus toward the Fallopian tube. If this were the case, however, this same sterile inflammatory reaction would certainly be toxic to the early embryo (called the "blastocyst") as well. Thus if an occasional sperm did manage to fertilize an egg, it is very unlikely that this fertilized egg would ever be able to implant. Because of the fact that children conceived when their mother had an IUD in place have no greater incidence of congenital abnormalities, it is clear that the IUD has no toxic effect on the embryo.

There are two major arguments for postulating that the IUD works instead by inhibiting implantation of the embryo on the uterine wall. One indication is that ectopic pregnancies, in which the embryo implants in the Fallopian tube, are much more frequent in women who get pregnant with an IUD in place than in the general population. Thus, the argument goes, the IUD prevents an intrauterine pregnancy but does not prevent fertilization and thus does not prevent ectopic pregnancies from occurring. Another argument is that the IUD is extremely effective in preventing pregnancy when inserted into a woman after she has been raped. In fact, in a group of 340 women who had a copper IUD inserted up to seven days after unprotected intercourse, no pregnancies occurred, even though statistically at least 25 pregnancies would have been predicted. But this latter argument does not necessarily mean that when used normally by a nonpregnant woman, an IUD works by interrupting a pregnancy, any more than the fact that birth control pills given over a short period of time in high doses after unprotected intercourse also prevent pregnancy. The birth control pill given in high dosage acts very effectively like a "morning after" pill and also is used for rape victims. Yet we know that the birth control pill does not work normally by interrupting an existing conception but rather by preventing ovulation from occurring.

The IUD does protect against ectopic pregnancies as well as intrauterine pregnancies. Although women who get pregnant while using an IUD have a higher risk of this pregnancy being in the tube rather than in the uterus, the overall risk of tubal pregnancy in IUD users is lower than in a population using no birth control. Consider ten thousand hypothetical Copper 7 IUD users: two hundred of these ten thousand (2 percent) will get pregnant in a year. Of those two hundred, 3 percent, or six women, will have an ectopic rather than an intrauterine pregnancy. Now consider ten thousand women using no contraception at all. About eight thousand will get pregnant in a year, and 0.3 percent of them, or twenty-four women, will have an ectopic pregnancy. Thus the use of the IUD has reduced the risk of ectopic pregnancy fourfold. This makes it clear that the IUD must work by a combination of mechanisms, including a toxic action on sperm that prevents them from fertilizing the egg, as well as interference with implantation.

As long as the complication of infection has not developed (you will learn later in this chapter how to safeguard against that), fertility returns as soon as the IUD is removed. Fifty to 60 percent of women become pregnant within three months after the IUD is removed, and 88 percent get pregnant within one year. This rate is no different from the pregnancy rate for women who have discontinued using condoms, diaphragms, or natural rhythm birth control. This is in marked contrast to the birth control pill, where return of fertility is somewhat delayed.

How and When Is the IUD Put in?

Proper insertion of the IUD is the single most important determinant of most of its potential complications. These include unwanted pregnancy, risk of expulsion, bleeding, pain, and perforation of the uterus. The IUD must be placed high up in the widest part of the uterus, called the fundus. If the physician inserting the IUD is too timid and inexperienced, he or she may not place it high enough for fear of punching it through the uterus, which would require emergency surgery to retrieve. Worse yet, if the physician didn't realize he or she had punched it through the uterus, you might get pregnant with an IUD halfway in your uterus and halfway in the abdominal cavity. But if your physician is careful and goes through the proper steps of inserting the IUD slowly and methodically, you will have no problem. It should be reassuring for you to know that the complications that may sometimes affect an IUD-wearer are, for the most part, preventable if you choose the right physician to insert it. If you choose a careful doctor, you will be assured a very minimum risk of difficulties with the IUD. The pregnancy rate with the older model TCU-200 copper IUD is as low as 0.9 percent in some clinics and as high as 3.2 percent in other clinics. This is clearly because of the difference in the ability of the physician to place the IUD properly high in the fundus. With correct placement, the likelihood of spontaneous expulsion is only 7 percent, no matter what IUD is used, and the chances for an unwanted pregnancy occurring are extraordinarily low.

I recently visited a very busy family planning clinic that is headed by two main physicians, with a number of rotating interns, residents, and other trainees. One of the physicians covering the clinic had only a small amount of experience putting in the IUD. The other physician had put in lots of them. The week before I came, the less experienced physician felt compelled to do the IUD insertions because the more experienced physician was on vacation. He told me that he knew something was wrong that day because the plunger he used to insert the IUDs was "stiff" and he had to "push hard" to get the IUD out of the plunger. The plunger was not really stiff, but rather he was pushing against the wall of the uterus. This is a sure way to perforate the uterus.

It's easy to avoid this problem. There are two basic techniques for insertion: withdrawal and pushout. The withdrawal technique is safe, and the pushout technique is dangerous. Make sure your doctor uses the withdrawal technique. It takes a matter of minutes in the doctor's office and should be brief and effortless.

With the pushout technique, the physician places the inserter through the cervix somewhere into the uterus and uses the plunger to push the IUD out into the uterine cavity. Then the inserter and plunger are removed. This is dangerous. With the withdrawal technique, the physician places the inserter into the uterus all the way up to the top of the uterine wall and then withdraws the inserter just enough so that the IUD springs out into its shape in the uterine cavity. Then the plunger and the inserter are both removed. The reason that this withdrawal method is so safe is that it is easy to feel the resistance of the back wall of the uterus when the entire inserter is being introduced. With the pushout method, however, when the physician pushes in the plunger to eject the IUD out of the inserter, it is difficult if not impossible for him or her to feel the resistance of the opposite side of the uterus.

Following is a detailed rundown of the steps that your doctor should take in inserting the IUD.

1. First he or she will do a pelvic exam to make sure your vagina, cervix, uterus, ovaries, and Fallopian tubes are normal, then will do a culture for sexually transmitted disease, and a Pap smear. He or she will then put what is called a vaginal speculum into the vagina to view the cervix. He or she will cleanse the cervix with Xephirine or Betadine antiseptic. These preliminary steps are taken to make certain you don't have a vaginal infection, so that no infectious organisms can be transferred from the vagina into your uterus.
2. Next your physician will grasp the top of the cervix (which has no pain sensation) with an instrument called a tenaculum and gently pull down on the uterus. This will not hurt. It is a critical step, however, because it reduces the angle between the cervix and your uterus, making it easier to slip the inserter in gently.
3. Your physician will then gently place a long, narrow instrument called a sound through the cervix into the uterus to determine how long your uterine cavity is. This will also indicate the exact angle of your uterine cavity so that he or she can precisely place the inserter in the right position. If your uterus is less than 6 1/2 centimeters (about 2 1/2 inches) long, which is very unusual, your physician will tell you that your uterus is just too small to allow an IUD comfortably.
4. After he or she removes the sound, your physician will introduce the IUD (loaded inside its inserter) into the uterus until resistance is felt (Figure 5–2).
5. He or she will then withdraw the inserter tube (not the plunger) enough to release the arms of the IUD, after which he or she will then withdraw the plunger as well (Figure 5–3).
6. Your physician will then place gentle pressure on the inserter (not the plunger) to make sure the IUD is properly seated. This step will not run the risk of perforating the uterus because it does not involve using the plunger, and it will assure proper positioning of the IUD against the top wall of the uterus. This maneuver will assure you an

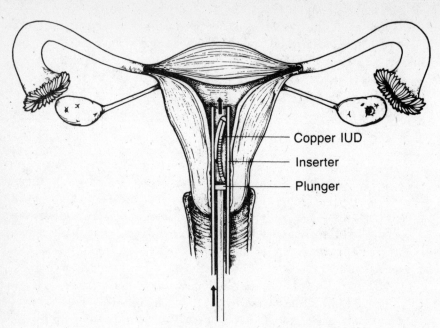

Copper IUD

Inserter

Plunger

FIGURE 5-2.

extremely low risk of expulsion, pregnancy, severe bleeding, and pain (Figure 5-4).

7. The inserter is then removed and the strings are cut right at the entrance to the vagina.

Usually no anesthesia is necessary for the IUD insertion, particularly if it is done at the time of menstruation, when the cervix is relatively open. But if the cervix needs to be dilated, the doctor sometimes may use a local anesthetic to minimize discomfort.

When should the IUD be inserted? Most doctors prefer to put the IUD in just at the end of menstruation. At this time the uterus is less irritable, the cervix is still wide open following the exit of menstrual blood, and perhaps most important, there is no chance of there being an unrecognized pregnancy. But although the end of menstruation is the most widely acceptable time for inserting the IUD, any time in the cycle is all right as long as you are certain you are not pregnant. Just recognize that if the cervix is closed at the particular time in the cycle when the IUD is being inserted, it may be a more uncomfortable procedure.

An IUD may even be inserted after an episode of undesired and

157

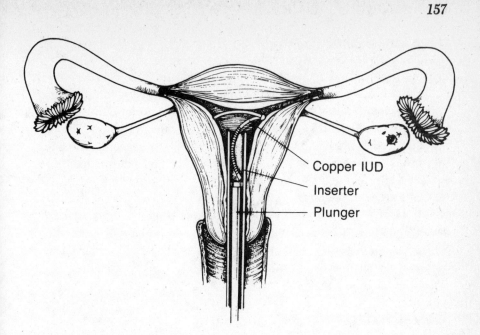

Copper IUD

Inserter

Plunger

FIGURE 5–3.

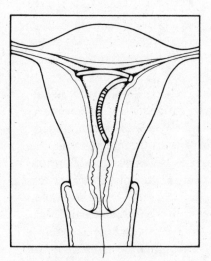

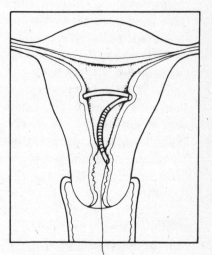

CORRECT Position
of Copper 7 IUD

INCORRECT Position (low)
of Copper 7 IUD

FIGURE 5–4.

unprotected intercourse, such as after a rape. So long as it is inserted within five to seven days after the rape, you are extremely unlikely to become pregnant. (Furthermore, unlike using the birth control pill in high dosages over a short period of time for this purpose, there are no agonizing symptoms such as unremitting nausea and vomiting, which high doses of the pill would create.) It is best not to put the IUD in just after delivering a baby. This used to be popular because it allowed the woman freedom to begin having sex without fear of pregnancy at any time after she left the hospital. But such early insertion leads to a much greater spontaneous expulsion rate and a greater risk of infection. It is best to wait until about six or eight weeks after delivery before having the IUD inserted. Thus you would need some other method of contraception (whether around-the-clock breast-feeding, barrier meth-. ods, or even abstinence) until such time as the IUD can be inserted.

Side Effects and Complications of the IUD

PELVIC INFECTION

The most controversial side effect of the IUD is pelvic infection with subsequent sterility. The IUDs available today are extremely safe from infection unless you are a young woman with multiple sexual partners.

Studies in the 1960s and early 1970s demonstrated that there are always some bacteria in the uterus within twenty-four hours after insertion of an IUD. However, within a day or two all of the bacteria are gone in 80 percent of the women, and by thirty days after insertion, there are no uterine bacteria present in any of the women. This means that the uterus is able to destroy completely the small amount of bacteria introduced into the uterus at the time of the IUD insertion. Furthermore, no new bacteria are able to migrate up into the uterus via the smooth monofilament tail of any IUD other than the Dalkon Shield, with its poorly conceived, multifilamented tail. The incidence of pelvic inflammatory disease after the first month of insertion among twenty-four thousand women using the IUD varied from 1 percent to 2.5 percent per year, which is no different from the rate of pelvic inflammatory disease (PID) seen in a normal population.

Since 1971, five separate studies have shown that the risk of pelvic infection in IUD-users was three to five times the risk of pelvic infection in those using other methods of contraception. But a large number of women in these studies had used the Dalkon Shield, many of them were under twenty-five years of age, many of them had never had children, and many had had multiple sex partners. This was a different group from those in the 1960s when the incidence of pelvic infection was no greater in IUD-users than in the normal population. If you looked at the details of the new studies you would find that the risk of infection with the Dalkon Shield was eight to seventeen times that of women not using IUDs, but the risk of pelvic infection in women using other IUDs was only 1.6 times that of women using other methods of contraception. Furthermore, the control group in these studies always included women who were either using birth control pills, diaphragm, or condoms, all of which protect the user from developing venereal diseases no matter how many sexual partners she has.

In one of these studies, the risk of infection was 6.2 times that of the control group when the IUD-wearer had never had children and was single, but only 1.7 times that of the control group when the IUD-wearer already had children. So these studies in the 1970s need not have scared away women who had already had children and were happily married with no other sexual partners. Yet the damage had been done, and as one lawsuit after another completely crippled the company that made the Dalkon Shield, the guilt by implication placed on IUDs in general led to hundreds of nonmeritorious lawsuits against the manufacturers of the safer IUDs.

The issue was really settled in 1985 with the publication of a large-scale study at Harvard. The study demonstrated that IUD-users who had only one sex partner had no increased risk of pelvic infection or tubal disease. Women who used the Dalkon Shield were eleven times more likely to get pelvic infection than the normal population. Women with a copper IUD had only a 1.6 times greater chance of having pelvic infection overall than women with no IUD. But women with a copper IUD who had only one sex partner were at no greater risk whatsoever of getting pelvic infection. This meant that the IUD would not be a good method of birth control for a twenty-one-year-old woman who experiments with sex with multiple partners, is unmarried, and is without children. But it would be an ideal contraceptive for married women in a monogamous relationship who already have had at least one child.

If you get a sexually transmitted disease, it is much more likely to result in a severe spread into the uterus and tubes if an IUD is in place. But in the absence of sexually transmitted disease, none of the IUDs presently available should cause an infection.

A good example of how quick people were to blame the IUD

unfairly was apparent to me when I saw a twenty-four-year-old woman at a birth control clinic. She had had two children already, was completely unable to take care of them, and had had a Copper 7 inserted. She came to the clinic a month later complaining of a rash on her palms and soles. She thought it was from an allergy to copper in the IUD, and had already contacted a lawyer to bring suit against the manufacturer. A simple examination and blood test demonstrated that this rash was not in any way an allergy to the IUD but rather was a symptom of syphilis. Rather than going home rich, as she had dreamed, she went home angry at one of her many boyfriends.

At the end of this chapter I will go into more detail on how the legal community's money-hungry attack on manufacturers has forced safe IUD models off the market and made it necessary for women who would be ideal candidates for it to plan a trip to Canada or another foreign country. But before you conclude incorrectly that I am recommending the IUD as a birth control method without any drawbacks, I need to go through some of its other side effects and complications.

Side Effects and Complications Other Than Infection

All of the major problems associated with an IUD can be minimized if it has been inserted properly. The biggest and most common problem with the IUD is increased menstrual blood loss and painful menstruation related to the presence of a foreign body within the uterus. During the first seven days after the IUD is inserted, menstrual-type cramps are common, along with spotting and sometimes even some dizziness at the time of insertion. These symptoms generally represent no problem, will be much better twenty-four hours later, and should be almost completely gone in a week. But the somewhat heavier and possibly more uncomfortable menstrual periods will continue in most women. If your menstrual periods become just too uncomfortable, or too heavy, you may have to choose another method of birth control. In most cases, however, these symptoms are quite tolerable.

A more important complication is perforation of the uterus at the time of insertion of the IUD. This occurs in less than one in four thousand cases and virtually never occurs in the hands of an extremely experienced inserter. It virtually always occurs at the time of insertion, even though you may not become aware of it until weeks or months later. The minute that you or the doctor suspects the possibility of perforation, you should plan on having it removed. Perforation is not an immediate emergency requiring a rush to the operating room, but it should be taken care of within several days. Often the IUD can be removed simply by laparoscopy, in which a telescope is placed through the belly button, the uterus is observed, and the IUD is removed through the telescope with a grasping instrument. If this should not prove possible, you may have to have a regular operation, in which your abdomen will be opened up, to remove the perforating IUD. If it is taken care of properly, this rare complication should not become a serious problem.

The inserter really should be aware of the problem when he or she first puts the IUD in because he or she should detect a sudden loss of resistance if the IUD has perforated the uterine wall. If perforation is not discovered until later, it could be very serious because you will find out only by virtue of the fact that you become pregnant. If you cannot feel the strings coming out of the cervix or if the strings suddenly feel shorter than they had originally (the doctor will explain what this will feel like), you need to have the doctor check the position of your IUD with a simple ultrasound test. This will assure both you and the doctor that the IUD has not gone through the uterine wall and is properly placed. As long as you know no perforation has occurred at the time of the insertion, you need not fear that perforation will occur later.

A relatively common problem is "spontaneous expulsion" of the IUD. On average in 5 to 10 percent of women the uterus simply will not tolerate having the IUD and will spontaneously expel it. You need to be aware of this possibility before you decide to use the IUD. Increased bleeding, uterine cramping, or persistent increase in pain probably means the IUD is being expelled. You need to learn how to check for the strings to see if they are protruding properly from the opening of your cervix. If you cannot feel the IUD coming through the cervix but just feel the strings coming out as they normally should, then everything is all right and the IUD is not being expelled. But if you have any doubts, you should check with your doctor.

If the IUD is being expelled, your doctor probably will finish removing it and then you have a simple choice. You can use another method of birth control, or you can have a different IUD inserted. The logic in trying again is that the most common reason for your IUD being expelled is that it was originally placed incorrectly, too low in the uterus. Proper reinsertion may result in it not being expelled the next time.

Generally speaking, all of these problems are most likely to occur in the first three months. If they haven't occurred by then, they probably won't occur later.

Another common problem is that of the "lost tail." Check regularly to make sure the strings still are properly protruding from the cervix, to be certain the IUD is in place. What happens if you don't feel the strings anymore? In 20 percent of the cases it means that you expelled the IUD from the uterus and weren't aware of it. In 80 percent of the cases the IUD still is properly seated in the uterus but the strings have migrated up. This can be ascertained by a simple ultrasound exam.

If the ultrasound exam shows that the IUD still is properly seated in the uterus, you have a simple choice. If you leave the situation as is, you have an advantage in that there is even less risk of infection than if the monofilament string were protruding from the cervix as originally designed. You can leave the IUD in, and whenever you decide to have it removed the doctor probably will have to use local anesthesia to dilate the cervix and pull out the IUD directly. A second possibility is that the doctor can give you local anesthesia now and try to guide the string down out of the cervix with a small instrument. The third possibility is that he or she can remove the IUD and reinsert another one. There is nothing wrong with leaving the IUD in place despite the fact the strings are not coming out of the cervix. In fact, this is the type of "stringless" IUD that forty million Chinese women are using today. But if you are unfortunate enough to get pregnant with the IUD in place and the strings are not protruding from the cervix, then you have a real problem.

Pregnancy with the IUD in Place

As we mentioned earlier, if you get pregnant while wearing an IUD it is a serious event. You must see the doctor *immediately* if that happens. In the first place, he or she has to make sure it is not an ectopic pregnancy by performing a pregnancy test and an ultrasound examination. Then he or she must remove the IUD. If the IUD is not removed there is over a 50 percent chance of your having a miscarriage, or spontaneous abortion, sometime around the middle of your pregnancy. Such a miscarriage is much more difficult than the more common miscarriages one sees within the first three months of pregnancy. It is very unpleasant. If the IUD is removed, you have only about a 20 percent chance of having a miscarriage, which is closer to the norm of women who get pregnant using no contraception. Perhaps even more important than saving the pregnancy is the rare but real possibility that if the IUD is left in, you might have an infected, or septic, miscarriage (or abortion) in the middle of your pregnancy.

Septic abortion is the deadliest complication of an IUD. This is what killed most of the women who had had a Dalkon inserted, and who later died as a consequence of serious infection. These women did not have ordinary miscarriages. They suffered from days or weeks of mild flulike symptoms that suddenly developed into overwhelming fever and collapse. The blood supply to a pregnant uterus is so incredibly abundant that the presence of a bloodborne infection at the time of pregnancy can be a death warrant. If your IUD is a safe one, the possibility of the pregnancy becoming infected is quite rare, but it is possible, and for this reason the IUD must come out.

You may worry that if the IUD is removed and the pregnancy in all likelihood goes to completion, there might be some abnormality with your baby. You can rest assured that studies have shown that there is no such danger. There doesn't appear to be an increased risk of developmental abnormalities or congenital problems in babies who were born as a result of a pregnancy with an IUD in place. The only reason for removing the IUD is to decrease the risk of losing the pregnancy, and to eliminate the rare possibility of having an infected pregnancy, which invariably would result in a spontaneous abortion and most likely the death of the mother. There seems to be no greater danger that the child of such a pregnancy would be any more abnormal than if you had gotten pregnant without an IUD in place.

If you see the doctor as soon as you think you are pregnant, he or she will most likely have no difficulty removing your IUD without complications. Often the IUD has been partially expelled anyway, and that is the reason you got pregnant. All your physician has to do is grasp the edge of the IUD that is coming through the cervix and pull it out. If the IUD is not being expelled, but you got pregnant simply because it had not been placed ideally high up in the fundus, your physician should still be able to see the strings coming through the cervix, and gently pull on them to remove it.

The problem is that if you wait until about the ninth week of pregnancy, the tail of the IUD will have been completely drawn up into the uterine cavity, and the doctor will have nothing to pull on to remove the IUD. This represents a very serious problem, much like the case of a woman who gets pregnant with a "tailless" IUD. You have the following difficult choices. To remove the IUD the pregnancy most likely will have to be terminated. It would be too dangerous for the doctor to probe the uterine cavity to try to remove the IUD in an effort to save the pregnancy, because this in truth would severely risk getting the pregnancy infected, which as you know by now would probably result in a septic miscarriage with all its dire risks, including your death.

Your other choice is not to do anything, to leave the IUD in place, and recognize that although there is a 50 or 60 percent risk of your losing the pregnancy at a difficult time between the third and the sixth month, the chance of it being a deadly septic abortion is very low as long as the doctor doesn't attempt to probe inside your uterus looking for the IUD. Very often the patient decides to leave the IUD in place and run the risk of spontaneous abortion, recognizing that her risk of a deadly, infected, spontaneous abortion is very low. But medically speaking, the smartest thing to ensure the future health of the mother is to terminate the pregnancy and remove the IUD.

So you can see that pregnancy is a serious complication with the IUD, and it is important for you to see the doctor as soon as you suspect you may be pregnant, at a time when it still is quite easy to remove the IUD with the least amount of threat either to you or the pregnancy.

Another reason to report to the doctor immediately if you become pregnant is that there is a 3 percent risk that the pregnancy will be ectopic—that is, in the Fallopian tube rather than in the uterus. Don't be confused into thinking that an IUD increases the risk of your having an ectopic pregnancy; actually, it decreases your risk. But if you do get pregnant with an IUD in place, the chances of it being ectopic are ten times greater than normal. An ectopic pregnancy requires surgery before it becomes an emergency caused by tubal rupture and bleeding. The earlier it is operated on, the less likely you are to lose that tube.

A pregnancy with an IUD in place is not a simple matter. It behooves you to choose the type of IUD, and the type of doctor inserting the IUD, that will afford you the lowest possible chance of this complication occurring.

What Are My Chances of Getting Pregnant with an IUD?

As you learned earlier in this chapter, there are a wide variety of copper IUDs available in most countries outside the United States.

Although some copper IUDs are clearly more effective than others, the most important step you can take in assuring a very low risk of pregnancy is to have the IUD inserted properly high in the uterine fundus. A properly seated IUD is very unlikely to be expelled and is very unlikely to allow you to get pregnant. Second, you should realize that the younger you are, the greater your chance of an unwanted pregnancy with an IUD. For example, using the most incredibly effective copper IUD available, the TCU 380A, if you are under twenty years of age there is a slightly greater than 1 percent chance of pregnancy. If you are over twenty-five years of age, the chance of pregnancy is less than 0.3 percent. With all IUDs most of the pregnancies occur within the first two years of its insertion. Pregnancies after two years are very unlikely because if you haven't gotten pregnant by two years, it probably means the IUD has been properly placed.

The virtual absence of any serious risk of pregnancy after you've had a successful first two years with the IUD argues for you making sure to use one that does not run out of copper and does not have to be replaced until you want it removed so you can have children. In this respect the older model TCU 200 and Copper 7 have the disadvantage of having to be replaced every three to four years. Furthermore, if you compare the pregnancy rate with these older copper IUDs in a variety of clinics, they simply don't give as great a sense of security as the newer ones, such as the TCU 380A (as well as the TCU 380AG, which lasts even longer), the Nova T 200AG, or the TCU 220C. These newer-model copper IUDs have a contraceptive action that lasts about ten years or longer, and a risk of pregnancy on average of less than 0.5 percent.

The pregnancy risk with non-copper-bearing IUDs such as the Lippes Loop, or progesterone-bearing IUDs such as the Progestasert, are roughly equivalent to that of the older copper IUDs.

Who Should Use an IUD, and How Does a U.S. Citizen Get One?

There are two bottom-line issues for making the IUD a safe and effective contraceptive: (1) proper insertion by the proper physician, and (2) the proper patient. Any woman with a history of pelvic infection (PID), a woman who has never had children before, or a woman with more than one sexual partner is an absolute "no-no" for any IUD. Having multiple sex partners or having a single partner who has multiple sex partners puts a woman at risk of getting a sexually transmitted infection, which, in the presence of an IUD, may march right up into the uterus and tubes.

Because women who have not had children, are under twenty-five, or unmarried, are likely to have multiple partners at some time, and are likely to have a small uterus that becomes very irritated by the IUD, they should avoid the IUD. The IUD is a better option for a happily married woman in a monogamous relationship who has already had at least one child. In a normal population of women aged twenty to twenty-four who don't use an IUD, there is a 6.3 percent risk of developing pelvic infection over a three-year period of time. For women over thirty years of age, there is only a 1.2 percent chance of pelvic infection. This simply relates to the increased risk that the younger sexually active woman encounters of contacting a sexually transmitted disease.

Women with an abnormal uterine shape (which can be determined on pelvic exam) also need to look for a different contraceptive because the IUD will not give them secure assurance from pregnancy. Women with painful or heavy periods will most probably not like the increasing bleeding and menstrual pain associated with the IUD. It is an ideal contraceptive only for older married women who already have had a child and who have a happy, monogamous marital relationship.

In the 1970s over one hundred million IUDs were inserted in women in China. At present China represents two thirds of the world's users of IUDs. Ninety percent of their IUDs are a stainless steel "tailless" ring much like the old device invented by Dr. Grafenberg in Germany in the 1920s. Thirty-five percent of married women in China use this. Sixty million people in the world now use the IUD, twenty million of whom are in the West. Two and a half million women in the United States and Canada use it. In developing countries other than China (where there is hardly any venereal disease), women rarely use the IUD because venereal disease runs rampant. In Africa, for example, in some communities as many as 47 percent of women are sterile as a result of pelvic infections. The IUD would be a disastrous birth control option for them. It may not be such a great idea in heavily populated cities with high rates of PID such as Los Angeles or New York City either, and certainly is a very worrisome choice for young women too undisciplined to rely on the pill, condoms, or a diaphragm. For such women, shocking as it may seem, sterilization with the idea of "reversibility" might be a better choice.

Why Can't I Have an IUD?

James and Carol were thirty-five and thirty years old, respectively, had been married for one and a half years, and couldn't understand why she had not gotten pregnant yet. They assumed that it was Jim's fault because he had a small testicle on one side, and a history of a hernia repair that they thought might have damaged the vas deferens. They also knew that Carol ovulated late in her cycle, which was easy to treat. She had no idea that her chances of ever having children had been destroyed by the IUD she had worn during her previous marriage.

She was twenty-three then and knew that she did not want to have any children in that marriage. But thinking ahead intelligently, she decided not to have a tubal sterilization, because she recognized that she might get remarried in the future and change her mind about having children. So she had a Dalkon Shield inserted in 1974, just before the Robins Company took it off the market. She then continued to use this IUD for the next seven years and was quite satisfied. She had no symptoms of infection, she was free from the worry of getting pregnant, and she believed that whenever she had it removed she would once again be able to have children. During these seven years that Carol wore the IUD, the A. H. Robins Company did nothing to inform her and three hundred thousand other women who were wearing their product that it was associated with some very serious complications. They simply took it off the market and said nothing.

Suddenly in 1981 Carol developed severe cramping and fever. She went to see the doctor. He immediately removed the Dalkon Shield and placed her on antibiotics. She got better rapidly, and thus assumed that everything was all right. She had no idea of the incredible amount of damage that little infection had done. Nor did she realize how lucky she was that she wasn't dead. Ironically, Carol had been referred to me by her next-door neighbor and friend who in the past had had a tubal sterilization that I had reversed two years ago. Because her friend got pregnant so readily after the tubal reversal operation, she sent Carol to me thinking that we could work the same wonders with her. What they didn't realize is that the infection Carol got after the insertion of the Dalkon Shield IUD turned out to be a permanent form of sterilization for Carol, whereas the standard tubal ligation that her friend had undergone was readily reversible with microsurgery.

You need to understand just how deficient the Robins Company was in informing patients about this disastrous risk in order to understand why the lawyers had such a field day. It wasn't until 1984, ten years after they discontinued their product, that they started a campaign to advertise in all major magazines asking anyone who had a Dalkon Shield in place to see a physician immediately, have it removed, and have the bill sent to them. They didn't take this step until they began to realize that all the lawsuits that were piling up against them totaled way over the $615 million they had tucked away for future legal expenses and damages. The company eventually had to file a Chapter 11 bankruptcy proceeding, which is basically a way of keeping it functioning and paying everybody off in a lump sum. There are three hundred thousand such women claiming a piece of these $615 million.

What this means is that James and Carol, whose only hope for pregnancy after their disaster was *in vitro* fertilization, cannot even get the company to pay for the cost of this treatment and will most likely collect only about $2,000 from the A. H. Robins Company. The cost of any medical attempt to help them achieve pregnancy could total as high as $50,000. Carol had worn the Dalkon Shield for seven years before she finally got her infection, and no one had warned her during all that time of what the company knew by 1974 and didn't share.

Why should that affect the availability of the safe IUDs? The safe copper IUDs are manufactured by a reputable company, G. D. Searle & Company. Because of the incredibly successful wave of lawsuits hurled at the Robins Company, which made the Dalkon Shield, makers of any IUD now appeared to be ripe for the picking. Lawyers unleashed one lawsuit after another on Searle, alleging that the Copper 7 or TCU 200 had caused pelvic infection or sterility. Searle successfully defended itself against most of these suits because, as you know from reading this chapter, studies have shown that the copper IUD does not cause infection, although it does allow sexually transmitted venereal diseases to do more damage than they would have if an IUD were not in place. Furthermore, Searle did not hide any of these data.

The cost of successfully defending the four most recent lawsuits in which G. D. Searle was found innocent was $1.5 million. Searle has already defended ten IUD lawsuits, eight of them successfully and two of them unsuccessfully. This is an enormous company whose total sales from the IUD amount to only $11 million per year and that isn't even profit, just gross sales. Their only intelligent reason for marketing the IUD would have to be humanitarian. For a company of this size, stature, and income, the IUD meant very little profit and a potential undeserved economic disaster. It is only in the crazy, litigation-happy environment of the United States that this could occur. Fortunately, the copper IUD will be available everywhere else in the world.

With this helter-skelter, OK-Corral-type legal liability system we are saddled with in the United States, it is a wonder that any methods of birth control, including the basal body temperature thermometer, are still available. For example, some people have idly speculated that "natural" rhythm birth control might increase slightly the risk of birth defects by making it more likely that an egg several days old will be fertilized rather than a fresh one. Furthermore there is no question that 3 percent of all children born by mothers using "natural" birth control will have birth defects, because that is the percentage of birth defects occurring in any normal population. Who will the lawyers sue for that one? Perhaps the makers of the basal body temperature thermometers, or perhaps the Catholic Church?

6

Barrier Methods of Birth Control: Condoms, Diaphragms, Contraceptive Foam, and the Sponge

Condoms and diaphragms are back in style. After having been regarded as virtual relics of sexual history, they have suddenly leaped back into popularity in the past several years. The epidemic of sexually transmitted diseases, particularly the uniformly fatal AIDS, plus the growing public concern over side effects of the pill and IUD, not to mention the surge in concern over this country's incredible teenage pregnancy rate (almost 20 percent of American girls have gotten pregnant by age nineteen), have brought back the diaphragm and the condom.

Although the sexual revolution is commonly thought of as being heralded in the 1960s with the availability of the birth control pill, in truth it had its modern origin in the late 1940s with penicillin. One of the major forces restraining widespread sexual promiscuity throughout history has been venereal disease. Syphilis and gonorrhea had their origin around the time of the Renaissance in the fifteenth century, a period of great revolution in sexual promiscuity. For the next five hundred years the threat of getting these deadly diseases served to restrain sexual practices. Before penicillin, the thought of getting syphilis or gonorrhea was just as terrifying as the thought of getting AIDS is nowadays. Both diseases had a high fatality rate and were absolutely incurable. But because of penicillin, today they are regarded rather casually. That is when the sexual revolution began.

The first hint that the sexual revolution might be dimming came with the widespread increase in herpes. Herpes is only an aggravating, nuisance of a venereal disease (unless passed on to an infant by a pregnant mother). But because it is a virus (for which no antibiotic is effective) everyone was, quite literally, painfully aware of the fact that it is incurable. Johnny Carson made jokes about when you should ask a date whether he or she has herpes. It is aggravating, and it is painful, but it comes and goes and is not fatal. With the advent of AIDS, however, a viral disease that is uniformly fatal and completely untreatable, a new sobriety has hit the sexual scene. Abstinence is once again becoming a legitimate method of birth control, monogamy is on the rise, and those who really want to be safe are going back to condoms and diaphragms.

But protection from sexually transmitted diseases is not the only reason for this increased popularity in "barrier methods" of contraception. They afford protection against development of cancer of the cervix, the second most common cancer in women. There are no hormonal side effects to worry about. There is no risk of developing increased complications from an infection, such as with the IUD. There is no surgical procedure involved, and there is no big upfront cost. It is hard to imagine a safer, more convenient method of birth control.

You don't have to take a trip to the doctor's office or to the clinic to buy condoms; you can buy them right at the drugstore. In fact, condoms now are so conveniently available that whereas ten years ago, less than 10 percent of condoms were purchased by women, today they purchase over 40 percent of them. In California, over 60 percent of condoms are purchased by women. Condoms are no longer found only in dirty-looking dispensers in men's rooms at the gasoline station. You can find them on colorful display in drugstores in light pastel boxes in the women's cosmetic sections. The woman can buy condoms, or diaphragms, or contraceptive sponges, along with her tampons and deodorant, throw it all into one bag and not be in the least bit embarrassed about it.

Then why have condoms and diaphragms been such a relatively unpopular method of birth control until recently, and why did they take such a backseat to the pill, the IUD, and sterilization? The reason is that they have some disadvantages also. In the first place, you have to remember to use a barrier method every time you have sex, and this may be just when things are beginning to get exciting. It requires some discipline and strong motivation to remember to use it each and every time. The condom and diaphragm should be extremely effective methods of birth control, with a failure rate of less than 1 percent. But in actual use the failure rate is as high as 10 to 20 percent because of nonuse. Perhaps more importantly, condoms (and to a lesser extent diaphragms) have had a social stigma associated with venereal disease and promiscuity still left over from before the 1960s.

Many people figure that condoms are a turn-off. But the Japanese experience shows that they don't have to be. Seventy-five percent of Japanese couples use condoms as their only method of birth control. For the Japanese couple it is an integral part of the lovemaking adventure and serves a role of almost ceremonial excitement. It is simply a part of the foreplay ritual. The woman may even put it on the man just to accentuate the tension that is building during foreplay. There is no "low class" stigma associated with the condom in Japan. There is no association with venereal disease or sexual promiscuity. This is simply a matter of public perception, and as public perception gradually changes, I see more and more wholesome couples, happily married for many years, going back to the safety and easy availability of condoms and diaphragms.

Nonetheless, these barrier methods are perfectly suited for singles with more than one potential sex partner, and particularly teenagers who shun the notion of abstinence. The very people for whom condoms in particular are most suited—teenagers who may have limited access to other methods of birth control, who have only sporadic sexual outings, and who often have more than one sex partner (or whose partner has more than one sex partner)—hesitate to use them because they are "uncool," or because they are afraid it will be insulting to the partner. After all, when you have seen countless movie after movie showing your favorite role models making explicit and passionate love on bigger-than-life screens, you are not about to do it any differently than they do. When have you ever seen Tom Selleck or Robert Redford stop for a moment in the middle of an explicit love scene, go to their drawer, and pull out a condom, or Meryl Streep tell her lover to stop for a moment while she goes into the bathroom to insert a diaphragm? Movie and television heroes are telling us that lovemaking must be effortless and spontaneous, and who can complain about that? It sure looks good the way they sell it. The fantasy they would have you believe is that you don't have to worry about getting pregnant, and you don't have to worry about contracting a disease that may kill you. But the emergence of AIDS has changed all that, maybe.

You can't effectively tell kids not to have sex and expect them to take you seriously when the movies you watch, the television you turn on, and the magazines you buy are all selling it. The purpose of sex education is not to sell sex. Society already is doing that. Your children will know the facts of life, and will most likely be pretty excited about them, long before you get around even to dreaming about telling them. So what you can give them, and hopefully what a sex education program can give them, is solid information and the truth, which they are not getting from the movies or television.

Even the Surgeon General of the United States, an otherwise conservative political figure, has now formally advocated sex education in our schools for children of almost every age to combat this. That includes birth control counseling and information on prevention of sexually transmitted diseases.

A Summary of Sexually Transmitted Diseases

"Sexually transmitted disease" is a new term. In the past these conditions were all called "venereal disease." But the term "venereal disease" was limited to the traditional five diseases of gonorrhea, syphilis, chancroid, lymphogranuloma venereum, and granuloma inguinale. The latter three of these diseases have been very common in Africa and Asia, but in Europe and North America the major two venereal diseases have been gonorrhea and syphilis. We now know there are at least twenty-four different diseases transmitted sexually, including the most common cancer of the female reproductive tract, carcinoma of the cervix. The term "venereal" just seemed too limited and had the stigma of being associated only with lower socioeconomic groups. The fact is that sexually transmitted diseases are found abundantly in all levels of society, as underscored by reports about the famous New York lawyer Roy Cohn and the movie idol Rock Hudson dying of AIDS. Over the past five hundred years there have been countless false rumors to the effect that you can catch syphilis or gonorrhea in a swimming pool, or from dirty toilet seats. The fact is that these diseases can be caught only by sexual transmission (with the exception of dope addicts using contaminated needles, or the unfortunate baby born of an infected mother).

Most sexually transmitted diseases are very weak invaders. If they were severely infectious, they would pass around the community like chicken pox and colds, or like mumps, polio, or smallpox of a previous era. Venereal diseases, or to use the modern term "sexually transmitted diseases," generally are carried by very puny organisms that couldn't possibly infect from one person to another with anything but the most intimate, direct contact. In a society that has little sexual promiscuity there would be little venereal disease. That is why evidence is pointing to the fact that AIDS really is not all that infectious and requires repeated, intimate contact for transmission (unless you are a dope addict, born of an infected mother, or receive an infected blood transfusion).

Sexually transmitted diseases include not only AIDS, gonorrhea, and syphilis, but also genital warts, hepatitis B, herpes, lice, scabies, nonspecific urethritis, and chlamydia. What has made this imposing list of sexually transmitted diseases relatively unworrisome in the past thirty years has been the ready availability of antibiotics, which overnight converted these deadly killers into mere nuisances. Instead of people having to worry about catching a venereal disease, all they had to worry about was remembering to go to the doctor or clinic to get treated properly. But long before AIDS came, those of us who knew the history of medicine had predicted that a deadly illness transmitted sexually, but too weak a germ to spread through the community in any other way, would eventually appear. You simply can't have a quarter century of complete sexual freedom with people engaging in sex with multiple partners each of whom have also had multiple partners without the emergence of a disease that would be transmitted through these vectors.

In case you are terrified by the specter of AIDS, or cancer of the cervix, or even the risk of sterility caused by gonorrhea or chlamydia, let me explain to you just how terrifying and deadly at one time was one of the weakest of all sexually transmitted diseases, syphilis. Syphilis emerged during the fifteenth-century Renaissance. The French blamed the disease on the English (they called it the "English pox"), and the English blamed it on the French (they called it the "French pox"), but in truth syphilis seemed to flower instantly everywhere in Renaissance Europe. Syphilis would begin with a small, painless sore somewhere on the penis or the vagina. Before you had much of a chance to worry about this ugly sore, it would usually heal and disappear on its own.

Then, about four to eight weeks later, you would get a rash almost anywhere on the body, including the palms of your hands and the soles of your feet. After several weeks, once again before you had much time to worry about this rash, it would also heal up on its own and disappear. These are the so-called primary and secondary lesions of syphilis, and they are completely harmless.

You would then feel just fine for about the next fifteen years, not realizing that all along the little syphilis germs, called spirochetes, were eating away at your heart, your blood vessels, your nervous system, and your brain. Fifteen to twenty years later, about one third of the people who contracted syphilis developed the terrible complications called tertiary syphilis and died. Up until 1945 there was virtually nothing you could do about it. The irony of it, much like modern-day AIDS, is that two-thirds of the people who contracted syphilis never came down with its deadly manifestations. So you can imagine the torment for fifteen to twenty years, after having had a painless sore on the penis or vagina, followed by a generalized rash all over the body, both of which went away on their own promptly, wondering what was going to be left of your brain or heart, or whether you would be one of the lucky ones who escape. Today a short course of antibiotics will kill these puny little spirochetes with little difficulty at all.

But antibiotics do not kill viruses, they kill only bacteria. So deadly diseases such as syphilis and gonorrhea, not to mention the bubonic plague (the famous Black Death), which killed a third of the European population in the thirteenth century, are easily cured with modern antibiotics. That is also true of some of the newer venereal diseases, such as chlamydia, nonspecific urethritis, lice, and scabies. Even warts, which don't respond to antibiotics, can be treated with cautery or a laser because they are localized. Cancer of the cervix can be diagnosed early with a Pap smear, and most such women are cured by surgery. But we can't treat viral diseases such as hepatitis, herpes, or AIDS, and because AIDS is fatal, people finally are beginning to take sexually transmitted disease seriously again.

There are somewhere between eight hundred thousand and two million new cases of gonorrhea every year in the United States, and even the weakling of all venereal diseases, syphilis, still manages to infect thirty thousand Americans every year. Nonspecific urethritis infects over two million men in the United States every year. Pelvic inflammatory disease (which usually leads to sterility) as a complication of either gonorrhea or chlamydia affects one million American women every year and hospitalizes three hundred thousand of them. The relatively benign but aggravating and sometimes painful venereal warts affect ten million men and women in America every year. Every time a woman contracts gonorrhea, she has a 40 percent chance of developing pelvic inflammatory disease—infection of the uterus and Fallopian tubes. Even with prompt antibiotic treatment, if she gets three such infections, she has over a 50 percent chance of becoming permanently sterile from them. Most men with just one episode of gonorrhea are likely to develop sterility. Both male and female sterility from these infectious diseases can now be corrected in many cases with very elegant microsurgical techniques. But the pain of surgery and the tremendous expense involved could have all been avoided by the use of a condom.

Every time a woman has sex with a man who carries gonorrhea, she has a 50 percent chance of getting it herself. Every time a man has sex with a woman who has gonorrhea, he has only a 25 percent chance of getting the disease himself. Since men transmit venereal disease more easily than women, you can see how what seems to have started out in Africa as basically a heterosexual disease (AIDS) was transmitted more rapidly in America via homosexual men with multiple sex partners, although AIDS occurs in the American heterosexual population as well.

You might be surprised to learn that cancer of the cervix is a sexually transmitted disease. The specific organism that causes cancer of the cervix has not been identified and certainly is not amenable to antibiotics. But cancer of the cervix virtually never occurs in nuns, or women with only one sexual partner. It is most common in women who had their first episode of sex under the age of twenty, who have had three or more sexual partners before age thirty-five, or whose sexual partner has had three or more partners. A variety of sexual partners means you are more likely to come across an infectious organism that gets into the cervix, leads to precancerous lesions, and eventually to cancer. However, women with multiple sexual partners who use a diaphragm, or whose partners always use a condom, are very unlikely to get cancer of the cervix.

In the chapter on the IUD, I discussed the case of a young patient with a rash all over her body who came into a birth control clinic I was visiting to complain that she was allergic to the copper in her IUD. She was already counting the money her lawyer would be able to get for her. She had already had two children by age twenty-three, she was unmarried, had multiple sex partners, and had no idea what to do with her children or with her life. When she found out that her rash was not an allergy to the copper in the IUD but rather a symptom of syphilis, she decided to keep her IUD, because it was certainly her safest guarantee against getting pregnant again and obviously wasn't the cause of her rash. The doctors left her IUD in place because they were so afraid that any other method of birth control that would require effort on her part might result in another pregnancy and the birth of a syphilitic baby. But what this woman really needed was either to use a diaphragm herself, or to insist on not making love with any man who didn't use a condom. She is getting no protection against any of the twenty-four different sexually transmitted diseases (including cancer of the cervix and AIDS) from her IUD.

In the chapter on tubal sterilization I refer to a young patient who went through a real contraceptive bind in what she called her "promiscuous period." She was afraid of the "dangers" of the birth control pill, and quite properly feared that if she were to contract a sexually transmitted disease, the IUD would increase her risk of developing the complication of sterility from it. So she decided to have a sterilization, which we were able to reverse successfully ten years later, when she found herself happily married. But was she really in such a bind that she had to take the extreme step of sterilization? No! In fact, in view of the wide variety of her sex partners at that time, the only reasonable contraceptives for her were condoms or the diaphragm. But she never entertained the thought. After all, what nice girl is going to go into a drugstore and purchase a pack of condoms from a sneering pharmacist? Well, all that has changed now, thanks to AIDS.

AIDS

There are over 21,000 Americans with classic AIDS. Unless we can find a cure, all of them will almost certainly die. By 1991 the Public Health Service estimates that 54,000 Americans will die from AIDS every year. By that time there will have been a cumulative total of 270,000 Americans who have contracted AIDS, and again, all of them either will have died, or will be about to die. This is only the tip of the iceberg. Ten times that many people get an "AIDS-related complex" caused by the same AIDS virus which is not quite as deadly as the classic AIDS. This is an epidemic of massive proportions that clearly is going to eventually affect both heterosexuals and homosexuals with multiple partners. There is at present no cure, and the only preventatives are abstinence or condoms.

About two million Americans actually have the AIDS virus, which is called the HTLV-3 virus. About 10 percent of those will get full-blown AIDS, but 25 percent of them will get one of the ARC, or AIDS-related complex. Classic AIDS presents with symptoms such as night sweats, fever, general feeling of tiredness and fatigue, loss of appetite, unexplained weight loss, and usually some enlargement of lymph nodes. This is associated with a positive blood antibody test to the HTLV-3 virus. Skin tests to a variety of irritants are all negative, indicating complete loss of immune activity. Finally, a rare type of cancer of the blood vessels called Kaposi's sarcoma presents itself as purplish sores on the skin. Alternatively, the person might develop pneumonia from a very rare organism called Pneumocystis Carini. Both of these illnesses—Kaposi's sarcoma cancer and pneumonia from Pneumocystis Carini—occur only in people whose immune system has stopped working. They are two of the common modes of death for kidney transplant patients who received too much drug to suppress their immune system to prevent rejection of the transplanted organ.

But this classic presentation is not the only way in which the AIDS virus can affect you. A good many more people get terribly ill from the ARC, the AIDS-related complex. These patients develop neurological diseases when the AIDS virus attacks the spinal cord, as well as brain damage. They may develop fevers, swollen glands, and mononucleosis-like symptoms, and possibly some form of lymph node cancer different from what was originally narrowly classified as AIDS.

In Africa more than 6 percent of the population is infected with the AIDS virus, which has spread almost everywhere across that continent. AIDS in Africa, unlike in the United States, started out as a strictly heterosexual disease affecting both men and women in equal numbers. Sixty percent of female prostitutes in Kenya carry the virus, while nearly 90 percent of female prostitutes in Rwanda are infected. By virtue of its spread through users of intravenous drugs, as well as through bisexuals and contaminated blood transfusions, it has spread to the heterosexual population of the United States. One study in New York reported fifty-seven cases of heterosexual partners infected with AIDS, 37 percent of whom caught that disease from purely heterosexual behavior. About ten million people in the world carry the AIDS virus at present but do not yet have symptoms. Within a decade 20 to 30 percent of these AIDS carriers will become AIDS victims. This is very reminiscent of the deadly course I described for syphilis, a disease whose birth came about five hundred years ago under conditions very similar to those now. The only difference is that today there are condoms.

Although we have no clear evidence that the diaphragm would protect against AIDS as much as the condom, it is clear that the diaphragm does protect against most other sexually transmitted diseases. Furthermore, protection from sexually transmitted diseases is not the only advantage of the diaphragm or the condom. As the Japanese have demonstrated, barrier methods are completely free of risk from dangerous side effects, are tremendously convenient in terms of availability, and really need not interfere with the joy of lovemaking if they become part of foreplay. Despite the safety of condoms and diaphragms, which is obvious to everyone, there always is someone who is going to spread scary rumors and point out the dangers inherent in anything we do, much like those who would claim that rhythm birth control creates an increased risk of having an abnormal baby.

"Risks" of Barrier Methods

You won't believe this one, but in 1980 a scientific paper was published speculating that reduced exposure to human semen might increase a woman's risk of breast cancer. The author therefore recommended against the use of condoms or diaphragms unless women were aware that by using them, they might be increasing their risk of contracting cancer. So here you thought you would be safe by avoiding the supposed risks of the birth control pill and IUD, only to find that someone is telling you the diaphragm or condom is dangerous because it reduces your exposure to semen! I have no doubt that after the lawyers have collected all of their money from lawsuits against the IUD, they may try their luck at the diaphragm-, and condommakers.

The effective use of the diaphragm, as I will explain a little later, requires the addition of a nontoxic spermicidal cream, foam, or jelly called nonoxynol-9. In over forty years of experience with this spermicide, no toxic effects have been found. Yet in 1981 a doctor named Jick was the first to suggest that there might be a link between spermicide use near the time of conception and the occurrence of a wide range of congenital fetal defects. Largely because of such papers, which come as an exception to over forty years of clinical experience, a lawsuit was actually won claiming that a baby was born with a limb defect because the mother used this spermicide around the time she conceived. The vast majority of studies before and since these papers have shown no effect at all of nonoxynol-9 on the fetus.

The study by Jick involved not a single patient he had ever seen, talked to, or examined. It was one of these statistical computer chart studies in which over four thousand women's hospital records at the time of delivery were checked to see whether they had had a prescription filled for a contraceptive spermicide somewhere within a two-year period prior to delivering the baby. There was no record as to whether the women had actually used the spermicide, or had indeed used it at any time around the time they conceived. Jick said that 17 of the 763, or an incidence of 2.2 percent, of the women who had filled a prescription for spermicide had children with some kind of birth defect. Only 39 of 3,902 women who had not filled such a prescription had a baby with a birth defect, an incidence of 1.1 percent. Jick concluded from this that women who have used the spermicide at any time within two years of having a baby have twice the risk of congenital birth defects.

Experts found his study flawed for many reasons, not the least of which was the fact that the national rate of congenital birth defects is 2.1 percent in women who have never used any contraceptive at all, which is not significantly different from the 2.2 percent that Jick reported in women who filled prescriptions for spermicides. Moreover, there wasn't a single well-defined syndrome or type of congenital defect in these women's children, who had a wide variety of birth defects no different from what is seen in a normal population. Finally, it was never established that the women had used the contraceptive spermicide at any time near when they conceived. Therefore, most experts in the field of genetics and birth defects feel that nonoxynol-9 is completely safe. But it may not be long before an avalanche of bloodthirsty lawyers swoops down on the companies making this contraceptive cream, foam, and jelly, forcing them to take it off the market. If they do so, then the diaphragm, as well as the new sponge, will be completely useless.

In fact, a jury awarded 4.7 million dollars to a couple who blamed their child's birth defect on this spermicide. The United States Supreme Court reviewed the case and upheld the verdict. It is inconceivable that Ortho will be able to keep this product, which has proven to be extremely safe for millions of women, on the market. So there goes the diaphragm and the contraceptive sponge.

The Diaphragm

For those of you who believe that the sexual revolution began in 1945 with the discovery of penicillin, or the invention of the IUD, it may come as a surprise to discover that its true origins were in Victorian England with the popularization of the "Dutch cap," or Mensinga diaphragm. Once again, as with the IUD, Germans deserve credit for the invention. Dr. Friedrich Wilde first invented the cervical cap in 1838, and it was mass-produced by the mid-1800s with the discovery of the process for vulcanization of rubber. The cervical cap (which will be discussed later) fitted directly over the cervix and had to be form-fitted specifically to each woman, so many couldn't wear it. Thus, even though it had the advantage that it could be worn for long periods of time without the need for changing, it had enough problems associated with its use that another German, in the 1880s, Dr. C. Hasse (using the false name of Wilhelm Mensinga to protect his good name), invented the much simpler diaphragm, and it immediately became a hit in Germany, Holland, and England.

The diaphragm, however, was not used in the United States for several decades because of laws against its importation. In 1923 Dr. Margaret Sanger, a founder of Planned Parenthood, smuggled them into New York and provided them for women in her clinic. Dr. Sanger's courageous efforts were aided in 1924 when Dr. W. A. Puesey, the president of the American Medical Association, officially endorsed contraception. From then on, modern birth control in the United States was on its way, and the diaphragm gradually increased in popularity year by year until 1960, when the birth control pill became available.

In 1934 only 3 percent of women used the diaphragm, but by 1955, 25 percent of married women used it, and 27 percent had their husbands use a condom. By 1965 the use of the diaphragm had gone down to 10 percent, and by 1974 it was down to 2.7 percent. Now with increased publicity about side effects of the birth control pill and the IUD, 13 percent of married women use the diaphragm, and 49 percent of young female students who are sexually active use it as their preferred method. Twelve percent of all of Planned Parenthood's services involve provision of the diaphragm. From Dr. Wilde's cervical cap and Dr. Mensinga's diaphragm in the 1800s, with its popularization in Holland and in Victorian England, came a method of birth control that has not changed much in almost 150 years except for one addition, which makes it exceptionally effective if used properly: spermicide.

In the 1950s nonoxynol-9 spermicides became available for use with the diaphragm, and this truly made it a potentially very effective method of birth control. A teaspoonful of the spermicide is squeezed from a toothpastelike tube into the dome of the diaphragm before inserting the diaphragm into the vagina to cover the cervix. In this way not only does the diaphragm block the flow of sperm toward the cervix, but also the few sperm that are able to get through are very efficiently killed before they can reach the cervical mucus. In a sense the diaphragm became not merely a barrier (which sometimes is not 100 percent effective as such) but also an efficient holder for spermicide through which any sperm had to travel first and be killed. Interestingly, it was as early as 1923 that Dr. Margaret Sanger originally advocated the use of a spermicide to make the diaphragm more efficient. And long before the invention of the modern diaphragm in the 1800s, women in antiquity would cut a lemon in half and insert it in the vagina with the acidic side toward the cervix. Thus for years, women who wished to avoid pregnancy were utilizing a system whose concept was no different from today's.

EFFECTIVENESS OF THE DIAPHRAGM

How effective is the diaphragm? The most carefully documented study, published in 1976 by the Sanger Institute, followed 2,175 women who were very thoroughly instructed on how to use the diaphragm with contraceptive spermicidal jelly. The study reported only a 2 percent failure rate. Twenty-two of the thirty-seven failures reported inconsistent use of the diaphragm as the reason for the failure. Thus, if the diaphragm is used correctly and consistently, the theoretical pregnancy rate could be as low as 1 percent. But the average pregnancy rate in actual use, among all of the women using the diaphragm, is 12.5 percent. Failure of the diaphragm is consistently related to inadequate training and incomplete instruction, poor fitting, or inconsistent use because of the trouble it requires to put it in before having sex. Various studies have shown a 2.4 percent failure rate, a 7.7 percent failure rate, a 17 percent failure rate, and a 19 percent failure rate, all depending on the motivation of the women, the fit of the diaphragm, and the quality of instruction they received from their physician or clinic.

In a recent large, multicenter study, the failure rate for married women was only 6.2 percent. The failure rate for unmarried women was 14 percent. The failure rate for women under twenty-five years of age was 16.8 percent, and for women over twenty-five it was 9.2 percent. The failure rate was higher for patients who simply wanted to postpone pregnancy for a little while to space their children than it was for women who did not desire any future pregnancy. Thus, how well the diaphragm works in preventing pregnancy for you depends a little bit on your risk-taking attitude, your motivation to prevent pregnancy, and how well you have been instructed. It may also depend a bit on how fertile you are. Older women are much more likely to find it effective than younger women.

HOW TO USE THE DIAPHRAGM

How does the diaphragm work, and how is it fitted? The diaphragm is a dome-shaped rubber cup with a flexible rim. It is inserted into the vagina before sex so that the lower rim rests in the bottom back recess of the vagina, and the top rim rests just behind the pubic bone. This is the bone that you can readily feel at the outlet of the vagina near the clitoris. When resting in this position, the dome of the diaphragm, if properly fitted, completely covers the cervix, and should not dislodge during intercourse. A teaspoonful of spermicidal jelly, foam, or cream is placed in the dome of the diaphragm before insertion, on the side that is to go against the cervix. (Many doctors also recommend lining the rim of the diaphragm with spermicide prior to insertion.) Thus the diaphragm works partly as a barrier and partly as a holder for the spermicide. Without the spermicide the diaphragm is not as effective a contraceptive. You must learn how to insert the diaphragm properly and should not leave the doctor's office or clinic until you are able to do this confidently.

You should plan to have sex within six hours of inserting the diaphragm along with the contraceptive jelly, cream, or foam. If more than six hours have passed since you inserted the diaphragm, the contraceptive protection of the spermicide will have dropped considerably, and you will have to remove the diaphragm, refill it with spermicide, and reinsert it. Therefore, most women wait until they are about to get ready to have sex before inserting their diaphragm. After intercourse, the diaphragm must be left in place for eight hours or longer. If you take it out before eight hours, it is still possible for sperm, however few, to reach the cervical mucus and get you pregnant. Furthermore, you should not leave the diaphragm in place for more than twenty-four hours, to avoid the slight risk of infection. The insertion of the diaphragm is protective only for a single episode of sex. For multiple acts of sex during the same period of time, you will have to insert more contraceptive cream, foam, or jelly into the vagina, since there will be more sperm to kill. This is easily accomplished with the use of an applicator into which you place additional spermicide. The tampon-shaped applicator can then be inserted into your vagina and the spermicide expelled when you press on the plunger. Whatever you do, however, *don't remove the diaphragm before eight hours* to put more spermicide inside the dome and reinsert it. After the eight hours have passed, and you remove the diaphragm, make sure to clean it well with a mild soap, but use no harsh antiseptics, because they could harm the rubber. When not in use, the diaphragm should be stored in its case to keep it clean and dry. The next time you're ready to use it, first hold the diaphragm up to the light and check to be sure it has no small tears or punctures.

It's important to note that when you are using the diaphragm, or any other spermicidal barrier method, you should not douche within eight hours of intercourse. Douching is *not* a contraceptive, and will interfere with the effectiveness of the spermicide.

CHOOSING THE DIAPHRAGM AND HAVING IT FITTED

There are four basic types of diaphragms designed to fit virtually any vagina, but the "arching spring rim" diaphragm is the most popular because it is the easiest for virtually all women to insert. It is made by Ortho and by Ramses. The Ortho model comes in sizes ranging from fifty-five to ninety-five millimeters, and the Ramses comes in sizes ranging from sixty-five to ninety-five millimeters. They cost about ten to fifteen dollars in a U.S. pharmacy. The number size of the diaphragm stands for the diameter of the rim in millimeters. When fitting the diaphragm, the goal is to get the largest rim size that is still comfortable. The physician must just make sure that the diaphragm will fit firmly in place and can only be dislodged either by the woman or her partner, using their fingertips. You can see how the diaphragm that was popularized in the late 1800s by Dr. Mensinga in Germany is so much easier to put on than the cervical cap, which was invented by Dr. Wilde in Germany fifty years earlier.

There are three other types of diaphragms. One is a "flat spring rim," which is very thin and delicate with a gentle spring and that has to be put in with an introducer and is especially suited for an extremely tight vagina. The "coil spring rim" is a somewhat sturdier rim, which works just fine for a somewhat looser vagina than the flat spring rim. The "wide seal rim" comes in both the arching spring variety and the coil spring variety. It is made by the Milex Company. It simply has, attached to the inner edge of the rim, a 1.5-centimeter flexible flange that supposedly holds the spermicide better and creates a better seal over the cervix. Again, the "arching spring" type is the most popular because it is easiest to insert.

The diaphragm must be fitted properly. This takes time and instruction, and may be done either by doctors or paramedicals such as nurses. The proper size diaphragm should fit snugly but comfortably between the deep lower recess of the vagina below, and the pubic bone above. Making sure the fit is right, and teaching the patient how to insert the diaphragm, simply takes time, and often a nurse is more likely to be able to give you this time than the doctor. The biggest error is to choose too small a size so that the diaphragm doesn't maintain its position over the cervix. Too large a diaphragm will cause some pain and discomfort. So you simply want to go for the largest size that doesn't hurt.

The doctor or nurse determines the size that will most likely fit you correctly in the following manner: First he or she inserts the index and middle fingers into the vagina until they hit the back wall. Next he or she uses the tip of the thumb to mark the spot on the index finger where it touches the pubic bone, then removes the fingers and measures the distance between the tip of the middle finger and thumb. This represents the proper size of the diaphragm. Once he or she has determined what the probable correct size of the diaphragm is, the nurse or doctor will insert a sample diaphragm of this size inside you and see how well it fits. If possible, you may have to go up or down a few sizes so that you get the largest possible size that fits snugly and yet is not uncomfortable.

You then need to learn how to insert the diaphragm yourself before leaving the doctor's office. First, you place about a teaspoonful of the spermicidal foam, cream, or jelly inside the dome of the diaphragm (see Figure 6-1), on the side that will be directed against the cervix (that is, going inside); you may also line the rim of the diaphragm with spermicide. Then you squeeze the two sides of the rim together and insert the diaphragm, with the contraceptive jelly on the inside wall, into your vagina (see Figure 6-2a). The diaphragm should guide itself into place after insertion with an additional push from your forefinger

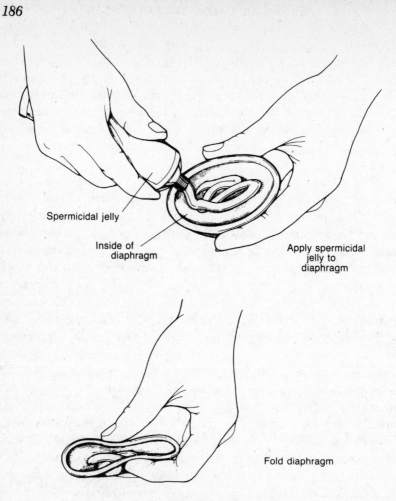

Spermicidal jelly

Inside of
diaphragm

Apply spermicidal
jelly to
diaphragm

Fold diaphragm

FIGURE 6–1.

(Figure 6–2b). The lower rim of the diaphragm should go all the way back into the lower recess of the vagina and then the upper rim should fit right under your pubic bone (Figure 6–2c). If you put it in properly it should not dislodge unless you specifically use your fingers again to push the two sides of the rim toward each other, or hook your forefinger over the rim to pull the diaphragm out of place.

You may find insertion a little tricky at first because the spermicide may make the diaphragm a bit slippery, but don't give up! You'll master the technique quickly with a little practice. The doctor or nurse should supervise your insertion and removal of the diaphragm in the clinic or office at least once before you leave.

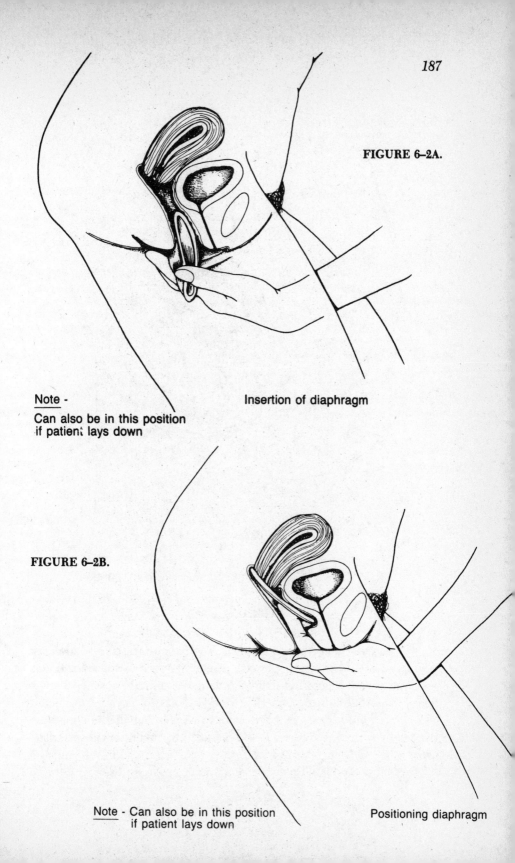

FIGURE 6–2A.

Insertion of diaphragm

<u>Note -</u>
Can also be in this position
if patient lays down

FIGURE 6–2B.

<u>Note</u> - Can also be in this position
if patient lays down

Positioning diaphragm

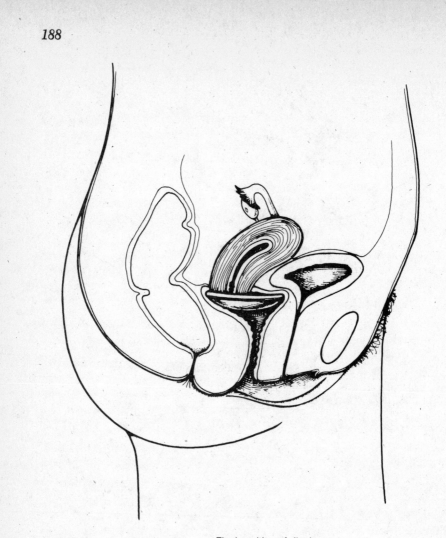

Final position of diaphragm

FIGURE 6–2C.

When you leave in the diaphragm (which can also be easily used when you are having your period), a small amount of spermicide may leak out of your vagina, so many women prefer to use a panty liner to guard against staining.

You should have your gynecologist check your diaphragm every two years or so to make sure it still fits well, and that the rubber hasn't worn out.

What should you do if your diaphragm becomes dislodged during intercourse? You should immediately add more contraceptive foam, jelly, or cream to kill any sperm that might be present, stop intercourse, and remove the diaphragm. You may then refill the diaphragm with fresh spermicide, reinsert it, and resume sex.

Some women complain that they can feel the pressure of the diaphragm against their cervix during intercourse, and this can be a source of discomfort for many. If this occurs, you should check with your gynecologist to see that the diaphragm has been properly fitted. Discomfort may also indicate that the shape of your vagina makes it difficult for you to accommodate a diaphragm, and you may have to opt for a different method of birth control.

It is also worth noting that the diaphragm may be slightly more expensive to use than other methods of birth control such as the pill or IUD, because of the cost of the spermicidal cream, foam, or jelly. You may find the costs lower at Planned Parenthood, university health services, and other facilities.

After reading all this you may be asking yourself: Why should I bother with this mess? Isn't it too much trouble? Well, remember that this contraceptive, unlike the IUD, does not give you any increased risk of pelvic infection and subsequent sterility. In fact, it reduces your risk of contracting gonorrhea despite the possibility of multiple partners. The spermicide is lethal not only to gonorrhea but also to herpes viruses and trichomonas. It is not known for sure whether the diaphragm plus spermicide protects against either chlamydia or AIDS, but there is a likelihood that it does. Certainly the safest protection against AIDS is the condom, but it is possible that subsequent studies will demonstrate good protection with the diaphragm plus contraceptive jelly. The diaphragm definitely decreases dramatically the risk of precancerous lesions, and cancer itself, of the cervix. Women who use the diaphragm have about one fifth the risk of getting cancer of the cervix as women who use any other method of birth control except for the condom.

Contraceptive Vaginal Sponge

Natural sea sponges have been used since antiquity for contraception. They are one of history's oldest methods for preventing pregnancy, and they date back to ancient Egypt. The woman would stuff the sponge into her vagina after soaking it with some oil or other solution that was toxic to sperm, and it worked in the same three ways that the modern sponge, first approved by the U.S. government in 1983, works. There are three modes of action. First, the sponge acts as a barrier (albeit imperfect) to sperm reaching the cervix. Second, the sponge absorbs the semen and in this fashion also helps to prevent it from reaching the cervix. Third, the sponge has in it one gram of the spermicide we have already talked about, nonoxynol-9. Without this spermicide, the sponge would be very ineffective.

The sponge is not truly an effective occlusive device like the diaphragm, the cervical cap, or the condom. Its major function is as a receptacle for the sperm-killing chemical. Its advantage over the diaphragm is that it is extremely convenient, and it lasts for a one- or two-day period. You do not have to inject more spermicide into the vagina for multiple acts of sex. The sponges come separately wrapped and three to a box, with full instructions for use. Each has a concave dimple that fits over the cervix so as to decrease the chance of the sponge being dislodged during sex. There is a woven polyester loop on the outside that you can use for a convenient pullout when you are done. One size fits all. The sponge is completely disposable. You simply throw it away when you are done. You do not have to be fitted for it, or even see a doctor. But despite all this convenience, it has a 10 percent failure rate no matter how properly it is used, and therefore it is not a terribly reliable contraceptive.

The contraceptive vaginal sponge's extreme convenience, lack of messiness (which is women's main objection to the diaphragm), and total absence of potentially dangerous side effects make it a very reasonable contraceptive for women who simply want to space their children, would rather not get pregnant right away, but who wouldn't really mind all that terribly if they did get pregnant.

To use the sponge you simply moisten it in tap water and insert it deep into the vagina (see Figures 6–3a, b, and c). It provides continuous protection for up to twenty-four or more hours. As with the diaphragm, the sponge must be left in place for at least six hours and preferably eight hours after sex. Removal earlier than that will definitely increase your risk of getting pregnant.

A May 1987 study published in the *Journal of the American Medical Association* suggested that the sponge offers some protection against Chlamydia and gonorrhea but may increase the wearer's likelihood of becoming infected with Candida. Other studies need to be done to prove or disprove other possible health benefits.

The sponge frequently is referred to as being equivalent in effec-

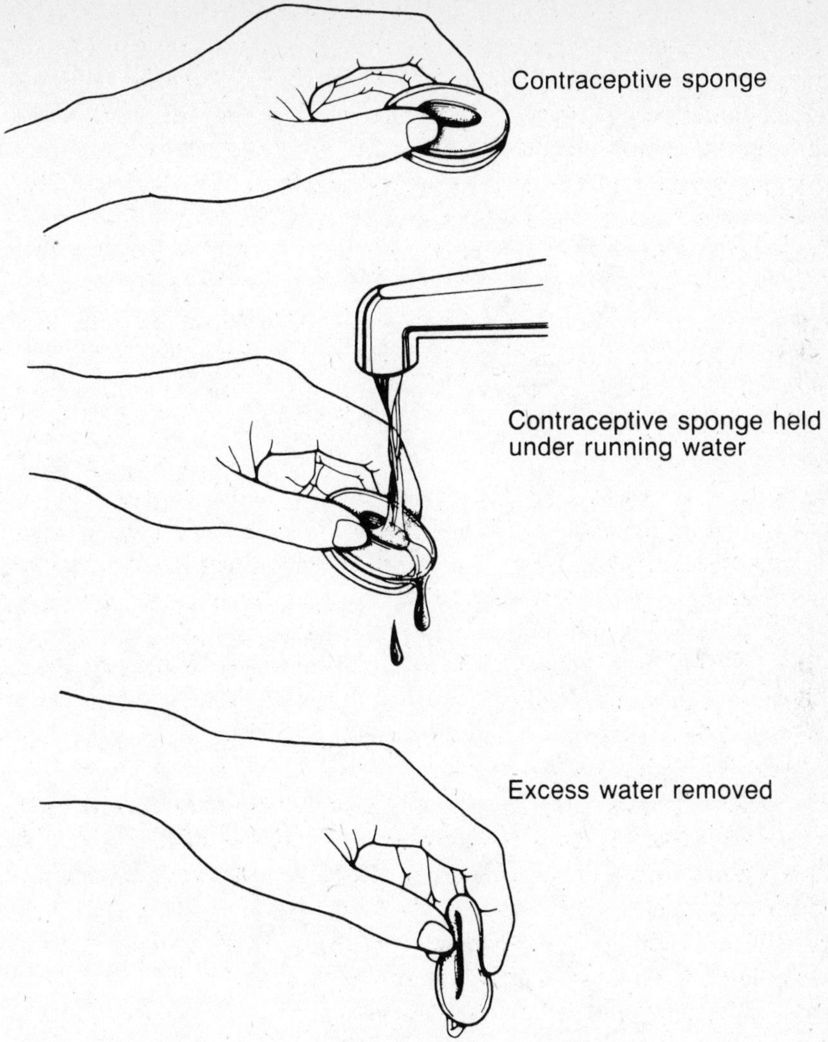

Contraceptive sponge

Contraceptive sponge held under running water

Excess water removed

FIGURE 6–3A.

tiveness to "other barrier methods," and this statement probably may be true, but is not fully documented yet. The condom, if used properly, has a theoretical failure rate of less than 1 percent, and the diaphragm with contraceptive jelly has a theoretical failure rate of less than 2 percent. But no study has shown the sponge to have a theoretical failure rate of any less that 8 percent, and almost all studies comparing the sponge to the diaphragm have shown the sponge to be inferior in con-

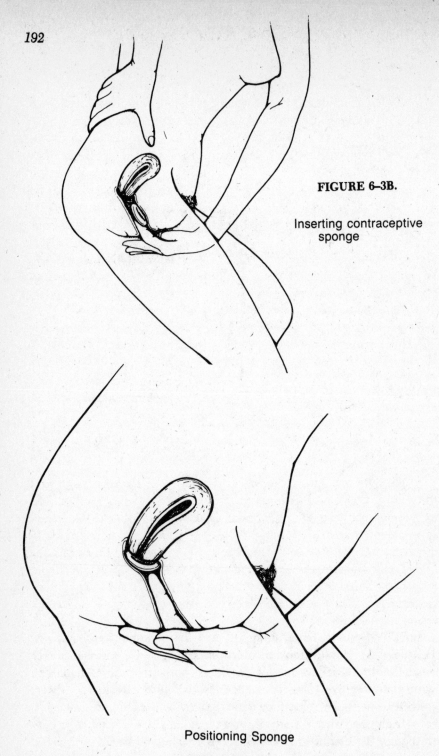

FIGURE 6–3B.

Inserting contraceptive
sponge

Positioning Sponge

FIGURE 6–3C.

traceptive effectiveness. But the diaphragm has a higher failure rate than the sponge if not used properly.

In a large randomized study among women who have already had children conducted by the National Institutes of Health, the sponge had a pregnancy rate of 28 percent, whereas the diaphragm had a pregnancy rate of 13 percent. This would suggest that in the narrower vagina of the woman who has never had a child, the sponge might possibly serve as a more effective barrier than in a woman who has already had a child. However, in a study performed in Britain, both in women who have had children and in women who haven't had children, the sponge performed considerably worse than the diaphragm, with a pregnancy rate of 27 percent and 23 percent respectively compared to the diaphragm's 16 percent and 9.6 percent. Furthermore, at least half of sponge pregnancies were not related to inconsistent or inadequate use of the technique.

In summary, the contraceptive spermicidal sponge is a marvelous idea that may in the future be a superb and completely reliable, simple barrier method of contraception. For the present, however, it is best used as a delaying device for women who really wouldn't mind very much if they eventually did get pregnant when they least expected it.

Toxic Shock Syndrome and the Diaphragm and Sponge

There is one rare, potential complication of the diaphragm and the sponge that you need to be aware of: toxic shock syndrome. You may remember reading several years ago about women who developed severe fever, diarrhea, vomiting, muscle ache, and rash—many of whom died—from using the new "superabsorbent" tampons and leaving them in for many days at a time without changing them. It was discovered that these tampons get soaked with blood, which is a good medium for bacteria to multiply in, and the normal bacteria, staphylococcus, which reside in the vagina, then multiply and release a toxin much the same as in food poisoning, but which produces much more severe symptoms. This problem virtually never occccurred before superabsorbent tampons, because before that women needed to change tampons more frequently. But if these women left tampons in for many days, as was soon discovered, they could become infected.

The same risk of toxic shock syndrome can occur if the diaphragm, or sponge, is left in for more than twenty-four to forty-eight hours, particularly during menstruation. The risk of this, however, is incredibly small. Ten of 100,000 users per year will develop toxic shock syndrome. Three percent of these women will die. That means that there is a death rate of 0.3 per 100,000, which compares to the normal death rate from pregnancy of 8.3 per 100,000. So you need to be aware of toxic shock syndrome and make sure not to leave one of these devices in for more than twenty-four hours. If you follow that precaution, then the diaphragm and the sponge are quite free of dangerous side effects.

The Cervical Cap

The cervical cap was first invented in 1838 and was the precursor to the more popular diaphragm, both of which were invented in Germany. Despite the fact that the cap was invented 150 years ago and is widely marketed in Europe, it is still unavailable in the United States. Like a forbidden fruit, it has become a rallying cry in women's health groups who are infuriated by our slow governmental machinery, which won't approve this perfectly safe contraception device. But once it does become available, don't get too excited. It has a lot of problems, and 50 percent of the women who start using it with enthusiasm, discard it within a year.

Actually, the concept behind the cervical cap was used four thousand years ago when women of Asia and the Middle East used various herbs and plants to occlude their cervix and create a hostile vaginal environment. The same concept of barrier plus spermicide is described in an Egyptian papyrus from 1850 B.C., which talks about three different types of vaginal pessaries, all made of a soft material that, when placed in the vagina, would then harden and occlude the cervix. One was made of crocodile dung, another of honey and bicarbonate, and a third of gum resin. Later women finally discovered the method of inserting a hollowed-out lemon half described earlier in my section on the history of the diaphragm.

The modern cervical cap is virtually the same as the one first invented by Dr. Friedrich Wilde in 1838 in Germany. They are custom-made rubber devices and are very popular in England today. Throughout the mid-1800s the demand throughout Europe was widespread for the cervical cap until the 1880s, when Wilhelm Mensinga (Dr. C. Hasse) popularized the diaphragm. Interestingly, the only reason the diaphragm is widely available in the United States while the cervical cap is widely used in England is that back in the early 1900s, the American pioneer Dr. Margaret Sanger preferred the diaphragm of Mensinga, and the British contraceptive pioneer Dr. Maria Stokes preferred the cap. Thus the cap-diaphragm controversy really has its basis in the early bias in the United States toward the diaphragm advocated by early American women's rights leaders.

The theoretical advantage to the cap (and the reason for its zealous endorsement) is that it can be left in place for longer than the diaphragm and therefore is not as inconvenient. In fact, women who used the early caps that were available in the United States forty years ago left them in place for weeks at a time. This was extremely convenient but led to a lot of infections, and the cap did not receive FDA approval. Nowadays we know that this practice can lead to some disastrous complications such as toxic shock syndrome, and the cap should not be worn continuously for more than two days.

Most studies show the cap to have a failure rate of 8 to 19 percent, which certainly is no better than the diaphragm, or for that matter the contraceptive sponge. The cap still has to be custom-fitted. Unlike the diaphragm, where specific measurements can be taken, the fitting has to be largely by trial and error. So what is the reason for this strong resurgence of interest in the cervical cap with a heavy political movement toward getting it approved in the United States? The major reason probably is the emotional one that it is perfectly safe, has been around for 150 years, and there is no good reason not to have it available. But when it does become available I would predict it will not be very popular or indeed very remunerative to the companies making it.

Thirty-seven percent of the women who use the cap complain that when they leave it in for more than two days there always is a problem with odor from retained secretions. Twenty-five to 30 percent of the women who tried it could not be fitted because their cervix was either too long or too short. Twenty percent complained of difficult removal and reinsertion. Eighteen percent complained of dislodgement during coitus. For all these reasons, there is generally at least a 40 to 50 percent dropout rate within the first year of use.

Vaginal Contraceptive Spermicides

Ever since women first figured out that a lemon had its own built-in spermicidal juices, sperm-killing techniques have been used for contraception. In fact, even the IUD is a sperm-killing device. The modern spermicide ingredient in almost any contraceptive foam, cream, or jelly is nonoxynol-9. This spermicidal agent has been used for over forty years, and hundreds of thousands of women in many studies have demonstrated its safety both to the wife and the future child. It works as a surfactant, which kills the membrane of the sperm cells. Because it is equally effective in killing the membrane of bacteria and parasites, it affords excellent protection against sexually transmitted diseases. When used alone, spermicide has generally been thought of as a rather insecure method of birth control, not to mention being somewhat messy. But it is crucial to the effectiveness of the diaphragm and is the major element in the popularity of the new contraceptive sponge. It is even available in a new condom called Ramses-Extra, the only condom on the American market that contains a spermicide.

When used alone as a contraceptive (not in conjunction with a diaphragm, a cervical cap, or a sponge), nonoxynol-9 is squeezed out of an applicator tube into the vagina as a foam rather than a jelly or cream. Foam would not be appropriate to use in a diaphragm because the contraceptive action will not last as long as a jelly or cream, which works for a good six to eight hours. But the foam does help to block the passage of sperm toward the cervix and so is the necessary form of spermicide to use if you are not using it with anything else. Since foam doesn't last as long as contraceptive jelly or cream, you should plan to have sex within thirty to sixty minutes of inserting the foam in the vagina, rather than the six hours you have with contraceptive jelly in the diaphragm. As with the diaphragm, you will need to insert more spermicide if you have intercourse more than once. Some couples have used this as a sole method of birth control with no failures for as long as five, ten, or fifteen years. Some have used it in combination with condoms. It seems that in certain couples it is an extremely effective method when used consistently. The failure rate varies widely from 1.5 to 29 percent. Yet recent studies have shown that in very well-motivated, intelligent couples, the method failure rate can be as low as 2 to 5 percent. This makes the use of such a vaginal spermicide not a bad adjunctive measure if you need some extra protection (for example, if you forgot your pill a couple of days during the month, or if your IUD comes out before you have a chance to embark upon a new method of birth control).

A new risk, however, has loomed on the horizon for nonoxynol-9, which may not only involve its being taken off the market, but also may involve taking diaphragms, cervical caps, and sponges off the market as well. As I mentioned before, early in 1986 a jury awarded $4.7 million to a woman who claimed that her child's birth defects resulted from her use of Ortho-Gynol contraceptive jelly (which is the jelly most recommended for use with the diaphragm). This case was appealed to the U.S. Supreme Court, and the company amazingly still lost. If the cost of litigation exceeds the earnings that Ortho makes from this product, it cannot possibly remain on the market. Lawyers whose cash flow has been severely injured by the Robins Company (makers of the Dalkon Shield) going into bankruptcy and stopping payments on all further claims, and who are doubtless disappointed by Searle taking the extremely safe Copper 7 IUD off the market, may well jump to nonoxynol-9 as a new potential gold mine.

But how can a jury not have sympathy with a child who is born without an arm or leg? We all want to blame someone for our misfortune and get some compensation. And when a big, wealthy insurance company can be told to pay $4.7 million to an unhappy mother with a tragically crippled child, what human being is going to turn her down? But society pays, because I assure you with this case having been lost on appeal to the Supreme Court there will soon be no more diaphragms, cervical caps, vaginal sponges, or any contraceptive jellies or foams available anymore in this country. You will have to go to Canada or another foreign country and go to any drugstore or grocery store, pick up a year's supply, and come back home with it.

The Condom, or Rubber

The modern condom is a thoroughly up-to-date device and is the safest of all contraceptives. For teenagers and particularly those with multiple partners, it is unquestionably the ideal contraceptive. It offers the best available protection against sexually transmitted disease. In fact, it was originally used not so much for contraception but to protect against venereal disease. As one doctor put it, it was used originally by rich men who cared less about what they might leave behind than what they might bring home. Although it is described in Egyptian papyruses as a decorative cover to be worn over the penis, the original condom was invented in modern form in A.D. 1564 by the great anatomist Fallopius, the same man who described the woman's Fallopian tubes in which the egg is fertilized. It was only natural that the condom would be invented after the Renaissance gave rise to the incredible epidemic of venereal disease of the fifteenth century, which I described earlier in this chapter. These early condoms were first made of linen sheets, and then later animal intestines, which were found to be superior. They were first called "condoms" in the 1700s and were popularized as a means of "protection from venereal disease and numerous bastard offspring" by the famous Casanova (1725–98). In the 1840s, with the vulcanization of rubber, mass production of "rubbers" was finally possible. Today forty million couples in the world use the condom as a sole method of birth control. It is the second most widely used reversible contraceptive method in the United States, only after the pill.

Ten million Japanese couples use the condom exclusively, which represents 75 percent of all Japanese using birth control. Seven million couples in Europe and three million couples in the United States and Canada use the condom. It is not just a birth control method for happy little kids to carry around in their wallets so they have something available when they hit it big some night. The concept of the condom as a legitimate method of birth control for happily married couples who want to avoid the messiness of the diaphragm and the dangers of the IUD and the pill is finally coming home.

I must confess that I, too, held the same stigma of associating the condom with promiscuity and venereal disease that most of you readers probably came to this book with as well. Many doctors don't even mention it as an alternative when women discuss family planning with them. In fact, you used to be able to get the condom only by purchasing it in a dispenser at a gas station, or by buying an embarrassingly obscene-looking package from your local pharmacist.

But all that is changing. The modern condom industry is a reputable, big business. American companies this time are actually copying the Japanese. For more than twenty years the condom has been the primary method of birth control in Japan's incredible population control program. For years Japan has made the thinnest, strongest, finest condoms on the market, packaged colorfully and attractively in a way designed to entice any purchaser to pick up a box. The condom in America alone now is a $250 million-a-year industry, and nearly 40 percent of them across America are purchased by women. In California 60 percent of condoms are purchased by women rather than men.

All condoms in the United States have to meet rigid government standards, and fewer than 0.4 percent are defective. Most of these defects have been shown not to be so severe as to result in a pregnancy.

American condoms now are thinner and stronger, and even have reservoirs at the tip to hold the semen. They come in packages that are much easier to open, even in the dark. You can imagine a bedroom scene of twenty years ago with a man in the heat of passion trying to open an impossible seal of a crinkly plastic container in the dark. It is no wonder that frequently he would throw care to the wind, resulting in a high pregnancy rate with this method of contraception. But as big business learns that condoms can be marketed as effectively as toothpaste and shampoo, they are going to become easier and easier to purchase without embarrassment, and easier to use without the fear of interference with spontaneity of the sexual act.

It is now becoming more and more accepted in society that men should participate in birth control. One third of couples in the world using birth control rely on methods that shift the responsibility to the male. Forty million have been vasectomized, and forty million use condoms. Furthermore, a great many use coitus interruptus, which is not very effective but still is a male method. One fifth of Americans use a "male" method of birth control, as do one half of Italians and four fifths of Japanese. As women become more independent and decide they don't want to mess with the pill, don't want to have the discomfort and heavy menstrual bleeding of an IUD, don't want to trouble with the messiness of the diaphragm, and don't want to take their temperature and check their cervical mucus every day, and are not ready to get sterilized, they are going to demand that their partner use a condom. Perhaps even more effectively, they will learn how to make it part of the excitement of sexual foreplay.

How effective is the condom? A British study showed a little less than a 1 percent failure rate when used consistently. The actual failure rate, however, in a broad spectrum of couples, some of whom may be motivated and others not so motivated, is about 10 percent. Well-motivated couples who simply forget to use the condom from time to time have a failure rate of about 3 to 5 percent. But couples who never fail to use the condom have a failure rate of consistently less than 1 percent. The only reason for condom failure, with the very occasional exception of defects or rips, is not using it. If a condom could become an accepted and inevitable part of the lovemaking routine, it would surely be the end of your search for an ideal contraceptive. It is cheap, it imposes responsibility on the male, and anyone can get it anytime without the need for a visit to a doctor or clinic. It's extremely easy to use; the condom should simply be placed over the penis before insertion. It provides the most effective protection for sexually transmitted diseases available with the exception of abstinence, and it prevents cancer of the cervix. It has no health hazards.

A study of Australian soldiers in Vietnam demonstrated almost complete protection against a wide variety of simply awful venereal diseases that were rampantly hitting other servicemen. In Sweden there was a widespread epidemic of gonorrhea until the government pushed its program of encouraging condom use. Now about 40 percent of Scandinavian couples use condoms, and there is very little gonorrhea anymore in that country.

But there are some problems. Some men have psychological hangups so that they simply cannot maintain an erection with a condom on. The only solution to this will be if women help make it an enjoyable part of foreplay. Other men complain that the sensitivity at the tip of their penis is decreased too much with a condom and it interferes with their pleasure. I have seen many married men who would rather abstain than have to put on a condom. But certainly for the hot young teenager or the young single who is most at risk for sexually transmitted disease or pregnancies he can't handle, it is very unlikely that anything including the necessity of wearing a condom would interfere with his erection.

There have traditionally been two kinds of condoms, "skins" and "rubbers." Prior to modern rubber manufacturing, the most comfortable and desirable condoms were "skins," made from collagenous natural "skin" or gut of animals. Now, however, with the special "dry" silicone lubrication introduced in the 1960s, rubber condoms give most of the same "feel" as the natural membrane product. Fourex is the classic expensive "natural" skin condom. Popular quality brands of rubber condom are Ramses and Trojan. Mentor is a new, high-quality product in this explosively expanding industry. The effectiveness of the various kinds of condoms is the same.

The risk of using a defective condom is very low now because of government standards and regulations, and the widespread practice of electronic screening for pinholes and weak areas. In 1939 in the United States, 75 percent of condoms were defective. By 1961, only 0.4 to 0.7 percent of condoms were defective.

Make sure to use a condom every time if this is your method of birth control. Use one with a reservoir tip to minimize the chance of bursting or overflow leakage, and also to allow an easy way of checking for an accident after you have finished intercourse. After sex, and before the erection goes down, hold onto the condom when withdrawing the penis from the vagina, taking care not to spill any semen.

One last word: convenience. Condoms all come in the same length (19 centimeters) and the same width (2.5 centimeters). You don't have to be embarrassed by asking the druggist for "big" or "small" sizes. There is no difference, and there is no need for a precise fit.

Coitus Interruptus, or Withdrawing Early

A time-honored technique of birth control, going back to the Old Testament, involves the male withdrawing the penis from the vagina just when he feels ejaculation is pending and ejaculating completely away from the female's vagina. According to the Bible, the man who committed this act was killed by God, but this punishment probably came not because he "wasted the seed" but rather because he failed to honor his duty to his brother's wife to "get her a child." In fact, because of the "moral safety" of this technique, it is used by about 29 percent of couples in Italy and 30 percent of couples in Poland, both highly Catholic countries. Unfortunately, the failure rate, even if used consistently—that is, the lowest possible figure—is 16 percent. In actual use the failure rate is closer to 25 percent. This means it is successful for a population at large in reducing the number of children somewhat, but it is not a reliable method for an individual family. Furthermore, the moment of ejaculation usually is the moment the male feels the strongest urge for deeper penetration, and therefore he may not withdraw soon enough. This is not a fun method of birth control.

Abstinence

At the risk of your closing this book and not going a step farther, I must say at least briefly, particularly for teenagers, that abstinence is a very acceptable alternative for birth control. As of 1976, 45 percent of unmarried teenagers in the United States still had not had sex by age 19. At present we have the largest teenage pregnancy rate in the civilized world. It is estimated that 16 to 20 percent of American girls have been pregnant at least once by age nineteen; the figure in large cities approaches 50 percent. If you include all fourteen- to nineteen-year-olds, over 10 percent have been pregnant at least once. Yet America is no different from the rest of the civilized world in the incidence of sexual activity among teenagers. Our teenagers are having no more and no less sex than teenagers throughout Europe. The only difference is that our teens are getting pregnant because they don't know anything about birth control. So the common solution to this problem is to teach birth control and encourage these teenagers to use it.

But there is another approach that is just so naïve that it may very well begin to catch on. There is no doubt that kids are having more and more sex simply because we are telling them to. The television programs we love to turn on, the movies we love to take them to, and the magazines we love to browse through all have the same message: Sex is great, it's easy, and there are no consequences such as pregnancy or venereal disease to worry about. If we admit that we as a society are telling thirteen-year-olds to have sex, then maybe we can begin to develop programs to help teenagers learn how to say "No." There is no insidious moralizing behind this suggestion. Thirteen-year-olds simply do not have sufficient maturity to take on gigantic responsibilities. They still are in a playful stage of life where they need to learn about emotions, caring, and respect through play. It simply is wise psychologically for teenagers to postpone sexual involvement. If they choose not to postpone it, you must understand it is simply because society has told them not to postpone it. In that case birth control education is critical. But I think it is quite possible to develop programs to help teenagers learn how to say, "I'm going to postpone sexual involvement until I have a better idea who I am and where I am going." Programs that have been most effective involve teenagers counseling teenagers. Peer counseling is extremely effective, and moralizing lectures from adults are completely ineffective.

7

Vasectomy

I realized on a recent trip to the Arctic that vasectomy and its reversibility touches on the central issue of life for most of the peoples of the world. I was traveling in the barren region of the magnetic North Pole, thousands of miles from any populated area, on a three-man expedition consisting of myself and two Eskimos. Kalook, my guide, had no idea that I was an expert on vasectomy. He looked sad as he stared at the floor of the igloo and said to me, "I made a very bad thing last year." I asked what happened. He said, "The government sends a doctor to our camp every year, and last year he gave me a vasectomy." Kalook already had five children. But Kalook deeply regretted that he could not have any more. He said, "I am so sorry I did that. I would like to have more children." I started to laugh, patted Kalook on the back, and said to him, "My friend, you have come to the right igloo."

Vasectomy Is Reversible

For reasons that will become apparent by the end of this chapter, I could assure Kalook a 99 percent chance of having his fertility restored, partly because the vasectomy was so recent, and partly because a delicate microsurgical operation I developed would enable me to restore the continuity of his vas deferens with over 99 percent assurance. But reversibility also is possible for men who have had a vasectomy many years ago. Vasectomy no longer is a simpleminded decision that requires an irrational conviction that no matter how life changes, one would never change his viewpoint about wanting more children. Vasectomy is a welcome relief for most of the four billion people who walk this planet and sometime in their life face the reality that their family probably is as big as they want it. Twenty more years of inconvenient, unsafe, or insecure methods of birth control do not seem as appealing as solving the problem with a simple ten- or twenty-minute operation. But the only drawback to vasectomy has been its irreversibility, and the hesitation of people who think they have had all the children they want, to "burn their bridges." I hope this chapter will help these people "come to the right igloo" also.

Even men with very low sperm counts, who at one time had difficulty getting their wives pregnant, eventually may need a vasectomy. For example, Dan was a patient of mine with severe infertility for five years. Every treatment failed to produce a pregnancy. His sperm count was extremely low, and the motility of the sperm was extremely poor. When he least expected it, however, his wife Alice got pregnant, and they were overjoyed that at last they could have a child. But two years later Alice got pregnant again, and they decided to start using condoms. Two children were quite enough. Then in April 1985 Dan forgot to use the condom once during intercourse, and sure enough, despite Dan's miserably low sperm count, his wife became pregnant again, with their third child. They came into my office begging for a vasectomy "as soon as possible."

Clarence was a patient with infertility for many years who after much effort was finally able to have a child, but then underwent a vasectomy, because he and his wife had decided they wanted to devote all their energy to raising the one child. That was enough for this "modern family." Yet five years after his vasectomy, Clarence wanted to undergo microsurgery to reverse it. So the tables can turn quickly on our views regarding family size.

Vasectomy is one of the most common operations performed in the United States today and certainly is the most popular method of birth control in the world. About ten million American men to date have undergone vasectomy, and almost half a million more undergo this operation every year. It requires ten to twenty minutes, can be done in a doctor's office under local anesthesia, and seems to be the simplest, quickest, safest solution to the problem of how to avoid an unwanted pregnancy. Yet despite careful counseling and warning that this procedure must be considered a "permanent" step, anywhere from 1 to 5 percent of men do change their minds at a later date.

Common causes for wanting to have a vasectomy reversed include divorce and subsequent remarriage; the death of a child; an improvement in financial stability; or simply a change of viewpoint. Almost all the men who regret vasectomy were well counseled, and the vast majority of them made exactly the right decision at that particular time in their life. But life is unpredictable, and that is the central issue around which this chapter revolves.

One patient of mine was working abroad and only got to visit the United States two weeks out of every year. He and his wife had several healthy children and decided that their family was complete, a reasonable decision in view of the tremendous amount of moving and shuffling around the world that they were forced into because of his profession. On one of their trips back to the United States to visit their parents the husband had a vasectomy performed. The day after the vasectomy his wife was killed in an automobile accident, and one child was in critical condition for several weeks. He knew then what a terrible mistake he had made the day before. But just one day earlier it seemed like exactly the right thing to do.

Our lives and our families are held together by such thin threads that it is hard to feel completely comfortable with a permanent decision to be sterilized. A patient of mine from the West Coast had two healthy children, a wonderful wife, a beautiful home, and just about everything anyone could want out of life. His third child, a boy, was born on Christmas Day and was the absolute culmination of all their desires. The patient waited several months to make sure the child would be healthy before having a vasectomy performed by his local urologist. One month after the operation he and his wife noticed a lump on the little four-month-old child's arm, which turned out to be a rare and incurable malignant tumor of the muscle. The child died four months later. The couple knew that having another child would not replace the one they lost, but they simply had to have another child. Ironically, this also was a couple who had experienced great difficulty in having children in the first place, but when they thought they had all the children they had wanted, he had the vasectomy performed.

But for most couples, even those who have had infertility problems in the past, vasectomy comes as a relief, and the great appeal of this method of birth control is its ease and permanence. An old friend from the South Side of Chicago paid me a visit several years ago. I hadn't seen him in twenty years and never knew his wife. For ten years they had tried unsuccessfully to have a baby, and were told by leading authorities on infertility they would never be able to have children. My friend had had several sperm counts that he was told were low, and his wife had gone through every test imaginable with considerable amount of expense and discomfort. Their fertility doctor was rather gruff and unpleasant. Under the pressure of his unnerving bedside manner and the many poorly explained tests she had to go through, her periods became even more erratic than they had been when she first went to see him. Despite much discomfort and many treatments costing a great deal of money, she still did not get pregnant. She finally became furious and decided the next month to give up any thought of ever having children and to pursue other interests in life. That month she became pregnant, and the next two children came in quick succession. Now, several years later, after they had tried the pill and had unpleasant side effects, then the IUD, which eventually gave the wife heavy, uncomfortable menstrual periods with unpleasant cramping, and after becoming totally annoyed with the notion of condoms or foam or diaphragms, my old friend from the South Side of Chicago wanted a vasectomy.

The goal of this chapter is to make you so knowledgeable about vasectomy that you should have little difficulty in deciding when the time has come to terminate all of the more complicated methods of birth control and take this simple, "final solution." But if you so decide, nonetheless, keep reversibility in mind.

What Is Vasectomy?

Sterilization is an operation for either a man or a woman that simply keeps the egg and the sperm from getting together. Sterilization is a terrible-sounding word and conjures up the notion of castration. But it is just a simple dividing of the sperm duct (vas deferens) in the male, or the Fallopian tube in the female. It is not like having your pet dog or cat spayed to prevent it from going into heat and having sex with all the other pets on the block. When your pet is spayed, it undergoes a castration operation in which all the reproductive organs are removed. Your pet literally becomes neutered and much more pleasant to live with. This is also true when a racehorse becomes gelded. With any of these operations on animals the goal is not simply to prevent the animal from getting pregnant, but rather to affect its personality so that it becomes easier to handle. That is not what happens when a human being undergoes sterilization. There is no discernible effect on sexual desire, personality, or any other aspect or functioning except for the fact that you can now no longer have a baby.

There are about one million sterilizations performed in the United States every year, and almost half of those are vasectomies. Most men who undergo vasectomy are over thirty years of age, have two or three children, have already used other methods of birth control with their partner, and have decided they want a quick, simple, safe, permanent end to their worry about having more children. In many cases their wives have suffered from ill effects from birth control pills, or have had painful cramping periods or infections from an IUD. Some have had failure of their method of birth control and so already have unwanted children, and some have already experienced the heartache of having an abortion.

Vasectomy is the most popular method of birth control in the world today. It is a simple operation that can be completed in a few minutes in the doctor's office under local anesthesia with just a handful of surgical instruments. It can just as easily be performed in a tent or a hut in developing world countries and therefore is the bulwark of massive population-control programs in countries such as China, India, Bangladesh, and those in Southeast Asia. It involves a simple severing of the duct called the vas deferens, which carries the sperm from the testicle into the ejaculatory duct. Because this duct can easily be palpated just underneath the scrotal skin, the operation requires only a tiny eighth-inch incision and can be accomplished simply in a matter of minutes. Once the sperm count goes down to zero, the vasectomized man has greater protection from causing an unwanted pregnancy than any other method of birth control would allow him. Furthermore, from then on this method requires no effort, no thought, and not the slightest inconvenience. He and his wife no longer have to take any drugs or chemicals. They don't have to remember to put on a condom. They don't have to do any planning for the fertile period during the month, they don't have to worry about dangerous side effects, and they generally have an improved sex life because they finally have a secure, thoughtless method of birth control.

There is no effect on the man's sex drive or sexual ability. The patient who has had a vasectomy notices no difference in his orgasm or the amount of fluid in his ejaculation. It simply is all fluid and no sperm. He notices no physical change in any aspect of sex, except that because of the absence of sperm in his ejaculate he is unable to impregnate a woman. The reason for this is that 95 percent of the fluid that comes out in the ejaculate issues from the prostate gland and seminal vesicles, which are at the base of the penis beyond the vasectomy site. At the time of ejaculation, normally, sperm are pumped from the epididymis, the delicate ductwork draining sperm out of the testicle, through the vas deferens, and up to the area of the ejaculatory duct at the base of the penis. There is very little fluid carrying the sperm to the ejaculatory duct. Most of what constitutes the ejaculatory fluid then meets the sperm at the ejaculatory duct and literally pushes them out, propelling them with tremendous force from the penis. When the vas deferens is interrupted by vasectomy, none of this changes except that the sperm never arrive at the ejaculatory duct. The ejaculation just takes place as though nothing were different.

The testicles produce the hormone testosterone, which provides men with their sex drive and secondary sex characteristics such as a beard, low voice, increased musculature, higher red blood cell count, increased facial oiliness as compared to women, and, even to some extent aggressiveness. Hormone production by the testicles as well as hormone levels in the blood are completely unaffected by vasectomy, because the hormones are released into the bloodstream directly from the testicle.

Why Is a Vasectomy Said to Be "Irreversible"?

Vasectomy has been considered irreversible in the past because of the difficulty of reuniting the tiny, delicate, inner canal, which is about one-seventieth inch in diameter, or smaller than a period on this page. However, with new microsurgical techniques I developed some years ago, vasectomy can be successfully reversed in the majority of cases. Unfortunately, the vasectomy reversal operation is very intricate. It takes only five or ten minutes in the doctor's office to do a vasectomy, because the outer muscle layer is very hard and the outer wall of the vas is a full eighth-inch thick. It requires no great surgical skill simply to palpate the hard outer wall of the vas and divide it. However, it takes over two hours in a sophisticated operating room with an expensive microscope to reconnect the vas accurately, using stitches that are literally invisible to the naked eye. But the operation is often much more difficult than just reconnecting the tiny inner canal of the vas. Here's why.

After vasectomy the tiny amount of fluid that carries sperm from the testicles begins to accumulate in the vas deferens. The pressure from this accumulation is not felt at all because the canal is very small. Yet pressure does build up, and sperm that otherwise would have gotten out, instead stagnate and die of old age (the longevity of the sperm in the vas deferens is about two weeks to a month). The sperm then gradually decompose, much as our bodies do when we die. Fluid and sperm accumulate in the epididymis, a tiny, coiled, delicate twenty-foot-long canal that carries sperm out of the testicle into the vas deferens. In this area the sperm ductwork is about one-three-hundredth inch in diameter and the thickness of the wall of the duct is one-one-thousandth inch. This twenty-foot-long tubule is all coiled up into a length of only one inch.

Although the amount of fluid from the testicle is tiny compared to the volume of the ejaculate, the pressure that builds up from its continuous production eventually results in microscopic ruptures or "blowouts" in this delicate epididymal duct, causing blockage in that region also. Thus sperm no longer can even get to the vas deferens. These blowouts then cause blockage in this much more delicate area, which requires tremendous microsurgical skill to repair. The good news is that with extremely refined microsurgical techniques, the damage in this area can be repaired or bypassed and the success rate for reversal of vasectomy can still be good. The bad news is that the technique requires so much practice and experience, that very few surgeons can perform it. Thus vasectomy, for practical purposes, still has to be considered a permanent procedure unless it is performed in such a way as to prevent pressure buildup, and I will discuss this new approach later in this chapter.

The only disadvantage to this extremely safe and simple method of birth control is the difficulty associated with making it reversible. For most couples it would be wise not to embark upon vasectomy unless you feel the decision is a permanent one. Yet because vasectomy is so appealing and because life is so changeable, the reversibility of vasectomy is very important, even for those who are "sure" they've had enough.

Should I Have a Vasectomy?

Despite my emphasis on reversibility of vasectomy, it is a good idea only for men who intend it to be permanent. Men who are most likely to regret having had a vasectomy are those who are under thirty, have no children, are suffering from marital problems (and see the vasectomy as a possible solution), and those who only recently have had a child. For example, several years ago I saw a very prominent businessman who had a happy, beautiful marriage and four gorgeous children, including a newborn. With the birth of the fourth child, he and his wife decided quite reasonably that this was it for them. He had a vasectomy performed by a very cautious and judicious physician who counseled them conservatively and wisely. There just seemed to be no question that this was the proper move for them.

Six months later the infant died of an obscure disease, and the parents, who were in their late thirties with three happy, healthy children, wanted another child desperately. They made sure to have careful genetic testing to see if there was any way that this death could have been predictable and whether there was any chance that they had a genetic predisposition toward having a child with such a malady. The answers to all of these exhaustive studies were that the child's death was unpredictable and that they had no genetic problem whatsoever.

The most dangerous period in a child's life is the first year, and particularly the first six months. Sudden infant death syndrome, known as "crib death," is so common that it probably is the biggest threat to our future existence when we are first born. Once we get past the age where crib death is a risk, the chances of dying prematurely from some other cause are comparatively low. The same can be said for the development of obscure and unpredictable diseases like the one to which this family's little baby succumbed. So no matter how complete your family has become in your own mind, wait until your youngest child is at least six months to one year old before you have a vasectomy.

Georgia was a schoolteacher who came to my office with her husband to have reversal of a vasectomy that had been performed ten years earlier just after the birth of their second son. In this case no child had died, but Georgia described what virtually all women will understand after having had several children. The discomfort of childbirth, the tremendous responsibility, and the time-consuming twenty-four-hour ordeal of taking care of a young infant, make this a time not of great wisdom and reflection but rather of exhaustion and intense devotion to an all-consuming job. Yet that's when this couple had decided to get a vasectomy. This was not the time to make a permanent decision, even assuming that no disaster befalls the child.

Georgia and her husband, an outstanding educator and headmaster of a religious school, had a beautiful, stable marriage with two impeccably polite, creative, and caring children, the youngest of whom was now ten. She had had an extraordinarily painful childbirth, and only now, ten years later, were they able to face their regret squarely. These people were just naturals to raise beautiful children. Any arbitrary limit that a "zero population growth" philosophy would make such as "two children per family" makes no sense when you see people like this, who are clearly capable of raising as many children as Nature will allow them. These people maintain that the Malthusian concept of population control applies only if we forget about the tremendous creative energy of human beings to make the earth provide. They maintain that if children are raised to respect their fellow human beings, to bend swords into plowshares, and to know love instead of hate, there clearly is enough room on this planet or beyond, if the human mind takes us in that direction through the development of space travel. This was similar to the view of Kalook, my Eskimo friend from the North Pole, who knew that with ingenuity and love he could support more than five children living on six feet of frozen Arctic Ocean ice.

Therefore, the number of children you have already had is not an absolute determinant of whether vasectomy is right for you. Although it is true that men who have had no children are more likely to regret having had a vasectomy, many of them plan on leading lives that just have no room for raising children. Similarly, many couples with more than the standard modern number of two or three children will feel that their lives have become empty because they cannot have more, and children from such large families need not suffer if their lives are full of love. One need only look at well-known families such as the Osmonds, coming from a religious Mormon background, or the Von Trapps from Austria, or Orthodox Jews for whom family is everything. It is a popular observation that these people raise large, marvelous families. But for others a large family can be a bitter sword that chops up into little pieces their chance for ever developing enough self-esteem and education to be productive members of society.

John was a forty-six-year-old Mormon man married to a thirty-five-year-old Mormon woman. In each of their previous marriages they had had one child, which was all their former spouses could handle. John underwent a vasectomy years ago because he knew that in that marriage more than one child would have been an intolerable burden. Now years later he is remarried to a wife who has a totally different philosophy. Because this vasectomy had been so destructive so long ago, he required a very complicated operation (which will be discussed later) to bypass microsurgically all the areas of pressure blowouts and damage in the delicate ductwork of the epididymis. It took several years for his sperm count to come up to a fertile range. In the meantime, his wife was developing infertility problems that frequently crop up in the late thirties in women who were perfectly fertile in their twenties. So they adopted one child after another, and by the time his wife finally got pregnant, four years after surgery, they already had a family of six. Two more natural children in no way interfered with the growth, development, or happiness of any of the children in that enormous family.

The two most clear-cut signals that vasectomy perhaps is inappropriate is if the man is under thirty or if the couple is suffering from marital problems. As I mentioned in the Introduction, many breakups of families that would have seemed to be good matches can be traced to the birth of the second or third child. The couple's entire life-style must make vast accommodations, and it requires a great deal of effort on the part of both marital partners to compromise, communicate, and work out their inevitable differences. Thus it would seem, superficially, that vasectomy might go a long way toward solving martial problems by keeping family size from exceeding tolerable limits. This would give the couple a chance to work things out without the increased stress of adding another child to an already faltering marriage, or to a faltering sex life. The problem with this approach is that very frequently such a faltering marriage finally breaks up and the husband may find himself several years later in a different marriage in which he can hardly believe how much he wants to have more children.

A good example of this is Mark. Mark was twenty-nine years old when he came to see me for a vasectomy reversal. He had no children, even though he liked them. His first wife was domineering, and he loved her, but she definitely did not want any children. So they had no children even though he would have liked to have some. Because vasectomy for him seemed much easier than tubal sterilization for his wife, and because of all of the disadvantages of the various other reversible methods of birth control, they both decided that vasectomy was a simple solution to some of their marital problems. Now, six years later, he has remarried a woman with a totally different view of life, and they want children. It is obvious that in Mark's first marriage his wife should have had tubal sterilization rather than Mark having a vasectomy.

Should the Husband Have a Vasectomy, or Should the Wife Have Her Tubes Tied?

Assuming that sterilization is the appropriate answer for a couple, how do we decide whether it should be the man or the woman? Legally a man's wife has nothing to say about what he does or does not do with his body, and therefore a wife's consent is not necessary for the vasectomy. Nonetheless, most physicians performing the vasectomy would try to get the wife's consent anyway, just to be safe. It would be difficult to imagine a husband wanting to have a vasectomy without the wife's approval in a healthy marriage. If he were doing it without the wife's approval, this would be legally quite permissible but probably would indicate marital discord, which as we mentioned earlier is one of the warning signs *not* to have a vasectomy.

More often the situation is in reverse. The couple needs permanent, convenient birth control, and the wife is pushing a reluctant husband into having the vasectomy. The reason may be that she feels she has gone through enough, having tolerated the pain of childbirth and having assumed most of the responsibility for childrearing. She may be tired of having been the only partner to take any responsibility for birth control in the past. She may have tried other methods of birth control with unpleasant side effects, and her husband may have been totally unwilling to take responsibility by using one of the few methods of birth control available to men, the condom. She may just feel that the time finally has come for him to do his part. Most of the time she is right.

But fairness and equality aside, I have found in thousands of cases that it is wisest for the partner who least wants another child to be the one who gets the sterilization. Thus if the wife is absolutely determined never to have another child, no matter what the husband says or thinks, and the husband is willing to go along with her decision, then it makes no sense for him to have a vasectomy. This was the case with Ralph and Betty. She was firm in her determination not to have another child, but her husband, while very happily married to her and quite willing to go along with her decision, was not as determined as she was. Both members of the marriage usually are happiest when the person who most wants the permanent birth control is the one who gets sterilized. Neither partner should be getting the sterilization under pressure from the other.

Often couples in this dilemma continue to put off sterilization, which in truth might be the best thing for them at this stage and use more conventional birth control with its attendant problems. Sooner or later if it becomes apparent that the time has come for a simple, permanent solution, and it is obvious that someone is going to get sterilized, whether it is the husband or the wife must depend on who is more motivated. Usually if the husband has no ambivalence about ending his childrearing days, then his fear of having surgery usually dwindles away and he steps forward out of a sense of responsibility to his wife who has put up with all of the birth control planning thus far. If he says he's just afraid, usually it means he really is ambivalent about becoming sterile. The husband should not get a vasectomy if his desire for birth control is not as strong as his wife's.

Banking Sperm for Insurance

Why not let the husband get his vasectomy but first have a sample of his sperm frozen in a sperm bank so that if he should change his mind at least he has some sperm available for future artificial inseminations of this or some future wife? There are two reasons why this is a terrible idea. The first is a technical reason. When sperm is frozen it undergoes a great deal of damage. The sperm of only one third of men in the population are capable of tolerating freezing and thawing without losing their fertilizing capacity. Even in the most fertile men (with sperm counts in the range of one hundred million per cubic centimeter with 90 percent vigorous motility), freezing and thawing leave half of the sperm sterile and the fertilizing capacity of the remaining sperm somewhat diminished. With one-third of men the sperm are so fertile that even such severe losses in fertilizing capacity are tolerable. But in two-thirds of men freezing just kills the sperm.

A few years ago in France a twenty-two-year-old woman was incensed when a sperm bank there refused to give to her her husband's sperm that had been deposited there and frozen in 1983 before he underwent an operation for cancer. The reason they had deposited that sperm in the bank was so that if he should not survive the cancer, she could still have a baby by him. But the sperm bank claimed after her husband's death that there was no legal way they could offer his sperm to her without his permission, and for that he needed to be alive. She was incensed, went to court and won her case. However, she failed to become pregnant after being inseminated with his sperm because, as any specialist knowledgeable in this area should have informed her, the chances of that sperm being able to fertilize her would be very low because of the damage caused by the freezing necessary to preserve it.

Furthermore, even with fertile sperm, the chances of pregnancy in any given cycle are generally no more than 20 percent. Thus, to assure a good chance for future pregnancies would require not just one but ten to twenty ejaculations. That is why frozen-sperm banks are so useful for donor artificial insemination for infertile couples but fairly worthless for preserving the sperm of men who wish to undergo vasectomy.

The nontechnical reason why banking sperm prior to vasectomy is unwise is simply that it indicates an ambivalence on the part of the man, and that ambivalence almost assures that he will have negative feelings about his sterilization procedure at some time in the future.

Other Faulty Reasons for Having a Vasectomy

You should not have a vasectomy because of some temporary emotional or economic stress, such as the loss of a job, marital problems, or pressure from anyone, including your wife. You should not have a vasectomy simply because you want to delay having your family, because other methods of birth control are easier to reverse simply by discontinuing them. For example, the new low-dose birth control pills are incredibly safe, often make women feel better rather than worse while they are taking them, and do not deserve all of the bad hype they have been getting. You should not be getting a vasectomy based on vague fears caused by bad publicity about birth control pills.

One final reason for getting a vasectomy that you should reject is a commitment to some abstract concept such as "zero population growth." These commitments, often strongly felt by couples in their early twenties, generally vanish by the early thirties. Life is generally a personal trip taken through the universe by you yourself, and a decision to avoid having children out of concern for the universe is ill-advised. The notion of having children is a deeply ingrained, intense human need, almost as strong as sex and hunger. But it is felt strongest as you get somewhat older and wiser.

Gary is one example of many. He had his vasectomy at age twenty-one, a brilliant college graduate with countless intense interests and a wife of similar background. He loved children but definitely did not want to bring any extra ones into the world. His wife was equally adamant in that view, and thus either one of them might have chosen to be sterilized. The issue here was the abstract goal of limiting world population growth, and it did not hold up ten years later. Gary and his wife simply did not want to make any major effort in their birth control in the heat of their youth, and fooled themselves into rationalizing a permanent position based upon demographic and philosophical grounds. So Gary underwent a vasectomy reversal ten years later (a new marriage, a new wife, a different viewpoint) and found out what he did not know before the vasectomy: He was a very infertile male all along.

To summarize, a vasectomy is intended to make you permanently sterile. You should not have it performed unless you and your spouse have carefully considered your other options for birth control and feel that you will never again wish to have more children. Men under the age of thirty, men who have no children, and men who are experiencing marital problems should be particularly cautious about taking such a permanent step. Having the vasectomy within three to six months of the birth of your last child is definitely not advised.

Despite all of the preceding precautions that you avoid a vasectomy unless your decision is permanent, you should strive to find a doctor who will perform the procedure so it will be most easy to reverse. Life can change in unpredictable ways, and no matter how certain you are today that you do not ever want children, there always is the possibility that you might regret this decision in the future. Furthermore, you should be aware of the fact that with delicate microsurgical techniques and very skilled surgical hands, a vasectomy can be reversed with absolutely superb success if attention was paid to the issue of reversibility according to the approach I will describe toward the end of this chapter.

Most surgeons performing vasectomy at present do not perform it in a reversible fashion. Fortunately, such vasectomies still can be reversed with good success in extremely skilled hands even when the vasectomy is performed in the worst possible fashion. But it requires a great deal of skill, and success cannot be guaranteed. Therefore, you would be foolish not to consider the possibility of reversal at the time of the original vasectomy. Most men who regret their vasectomy never would have predicted that they would feel the way they do when they originally were sterilized. If all of these factors have been taken into account, vasectomy is one of the simplest, safest, and most secure methods of birth control.

How Is the Vasectomy Performed?

Vasectomy is one of the simplest, safest, and most common operations performed in the United States. It is performed right in the doctor's office using local anesthesia only. It is much less painful than a simple dental extraction. The surgery requires only ten minutes, although somewhat more time may be needed for various preparations, such as washing and shaving the scrotum. The incisions are in the scrotum (not on the penis) and generally are only one-eighth to one-quarter inch long, one on each side. They will hardly be visible to you postoperatively. You will generally feel pain for about three seconds on each side when the local anesthetic is first injected. The doctor frequently forgets to mention this, or may underestimate it by referring to it as a little mosquito bite. The fact is that the local anesthetic stings sharply for a few seconds before it makes the area completely numb. I have found that if the patient knows about this ahead of time, it really does not bother him.

In fact, if the doctor warns you just before injecting the anesthetic that you are about to have your three seconds of pain, and tells you ahead of time that he is going to warn you just before he injects it, then most patients look upon the pain quite objectively and literally do not mind it. Before and after that three-second injection of anesthetic you should be completely comfortable. The vasectomy area turns numb very quickly, and from then on you should not feel anything the doctor is doing.

You will not believe how quickly it is all over. When the procedure is completed, the doctor usually will ask you to remain lying down on the examining room table for anywhere from five to fifteen minutes before getting up. Many patients would faint if they were asked to get up too quickly. In fact, a few patients come close to fainting during the operation, not because of any physical harm inflicted but simply as an emotional reaction to the thought of having surgery. If you are one of these few patients who would feel faint like this during the vasectomy, I assure you that after five minutes of lying down you will feel much better.

Normally you and your wife would come to the office together, and you should plan on having her drive you home. You should go directly home after the procedure and lie down for twenty-four hours. It is best not to plan any important business for the day of, or the day after, the vasectomy. For this reason most couples like to have the vasectomy on a Friday and plan on not going back to work until Monday.

Despite all you have read and know about vasectomy, you should not have the procedure until you (and preferably your wife as well) have had a thorough discussion with the physician and feel comfortable with him. Despite all you have read and heard elsewhere, you must go by whatever the physician tells you, and if you are not comfortable with the physician or his approach, then look for a different one.

Bring an athletic supporter with you. You will need this to support the gauze dressings for the first day or so and to reduce discomfort by giving support to the testicles so they do not hang down and pull on the incision area. Following the vasectomy and before getting up off of the examination table, the doctor will help you put the athletic supporter on and show you how it can be used to hold the gauze dressing in place. Without the supporter you would be much more uncomfortable postoperatively. Continue to wear the supporter simply for comfort until you no longer need it for that purpose. With some men, the athletic supporter is no longer necessary in a matter of days; and others wear it for a couple of weeks. The termination point is when the discomfort stops, which is highly variable from one man to the next.

You will need to visit your doctor six to eight weeks after the operation so that he can check your semen to be sure there are no sperm present.

THE SURGICAL TECHNIQUE

The details of the surgical technique are important in helping you decide whether the doctor you have seen is the right one to do the procedure for you. The incision is only one-eighth to one-quarter inch long because the vas can be felt so easily between the surgeon's fingers just underneath the scrotal skin. You could try this yourself. Despite the incredibly delicate, thin, inner canal and lining of the vas deferens, the outer muscular wall that pumps the sperm up into the ejaculatory duct region is thick and tough. That outer wall is about one-eighth inch thick and feels like a copper wire underneath the scrotal skin. It is as though Nature planned this unusual anatomical feature just to make vasectomy easy.

The surgeon will feel the vas and hold it between his thumb and forefinger (believe it or not, this does not hurt) and then inject local anesthesia over the area of scrotal skin under which the vas is lying (this does hurt). The vas can be mobilized painlessly by the surgeon's fingers to any area of scrotal skin where he wishes to make the incision. Once the local anesthesia has been injected and the area is numb, the surgeon then clamps the vas deferens to the scrotal skin. This secures it just underneath the skin in that particular region where the anesthesia was injected.

A one-eighth-inch incision then is made just over the vas. The tiny incision goes through multiple layers of connective tissue that have all been squeezed between the vas and the scrotal skin by the clamp. The surgeon knows he has reached the surface of the vas deferens when these layers of shiny connective tissue are no longer seen and the surgeon is directly facing the more dull surface of the vas deferens. The physician then grasps the vas deferens through this incision with another clamp, which allows him to pull the vas deferens right out of the incision (Figure 7–1).

The surgeon then either divides the vas with a scissors, or cuts a piece of it out. The reason for removing a piece of vas is to ensure a large enough space between the two cut ends so they are less likely to heal together spontaneously, allowing sperm to get through to the other side. The gap created by removing a large area of vas at the time of vasectomy can *always* be bridged (and I emphasize always) during a reversal operation. There are more important things to consider in the issue of making vasectomy easily reversible, mainly preventing pressure buildup. I will get into that in more detail toward the end of this chapter. Suffice it to say that a large area of vas need not be removed, but often is, and should not be a problem for reversibility.

If the vas were simply cut and nothing further done, sperm would continue to leak out of the end of the vas coming from the testicle and form an inflammatory little cluster of scar tissue known as a sperm granuloma. Sperm are incredibly corrosive, anxious little fellows that grind their way mercilessly through short distances of scar tissue and seem to be driven by a need to reach the other side of the vas. They bridge the gap on their own and continue on their way into the ejaculate. So if one were simply to cut the vas and do nothing else, there would be a seemingly miraculous failure to achieve sterility in some patients. But a long area of scar will stop the sperm dead in their tracks because they only have this ability to fight their way through to the other side if the distance being bridged is extremely short.

A better way to prevent this spontaneous "recanalization" is to seal the ends of the vas properly. In the late 1960s and early 1970s, when vasectomy was beginning to surge in popularity, the two ends of

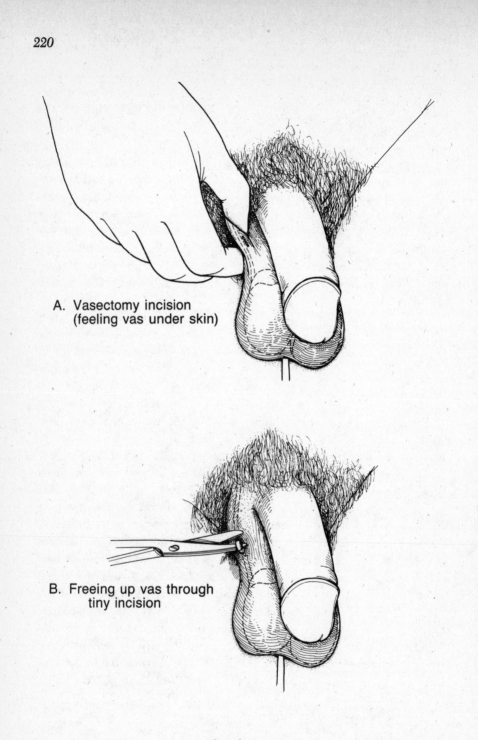

A. Vasectomy incision
   (feeling vas under skin)

B. Freeing up vas through
   tiny incision

FIGURE 7–1.

the vas were sealed simply by tying surgical thread around each end. This probably is the least effective way of sealing the vas, and yet it still is used by many surgeons. As I'll discuss in detail later, the problem is that when the surgical thread, or suture, is tied, the stump on the other side of the tie loses its blood supply, dies, withers away, and then sperm begin once again to leak out of the stump. This problem was not at first appreciated by surgeons, because this method has been used successfully for a hundred years to occlude blood vessels. However, from the mid-1970s to the mid-1980s, another method of sealing the vas became more popular because it was so much more reliable: cautery.

Cautery simply means burning. When the vas is cut, a little wire (or needle electrode) is slipped into the opening down a distance of about one-half inch into the vas canal. A button is pressed and the wire heats up, thus burning the delicate mucosal lining but leaving the outer musculature of the vas unburned. The needle electrode or wire then is removed and the vas is thus very efficiently sealed. The inside of the vas becomes sealed solidly and the stump of the outer muscular wall cannot fall off and allow sperm to leak.

The only problem with cautery is that it is too good. Since its widespread adoption, there has been a much greater (and earlier) increase of pressure on the testicular side of the vas deferens after vasectomy. This has resulted in an earlier occurrence of blowouts in the more delicate epididymal duct near the testicle. Thus we have had to perform much more delicate microsurgery to reverse this type of vasectomy. This greater pressure buildup from cautery also causes more postoperative pain. Nonetheless, cautery is very appealing because it so efficiently seals the vas that the chance for spontaneous recanalization, and thus failure of the sterilization procedure, is extraordinarily low.

My approach is to utilize the efficiency of cautery without creating the pressure problem by sealing only the side of the vas going toward the ejaculatory duct (so as securely to prevent sperm from bridging the gap), leaving the testicular end of the vas open so that sperm can continue to leak and thus prevent pressure buildup (Figure 7–2). But if this "open-ended" approach is utilized, a full inch should be cauterized on the end of the vas going toward the ejaculatory duct. Otherwise, open-ended vasectomy would create too great a risk of spontaneous recanalization, with sperm forging their way through to the other side.

There need be no stitches at all with the vasectomy. The incision in the scrotum is so small that stitches are not necessary. Furthermore, without stitches the bloody fluid can drain out of the tiny incision site

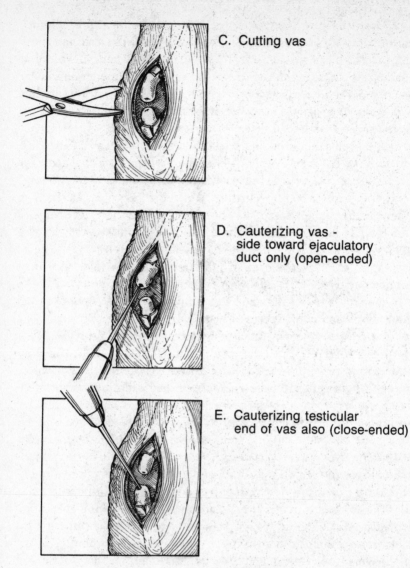

C. Cutting vas

D. Cauterizing vas -
   side toward ejaculatory
   duct only (open-ended)

E. Cauterizing testicular
   end of vas also (close-ended)

FIGURE 7–2.

into dressings that you can wear for a day or two after the vasectomy. This reduces the amount of swelling dramatically. When the incision on each side of the scrotum is closed with a stitch or two, bloody fluid cannot drain out, and the scrotum can swell, sometimes enormously. The incision seals rather quickly and within a day or two there no longer is any bloody drainage. You literally cannot find any sign of where the operation was performed.

Despite the fact that vasectomy is an extraordinarily simple operation that could be performed in a hut with a flashlight by a "barefoot" doctor in any little remote village in the developing world, it is possible for some disastrous complications to occur if performed incorrectly. There have been several patients who actually lost one of their testicles because the spermatic blood supply was accidentally tied off. This is a rare occurrence, and is likely to happen only if the doctor is having difficulty locating the vas. The reason that this would be such a rare complication is that, as we mentioned earlier, the vas has a characteristic "feel" to it that is unmistakably like a copper wire underneath the scrotal skin. The blood vessels to the testicle always are soft and pliable. That is why it is so easy to isolate the vas through a tiny little incision and not to have to visualize any of the other important structures in the scrotum when doing a vasectomy.

DISAPPEARANCE OF SPERM (AND RISK OF REAPPEARANCE)

Your first ejaculate after vasectomy should have a sperm count of about 35 percent of what it was before the vasectomy. Your next ejaculate after that will have a sperm count of about 35 percent of the previous ejaculate. After about ten or twelve ejaculations there should be close to zero sperm in the ejaculate. For example, if you started with an average count of about 60 million per cubic centimeter, your first ejaculate after vasectomy would have a sperm count of about 21 million per cubic centimeter. Your second ejaculate after vasectomy would have a sperm count of about 7,350 million per cubic centimeter. Your third ejaculate after vasectomy would have a count of about 2.5 million sperm per cubic centimeter. Your fourth ejaculate would have about 900,000 sperm per cubic centimeter. Your fifth ejaculate would have about 300,000 sperm per cubic centimeter, and you can see how by the tenth to twelfth ejaculate you would be approaching zero. This, in fact, is exactly what we observe in vasectomy patients. If spontaneous recanalization has not occurred by the twelfth ejaculate, the vast majority of patients no longer have any sperm whatsoever in their ejaculate (Figures 7–3a, b).

Even before the sperm count has gone down to zero, you could be sterile once your sperm are no longer motile—alive and swimming. Even in men who have not had any ejaculations after vasectomy to empty out the sperm, we find that the motility of the sperm is zero in the vast majority after two weeks. This means that without a continuing supply of fresh, healthy sperm coming up from the testicle and epi-

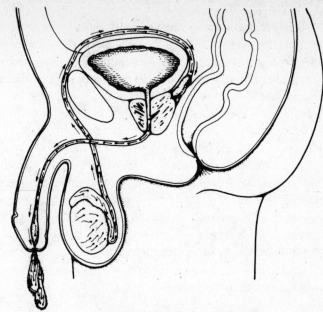

FIGURE 7–3A. Before Vasectomy.

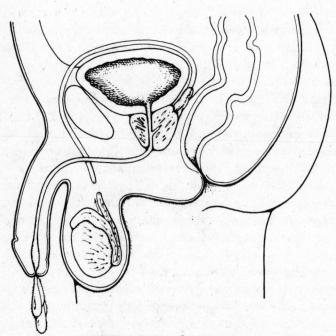

FIGURE 7–3B. After Vasectomy.

didymis, the sperm in the vas deferens die of old age after about two weeks. If there still are live, motile sperm in the ejaculate by one month after the vasectomy, in most cases either the vas was not cut, or there was a spontaneous recanalization, in either case a failure of the vasectomy.

SO WHEN IS IT "SAFE" TO HAVE SEX?

So when do we tell a patient that he is safe to have intercourse without using other methods of contraception? The safest approach is to wait until there is absolutely zero sperm in the ejaculate. For the patient's convenience (so he does not have to bring in a multitude of samples until he has emptied out), we generally ask that he simply bring in a semen specimen after he has had about ten or twelve ejaculations. From a practical point of view, this usually occurs at about six weeks postoperatively, but in some patients it occurs in three weeks and in others it occurs in six months. Theoretically for the patient who has had no ejaculations for one month after the vasectomy, the absence of any live, motile, swimming sperm would be enough to secure that he is safe, but this is only theoretical, and absolutely no doctor regards this as a safety point but rather just a point of interest. To be absolutely as secure as possible, you should wait until you have emptied out all of your sperm and the semen analysis documents that there is *no sperm at all left*.

If any sperm remain in the ejaculate after twelve ejaculations, or after one month has passed, the critical remaining issue is whether the sperm are motile or not. If the sperm are motile, then that means that the operation failed and may need to be repeated. There might be no point in waiting and wondering how long it will take for the remaining sperm to empty out, because if there are motile sperm, they will never empty out because the vas has recanalized. However, if all of the sperm are dead, it would be worth waiting another month or two and then having the semen checked again for sperm. In most instances in this case, the semen shows zero sperm several months later. It is only at that point, *when the semen shows zero sperm*, that you can feel secure in having unprotected intercourse.

Many years ago a patient named Hal came to my office for a vasectomy reversal. The operation went beautifully, but by two months postoperatively, his sperm count was only 500,000 per cubic centimeter. Yet the motility of the sperm was quite good. I figured that eventually his sperm count would come up to a nice, normal range of over 20 million per cubic centimeter, and he should be able to get his wife pregnant. But at six months postoperatively his sperm count was only 740,000 per cubic centimeter, but the motility was still very good. He was very depressed, and I was somewhat confused because the reversal operation had gone so beautifully. I did not see how his counts could be so incredibly low and yet the quality of the sperm so good. I assumed that the chances for Hal getting his wife pregnant were very remote.

What neither Hal nor I realized is that before he had had his vasectomy, his sperm count was also this low, and yet he had fathered three children. In fact, about ten months after the vasectomy reversal operation, Hal's wife became pregnant and they have had several more children since then. Let me explain to you just how low a sperm count of 740,000 sperm per cubic centimeter is. If you take a normal sperm sample with about 60 million sperm per cubic centimeter and you put a drop of it on a slide under the microscope, you would see about 50 or 60 sperm swimming around frantically within every field of view. If you put a drop of Hal's sperm on a slide and looked at it under the microscope, you would see an occasional sperm swimming across the microscopic field, very, very lonely and depressed-looking. In fact, if you looked too quickly without observing for a while into the microscope, you might even falsely conclude that Hal had no sperm in his ejaculate.

A more striking example is the patient I referred to at the beginning of the chapter, a man who suffered years of infertility caused by a low sperm count and terrible sperm motility. Yet this "hopelessly" infertile man got his wife pregnant three times before he finally came in begging for a vasectomy. There was also the case of Barry, who had a sperm count so low after vasectomy reversal that he and his wife had signed up for donor artificial insemination. But the day they were supposed to go in for their first artificial insemination with donor sperm, a huge storm hit their city, and they could not travel to the medical center to have it done. So, disappointed, they figured they would have to wait until the next month. But they never had to wait because that month his wife became pregnant, naturally, from his few sperm. So remember that you cannot consider yourself safe just because your sperm count is low. It has to be *zero*.

Why is it so easy for some men with a very low sperm count to get their wives pregnant, while others have an extraordinarily difficult time? Why is it that so many men with poorly done vasectomy reversals cannot get their wives pregnant because of a low sperm count, even though others despite an occasional low count seem to get their wives pregnant quite easily? The reason is that the number of sperm itself is not that important in making a man fertile. What matters most is the *quality* of the sperm. If there is a partial obstruction causing the count to be lower than the amount of sperm his testicles are producing, the pressure buildup within the system makes the sperm less healthy and slows down all the enzyme processes that help the sperm to mature in the male tract sufficiently to make them fertile. If there is no partial obstruction, and the sperm count is low simply because that testicle does not manufacture a lot of sperm, then fertility can be quite good despite a low number of sperm. That is why after your vasectomy you are not really safe until your sperm count is zero. That is why after a vasectomy reversal some patients are quite fertile with a low count, while others are extremely infertile with a low count and require a reoperation to correct partial obstruction. The bottom line is: Do not consider yourself secure after a vasectomy until you are certain that your count is zero.

Postoperative Complications

SCROTAL SWELLING

The most terrifying-looking complication after vasectomy is the so-called swollen scrotum. It occurs only within the first twenty-four hours. It will not occur later. The chances of it occurring are very low. The medical term is hematoma, which means "full of blood." Because the vasectomy is performed through a tiny incision, in most cases there will be virtually no sign of any surgery having been performed. But if you are unfortunate enough to have a hematoma, your scrotum will swell up to the size of a grapefruit or possibly even a football, it will turn black and blue, and the pain from this will be difficult to describe. Now that you have recovered from this description of a hematoma and have pulled yourself up from the floor and resumed reading, I need to explain to you why a hematoma occasionally forms, how to prevent it from occurring, and assure you that despite grim appearances, it is harmless and will go away. It should not drive you away from this otherwise very safe and simple operation.

This is what my consent form for patients undergoing vasectomy says about hematoma:

> Vasectomy is one of the safest and most common surgical procedures performed. Yet *any* surgery involves some slight risks, and modern medical practice requires that you be informed of them. As a part of the design of the operation (to minimize swelling), a small amount of bloody drainage normally is allowed to occur at the tiny incision, and this eventually seals off on its own. There is likely to be a very small degree of swelling near the tiny incision site, which should resolve in one day to two weeks.
>
> Very rarely the scrotum could become temporarily quite swollen. This is called a "giant hematoma." If it were to occur, it could be temporarily painful and result in a few days' hospitalization and possibly several weeks off of work. The scrotal appearance after such an unhappy complication returns to normal in two to eight weeks. Though a very aggravating complication, a hematoma has not been known to cause any permanent harm and is very unlikely to occur.

The scrotal tissue is unique compared to that of any other part of the body. It is loose and incredibly expandable. It is like a little rubber balloon that could be blown up to enormous proportions. With most tissue in the body—for example, a cut on the finger—you put on a Band-Aid and the rigidity of the tissue itself stops the bleeding and minimizes the swelling. In the scrotum the tiniest little "bleeder" that would be inconsequential in any other part of the body (except perhaps the brain) just keeps on bleeding, and the scrotum just keeps on expanding as it fills with as much as a pint of blood.

Despite the terrifying painful image that a scrotal hematoma presents, it is truly not a dangerous complication, and if left alone, it eventually will resolve completely over the next three months, and the scrotum and testicles will look and feel as though this never happened.

But what a miserable three months this could be. Therefore, it is important that you and your doctor take measures to ensure the lowest possible risk of hematoma. First you should realize that if a hematoma is going to occur, it will be only in the first twenty-four hours after the vasectomy. Do not fear that two or three days later, or a week later, you are suddenly going to develop a massive swelling in the scrotum. If you get over the first twenty-four hours without a hematoma, you are safe. So the most important thing for you to do is to go right home after the vasectomy. Do not stop to go to a movie, eat dinner out, or go to a dance. Do not stop by the nearby driving range or batting cage to prove that your macho has not left you. In fact, do not even insist on being the one who drives home, but have your wife drive. When you get home, do not help move the furniture, or catch up on your gardening. Simply go straight to bed and put your feet up. Do not move from that position (except to go to the bathroom) until the next day. The less activity you engage in during that first twenty-four hours, the less likely you are to develop a hematoma.

The reason for this is that any physical activity you engage in, including just walking around or standing erect, increases your venous pressure. Blood comes back to your heart via veins. When you stand up, the pressure in these veins increases because they are carrying blood back to the heart against gravity. When you take a deep breath or strain during any muscular activity, the pressure increases in both the veins and arteries. You can easily go home with a simple vasectomy that produced remarkably little pain, jump for joy, and get out the baseball bat to play with your kids all afternoon, only to be miserable in the evening with a giant black-and-blue scrotum.

What can your doctor do to minimize this risk? He should be a good technical surgeon and should make sure to stop all bleeders. He should not put you on pain killers such as aspirin that act as anticoagulants. He should leave the tiny incisions in the scrotum open, because if the little incision is closed with a stitch, there is no escape route for blood to drain if bleeding should develop. Leaving the incision open may appear to be sloppy, because of the bloody drainage that spots your gauze dressings. But any blood that drains into those dressings should be viewed as a blessing rather than an inconvenience. If the blood did not drain out, it would stay in and just lead to more swelling.

You will use an athletic supporter postoperatively, with some gauze dressings. Just insert the gauze dressings into the athletic supporter over the tiny incision sites in the scrotum. When the drainage stops (usually within twenty-four hours), you need no longer use dressings. The athletic supporter reduces the discomfort considerably by keeping the testicles from hanging down. Continue to wear the athletic supporter until you no longer need it for comfort. This may be a few days to a week.

A little bit of swelling and a small amount of black-and-blue discoloration to the scrotum is common and should be of no concern to you. It should not be confused with the hematoma that you are trying to prevent during the first twenty-four hours. If you have your vasectomy on a Friday and plan not to go back to work until Monday, you should have minimal discomfort and will be one of the hundreds of millions of men talking about how simple and painless your vasectomy was.

OTHER PROBLEMS AFTER VASECTOMY

The other possible problems of vasectomy are not as scary as hematoma. My operative consent form summarizes them:

> The vasectomy causes blockage, dilation, and congestion of the sperm duct going back to the testicle. This should not usually cause significant discomfort except in some patients. Though quite rare, infection could occur at the vasectomy site. If it were to occur, it might require antibiotics or drainage. A "sperm granuloma" frequently occurs either at the vasectomy site or in the epididymis. This is a very small lump in the scrotum caused by leakage of sperm from the duct. There can be minor but aggravating pain related to such a granuloma, and another operation could be required to excise it. The operation may fail and you might remain fertile. This is very rare, but it unquestionably can occur. YOU MUST USE OTHER BIRTH CONTROL METHODS UNTIL YOUR POST-OPERATIVE SEMEN ANALYSIS DEMONSTRATES NO SPERM. If your sperm count does not go down to zero (this very occasionally occurs), you may need to have the vasectomy performed again. Furthermore, even after your sperm count goes down to zero and you are "safe," there is still the remote possibility that the vas (duct) could "recanalize" at a later date and you could become fertile again without realizing it. Despite all of these warnings, vasectomy still is one of the safest and surest methods of birth control. I do not know of any patients who have complained of sexual impotence after vasectomy, but any operation in that area could have unforeseen psychological effects that might conceivably cause impotence.

LOSS OF TESTICLE

The greatest risk of vasectomy, of course, would be the loss of a testicle or both testicles. I just cannot imagine this happening, but there are cases on record where it has happened that have reached the law courts. There is a famous case from 1979 in Louisiana. The patient called the doctor several days after his vasectomy complaining of severe pain and swelling. Antibiotics did not correct the problem, and the doctor elected to remove the infected testicle rather than drain it, relying on the other testicle to provide the man's hormone production. But that testicle, which was supposed to provide him with all of his hormone function for male sex drive, was, to the horror of the patient and the doctor, shrinking. Three months after the vasectomy that was supposed to provide this happily married man and his wife with a new degree of sexual freedom, it had instead made him an impotent eunuch.

SPERM ANTIBODIES

I do not mention the loss of a testicle in my consent form because I consider it such a bizarre event. I also do not mention the risk of disease from sperm antibodies because despite all of the scare publicity, a whole variety of very carefully performed studies has disproven that there are any general health risks caused by vasectomy, or by the production of sperm antibodies in people who have had a vasectomy.

To make it clear where this scare publicity came from and why people were worried about it for a while, I should relate the story of a patient I saw in 1978 because of severe arthritis, presumably caused by his vasectomy. This was a terrifying case of an otherwise young, healthy, happily married man who did not want to have any more children despite his wife's interest in having more. After the vasectomy he began to develop severe pains in all the joints around his body. His knees, his elbows, his ankles, and even his finger joints began to ache, and he became disabled. His regular doctor was confused by this peculiar arthritis occurring in such a young man right after he had a vasectomy, and so he ordered sperm antibody tests. This man was found to have high levels of sperm antibodies in his blood, and his doctors feared that these antibodies were causing a so-called autoimmune disease.

Autoimmune diseases are rather uncommon. They occur when an immune response to something foreign creates a peculiar type of chronic allergic reaction, and the antibodies so produced actually damage your own tissue. To understand this sperm antibody controversy better, let me first give you a little introduction to what you need to know about your immune system in general.

We live in a hostile world surrounded by an infinite swarm of bacteria, viruses, parasites, and microscopic creatures of the most hideous varieties that would like nothing more than to feast upon us. Our constant protection against the eternal threat of invasion by these infectious organisms is our immune system. Any living thing that our body recognizes as foreign to our own tissue stimulates the production of antibodies, which specifically attack the invading organism and kill it. Our white blood cells then move into the area to dispose of the dead carcasses of bacteria and viruses. Frequently, bacteria and viruses do get a temporary foothold (such as flu, a cold, or even a case of pneumonia), but it takes very little time for our immune systems to overwhelm them. Occasionally we need a little help from antibiotics, but without the help of that remarkable antibody system designed to overcome any foreign invader, no antibiotic medication would be of any use.

Occasionally the immune system may produce adverse rather than beneficial effects. If the patient has a kidney transplant, the immune system may recognize the kidney as a foreign enemy and attack it. You can see how easy it would be to wonder whether after vasectomy, a man's sperm (which are slightly different genetically from all the other cells in his body) wouldn't be thought of as foreign invaders and stimulate an antibody response. Could this autoimmune response after vasectomy be harmful, or are we protected from it just as the fetus is protected against the mother's immune system.

Somehow the body seems to have a remarkable and as yet totally inscrutable mechanism for recognizing that a new baby living within the mother's womb is not to be rejected or attacked by antibodies. The same protection appears to be conferred upon sperm so that usually they do not stimulate an antibody response in the woman with each episode of intercourse.

Going back now to the patient of ours who experienced joint pains all over his body and high sperm antibody levels after vasectomy we had some cause to worry. He was sent to St. Louis for a vasectomy reversal operation in the hopes that it would bring his sperm antibody levels down and correct the arthritis. When this young man arrived in St. Louis with his wife, it did not take a lot of insight to observe immediately that he was very high-strung and somewhat neurotic. His wife clearly was interested in having more children, and he clearly was not. Yet in a sense he felt that she had made him get the vasectomy because she had told him that if he did not want children it was up to him to have the operation, not her. He felt that if he did not want more children, she should have the operation. He was a very macho-type fellow who felt threatened by being sterile, despite his desire never to have children.

We performed a vasectomy reversal on him and achieved a beautiful result. His sperm count went up to normal, and his sperm antibody level gradually went down. He felt psychologically relieved, and his wife then had her tubes tied. He remained virile and fertile and he continued to be catered to by his wife just the way he wanted. Not surprisingly, after a couple of years his joint pains completely went away and his "arthritis" was cured.

Clearly this man had psychosomatic pains related to poor counseling and poor decisionmaking in having the vasectomy. He may have had elevated sperm antibody levels, but this was not the cause of his joint pains. The joint pains went away after he was told that he was no longer sterile. It is this kind of isolated, rare case that can create hysteria and dreaded fear of a medical procedure that has been performed on over one hundred million men in the world and clearly demonstrated not to affect health adversely.

Large-scale Studies Prove Vasectomy Is Safe

How sure can we be that the rare case of illness occurring after vasectomy might not in truth be caused by it? The only way to find the answer is to have large-scale population studies involving hundreds of thousands of people, some of whom have been vasectomized and some of whom have not, to see whether there is any difference in their health. We do not have to get alarmed if a certain percentage of men get arthritis or heart attacks after their vasectomy, if the same percentage of men get arthritis or heart attacks after they start using a condom. The fact that a man may have had a vasectomy prior to developing a health problem does not mean that the vasectomy caused it. Rather it simply means that a certain percentage of men in any population at any time, whether or not they have had a vasectomy, are going to develop heart disease, arthritis, and any number of other diseases.

About one half to two thirds of men will develop sperm antibodies following vasectomy. Widespread publicity of this finding created almost hysterical fears that vasectomized men would not only develop autoimmune disease but also have no possibility for restoration of fertility. Both of those notions have now been disproven. We can return fertility to the great majority of men who have had a vasectomy, and epidemiological studies have proven that vasectomy results in no autoimmune disease such as arthritis.

But what about the monkey scare? In 1978 and in 1980, studies suggested that vasectomized monkeys on a high-fat diet developed arteriosclerosis (and presumably heart disease) at a much greater rate than monkeys who were fed the same high-fat diet but who had not been vasectomized. A new wave of hysteria developed, not because physicians seriously believed that vasectomy could cause heart disease, but rather because such a study in monkeys created a legal liability risk if patients were not so informed. Yet very few physicians I talked to had any realistic concerns that vasectomy did any damage whatsoever to the heart or blood vessels. The theory went that sperm antibodies created by vasectomy could lodge in the inner wall of the blood vessels and cause arteriosclerosis to develop. What we needed was a huge, properly controlled, scientific, epidemiological study of thousands upon thousands of patients so we could know once and for all whether vasectomy should be abandoned as a method of birth control, or whether it could be performed safely without risk of endangering health. Because of a few sick monkeys, an enormous amount of work was needed, and your tax dollars paid for it.

Five separate, large-scale epidemiological studies were undertaken. The results, which were just recently published, showed that vasectomized men had absolutely no increased risk of heart disease, arteriosclerosis, strokes, arthritis, or any other major health disorder. Why did those monkeys get sick? One possibility is simply that monkeys may be different from humans. The other possibility is that these monkey studies were done with very small numbers, and since the "control" monkeys were not randomly alternated with the vasectomized monkeys to make sure that all other factors were the same, it could very well be that the vasectomized group was at greater risk for other reasons, such as diet, or even life-style in the cage. In any event, we can all breathe a sigh of relief, because vasectomy is safe.

What Is the Risk the Vasectomy Will Fail and My Wife Still Will Get Pregnant?

The major risk of vasectomy is, of course, that it will fail. That means that you would have your vasectomy, and after twelve ejaculations (or six weeks) have a sperm count that still showed sperm present. As we have already discussed, if there is even a small number of sperm in the ejaculate, there is a risk of pregnancy, and so the operation has failed unless it reduces your sperm count absolutely and unquestionably to zero. Urologists are literally terrified of this complication. It is the largest single cause of lawsuits against urologists, particularly if a defective child is born as a result. This is the "wrongful birth" lawsuit.

In such a lawsuit, the child "sues" the doctor for being born, and the parents are initiating the suit on the child's behalf. The child sues the doctor for the entire cost of raising him. Fortunately for the doctor, the courts have generally found that no one is being done a disservice by being born, and no parent should expect anyone to pay for the rearing of their child, since according to the courts a child is a precious gift whether expected or not expected. The courts have said that the mother of an accidental pregnancy after vasectomy may be entitled to recover some money for the "physical pain and suffering" resulting from her unanticipated pregnancy and delivery, but she cannot sue the doctor for the cost of caring for and raising a normal, healthy child.

But what if the child is deformed or defective or has some congenital illness? Here is where the courts' wisdom is a little exasperating. The courts have already ruled that the doctor does not have to pay for the cost of raising a normal child. But if by some chance the child happens to have a birth defect, then the doctor can be liable for paying for the entire cost of rearing that child over and above what it would cost to rear a normal child. About three of every one hundred births involves some congenital abnormality, and about one in five hundred are serious, heartbreaking deformities. So whenever you decide to have a baby, you are taking a one in five hundred risk that your baby will have a severe, terrible deformity. This has been true during the entire history of humanity. Yet the courts have decided, on what seems to be a purely emotional basis, that when a defective baby is born after a vasectomy that failed, it represents so much heartache that someone has to pay.

Whether it involves the doctor, the doctor's insurance company, or the doctor's life savings, you can readily understand how this kind of legal system can severely influence the availability of any improved method of birth control that might deviate slightly from traditional methods. When we talk about how your vasectomy should be performed, open-ended or close-ended, to give you the greatest likelihood of reversibility, you will understand how our crazy legal system has drastically reduced your options and made it difficult for you to obtain a more easily reversible type of sterilization.

What causes a vasectomy to fail? The first and most obvious reason might be that an inexperienced doctor did not actually cut the vas even though he thinks he has. This used to be more common fifteen years ago, but nowadays doctors are getting so experienced with vasectomy that they rarely commit this error. The second more common cause of failure is that sperm manage to leak out of the testicular end of the vas and grind their way through the small amount of scar tissue to get to the other side. When it occurs, this spontaneous recanalization almost always happens within six months after vasectomy. It would be extraordinarily rare for a recanalization to occur suddenly after there were zero sperm for six months.

Vasectomies performed by different doctors have different rates of spontaneous recanalization. For example, if the doctor simply cuts the vas and ties it off with a surgical string called a suture, 3 percent of the patients will continue to have sperm postoperatively because of recanalization. If the doctor who is using this method takes out a large segment of vas, then the added space between the two cut ends will reduce that risk of recanalization to less than 0.5 percent. If the doctor seals the inside opening of the vas by burning it with an electrocautery needle rather than "tying it off," this is much more secure and leads to a recanalization rate of less than one in one thousand. That is why the safest approach to having permanent sterilization with no spontaneous recanalization is to seal the inside of the vas with cautery, or to take out a large section. Unfortunately, both of these approaches make the vasectomy more difficult to reverse and will require much more microsurgical expertise to reverse than the open-ended approach I recommend.

Open-ended vs. Conventional Vasectomy

LONG-TERM SCROTAL PAIN AFTER CLOSE-ENDED VASECTOMY

There are two reasons I developed the concept of open-ended vasectomy. One is to reduce the risk of long-term aching scrotal pain caused by the inevitable pressure buildup that always occurs after regular vasectomy. The other is to increase the ease of subsequent reversibility. When you go to the doctor inquiring about vasectomy, you virtually never hear anything about the pressure buildup that occurs after vasectomy, or about the consequences of that pressure buildup. In most cases the doctors are not willfully concealing anything from you; they just are not up-to-date on the basic science of the testicle and vas deferens. Last month I received a call from a urologist who has done over a thousand vasectomies and never believed his patients' reports about lingering mild, aching pain until he had a vasectomy last year and now has pain from it himself. He had no prior scientific knowledge of this problem, but he called me when he experienced it himself.

Two years ago I received a call from a law firm that was defending an osteopath who was being sued for a vasectomy he performed. The patient developed in his left testicle a mild, chronic, aching pain that would not go away despite aspirin, Tylenol, sitz baths, and anti-inflammatory drugs. The osteopath presumed that the pain had to be caused by a sperm granuloma at the vasectomy site, but physical examination revealed there was no sperm granuloma present. Classical medical teaching is that when anyone has pain after vasectomy it is caused by this sperm granuloma. More recent studies, well documented in the scientific literature, clearly prove that that is not the case. Sperm granulomas are for the most part painless, and indeed they allow a release of the pressure buildup that would otherwise extend all the way back to the epididymis and testicle. Thus sperm granuloma minimizes the risk of pain that, in truth, is caused by pressure buildup in the epididymis.

The osteopath had no comprehension of this situation, and the patient went to an M.D. thinking that he would understand it better. The M.D. had no greater understanding of this confusion than the osteopath, but unfortunately he was much more aggressive at treating it. He simply removed the painful testicle. Now the patient had only one testicle left, on the right side, and when a different M.D. saw the patient later, the doctor was really in a quandary because the patient had developed the same pain on the other side. The pain was so aggravating that the doctor decided to "explore" the scrotum of the remaining testicle, and through a series of poor judgments, wound up removing it also.

The prestigious law firm that called my office was suing the osteopath who originally performed the vasectomy and the two M.D.s who had separately removed each of the testicles. I refused to testify because I did not feel any side in this party was interested in the truth but simply was interested in winning some money or saving some money. But I will tell you, the reader, what neither the lawyer, the osteopath, the two M.D.s, nor the patient understood.

After vasectomy the testicle continues to produce sperm and fluid at the same rate as before the vasectomy. The testicle produces only a small amount of fluid compared to the rest of the ejaculate volume, making up only 5 percent of the fluid we ejaculate. Otherwise, vasectomy would cause incredible amounts of congestion and pain. As it is, however, this continual production of fluid from the testicle, with no place to get out, causes a gradual pressure buildup within the vas and the twenty-foot-long microscopic epididymal tubule. A valve prevents this pressure buildup from going back into the testicle, and protects the testicle from any damage, but the epididymis remains vulnerable. Eventually there are blowouts and perforations in this delicate epididymal tubule, and this relieves some of the pressure. It is this dilatation and "blowing up" of the epididymis that results in the mild but aggravating pain that occasionally bothers a small percentage of men who have had vasectomy. Usually it is referred to as epididymitis, and although epididymitis is not an uncommon condition for urologists to treat, no one ever associated it with the vasectomy before.

Epididymitis—inflammation and dilation of the epididymis—occurs in virtually every patient who undergoes vasectomy but usually produces no symptoms. Pain from epididymitis occurs in only about 8 percent of patients. In a small percentage of these men the discomfort can be extremely irritating and aggravating.

For example, Cal came to me for a vasectomy reversal simply to get rid of the chronic epididymitis he had had ever since his vasectomy. Right after the vasectomy his right scrotum had swollen up dramatically, with severe pain for about two months. The swelling eventually subsided, but the pain remained. The pain was mild and he could tolerate it. It was aggravated by intercourse, and sometimes was just a sense of dull aching. Then, about six months later, the pain became quite severe. Cal was treated in the emergency room with antibiotics for epididymitis, and he continued to have intermittent attacks of it over the next several years. Finally he saw a urologist who told him he had seen epididymitis more commonly after vasectomy than in the normal population of men, and finally recommended a reversal. So he was sent to our clinic at St. Louis.

Another such patient had pain that was so aggravating that he wanted his vasectomy reversed even though he was extremely satisfied with it as a simple and safe method of birth control. In both of these patients we successfully performed a microsurgical reconnection of the vas and relieved the pain. In Cal's case, he was happy to have his fertility restored. But the other patient was unhappy because he would have preferred vasectomy as a method of birth control, if only he did not have to deal with the uncomfortable symptoms of pressure buildup. He should have originally had an open-ended vasectomy.

Pain and Epididymal Damage from Close-ended Vasectomy

Another example of the ignorance of most paramedical personnel dealing with vasectomy is what happened to a major administrator with a family planning center. Jack had two children, was happily married, and had a close-ended vasectomy performed in such a way as to get the tightest possible seal of the vas and to remove a large segment, to be as safely permanent as possible. Jack assumed that the standard method of cauterizing the inside of the vas canals on both sides of the cut vas to get as tight as possible a seal would give the lowest risk of spontaneous recanalization, and the least risk of a "painful" sperm granuloma at the vasectomy site. We have already discussed the fact that sperm granulomas at the vasectomy site do not cause pain, but, if anything, relieve it. What nobody predicted was that his two-year-old daughter would die several years later.

At that point, Jack contacted us for a vasectomy reversal and thought that it would not be too difficult because the vasectomy was so recent. Despite the fact that he was in the vasectomy-counseling business, he really had no understanding of the pressure increase after vasectomy and what it does to the epididymis. When we operated on him we found that he had extensive blowouts throughout the epididymis, and in fact on one side the epididymis was completely destroyed. On the other side a very difficult microsurgical hookup was required to restore his fertility. This man did become fertile after surgery and now they have another child, but because of the vasectomy method that was used on this vasectomy counselor, one epididymis was destroyed, and he had almost permanently ruined his chances for reversibility.

We have quantitatively studied sperm production in the testicle in literally thousands of men after vasectomy, and it is unequivocally clear that vasectomy produces no change in hormone or sperm production of the testicle. In fact, this complete lack of effect of vasectomy on the testicle itself is what creates the problem. The testicle continues to produce fluid and sperm that are transferred into the epididymis and from there into the vas deferens, which is now completely blocked and unable to let any of that fluid out. The big question should not be why a small number of patients have pain after vasectomy, but rather why everybody doesn't have constant, chronic pain after vasectomy. With all of that pressure buildup, why doesn't everyone hurt? The answer to that question is simpler than it may seem.

The reason is that with complete blockage, the tubules of the epididymis dilate up quickly, and the muscle wall thins out. As it becomes thinned out and more able to expand, there is less pain from pressure within it. The initial pain is masked by the pain that the patient feels because of the surgery, and within a week the epididymis has dilated so much that it no longer hurts. But 8 percent of the time it does hurt.

SPERM GRANULOMA, THE HELPFUL LUMP

What exactly is a sperm granuloma? It is a lump at the vasectomy site caused by sperm leakage. In the early days of vasectomy, over fifteen years ago, sperm granuloma occurred in 33 percent of men after vasectomy. It is caused by a "sloppy" vasectomy. It represents continual sperm leakage at the vasectomy site, thus preventing pressure buildup in the epididymis. If leakage at the vasectomy site were ever to stop, the sperm granuloma would disappear within weeks. The presence of this lump at the vasectomy site does not represent a permanent glob of scar tissue, but rather a dynamic pressure-releasing valve. The sperm leak into the space just outside the cut end of the vas, and this space automatically surrounds itself with granuloma cells, which absorb fluid and sperm. Outside this surrounding wall of cells is a small "fence" of scar tissue that prevents the sperm from leaking into surrounding tissue of the scrotum and forces it to be reabsorbed dynamically by the cells inside the granuloma. The reason we can feel so confident that such a granuloma is not harmful is that it is present in literally millions of men who had vasectomies in the early days, when the vasectomy was performed more sloppily. Over the course of twenty to forty years these granulomas have caused no harm.

Why did the sperm granuloma occur more frequently in vasectomies performed with older techniques than they do now? The common technique in the past was to divide the vas and put a "tie" of surgical string, or suture, around each end. This tie was meant to seal the two ends of the vas to prevent sperm from leaking out of the testicular side. In case sperm did manage to leak out of the testicular side, the tie on the other side would prevent the sperm from getting into the end of the vas going toward the ejaculate. But this method of sealing the vas proved to be very poor. Once the vas is tied off, there is no longer a blood supply going to the stub of vas on the other side of the tie. Thus the little stub on the other side of the tie withers away and falls off, leaving behind a raw end of vas that is able to leak sperm freely. The more modern method of sealing the vas with cautery is to burn the lining of the canal so that it fills up solidly with scar, forming a permanent block. With this technique for sealing the vas, sperm granulomas almost never occur.

The risk of sperm creating a bridge to the other side and making the vasectomy fail was much greater with the old, inefficient techniques of sealing the vas. The fear of recanalization prompted a movement toward the cautery technique of vasectomy. What was not anticipated is that while reducing the failure rate almost to zero, cautery created such a rapid and complete pressure buildup that the risk of painful, congestive epididymitis increased, and reversal became more intricate. For example, Marvin was a pilot with six children from a previous marriage. With his wife's demise, he remarried a younger woman and wanted to have just one more child, with her. His vasectomy, performed in the "modern" way with cautery, established such a rapid, high-pressure buildup that he had rock-hard blowouts in the epididymis all the way up to near the outlet from the testicle. It required extraordinarily intricate and difficult, time-consuming microsurgery to restore his fertility. Such intense microsurgical effort might not have been necessary had he undergone the "old-fashioned" sloppy method.

Another example is Charles, a fifty-year-old man who was one of the first to undergo vasectomy with the new cautery technique of sealing the vas, over twenty years ago. He developed such painful congestive epididymitis that he required an epididymectomy in a subsequent surgical procedure fifteen years later after enduring chronic, aching pain on one side. The epididymectomy (removal of the whole epididymis) meant that on that side there was no chance ever to restore fertility.

The amazing fortune in Charles's case was that on his other side, the new cautery technique had failed, and he had formed a sperm granuloma on that side. Naturally, that was the side that did not hurt him, and therefore the side that did not require an epididymectomy. In fact, it did not even require very difficult microsurgery to reverse because of the completely intact epididymis. He is now a happy, fertile man raising a family thanks to the ineptitude of his doctor over twenty years ago in doing the vasectomy on one side so sloppily that a sperm granuloma had formed! So although a sperm granuloma increases the risk of recanalization and failure of the vasectomy, it results in lower pressure with greater ease of reversibility, and less risk of congestive epididymitis pain.

There are rare men who will have some discomfort and tenderness at the site of a sperm granuloma. Of the literally thousands of vasectomy patients with sperm granuloma I have examined, pain is a rare occurrence. It happens when, by chance, the granuloma is touching on a small filament of a nerve fiber. There is a relatively simple solution if you are unfortunate enough to be one of the rare persons who has a painful sperm granuloma. The vasectomy can be redone just as simply as it was done the first time, requiring no more than a few minutes in the doctor's office. But this time the cut will be made slightly below the level of the sperm granuloma. Sperm will no longer reach the painful sperm granuloma. Within a matter of weeks that granuloma will disappear and cease to produce pain. If the vasectomy is performed to allow another sperm granuloma to form at the new vasectomy site, most likely this will be like the usual sperm granuloma, and not be painful because it will most probably not touch a nerve fiber.

A SPERM GRANULOMA HELPS REVERSIBILITY

Some doctors have wanted to prevent sperm granuloma at the vasectomy site out of fear that sperm antibodies would be caused as a result of the sperm leakage, and they would make subsequent fertility after vasectomy reversal less likely. This is a severe misconception. We found no difference in pregnancy rates among those patients who had sperm antibodies vs. those who did not have sperm antibodies. In fact, the patient with the record for getting his wife pregnant the earliest after vasectomy reversal (four weeks) had the highest sperm antibody titer.

Some patients do not get their wives pregnant right away, and doctors get worried that sperm antibodies may be the cause. They recommend all kinds of treatment to suppress the immune system, very much like kidney or heart transplant recipients. These medications can be extraordinarily dangerous. Several such men, inappropriately treated in this way, have developed severe infections, destruction of the hip joint, or premature cataracts and blindness as a result of this rather dangerous effort to suppress the immune system under the notion that sperm antibodies are interfering with fertility.

A good example of a man who wisely avoided this recommendation is Rusty. Three years after his vasectomy reversal operation, Rusty's wife, Diane, still was not pregnant. His sperm antibody levels were elevated, as is the case with half of all men who have undergone a vasectomy. The motility of Rusty's sperm had been low, but the sperm count was very high, indicating that there was no partial blockage and that the reconnection had been surgically quite accurate. His doctors at home recommended that he go on high doses of Prednisone to try to suppress antibody formation, and he called me to ask my opinion. When I told him about the risk of going on that medication in such high doses, and relayed the fact that we had no evidence that sperm antibodies interfered with fertility, he decided not to take the risk and just wait it out.

When Diane still did not get pregnant, he had her evaluated, too. He had what appeared to be a normal, fertile sperm count, but everyone was telling him he was infertile because these sperm antibodies were, in some obscure way, preventing the sperm from working properly. It did not make common sense to him. As it turns out, he was correct. Diane, after all these years, was found to be a poor ovulator, was placed on Clomid, and became pregnant soon thereafter.

His case was similar to that of a patient I had never even met but who had read my first book, *How to Get Pregnant*, and sent me a letter with her "antibody story." Her husband had never had a vasectomy. They were simply a couple who had been trying hard for many years, unsuccessfully, to have a baby. She was diagnosed as having sperm antibodies. They used condoms for eighteen months, but the antibody level did not change. Eventually they gave up using condoms, took no fertility drugs, tossed out their temperature charts, and adopted a child. Much to this woman's surprise, five years later she became pregnant. Her gynecologist could not explain this "spontaneous remission." In truth, antibodies seem to be blamed for infertility whenever no more obvious explanation is found. Numerous attempts to prove scientifically a correlation between the presence of sperm antibodies and infertility have just not been successful.

The presence of sperm leakage at the vasectomy site does not increase the likelihood of having sperm antibodies anyway. The incidence of sperm antibodies in patients who have and those who don't have a sperm granuloma is about the same. The reason is that once you have a vasectomy, you simply physically have to have sperm leakage somewhere. The leakage is going to occur either at the vasectomy site, forming the sperm granuloma, or from blowouts in the epididymis. It is a closed sperm transporting system, and thus vasectomy means there must be sperm leakage. Therefore, no matter how you do the vasectomy, the risk of formation of sperm antibodies is the same.

In summary, a sperm granuloma represents a continual tiny leakage of sperm from the vasectomy site that protects against pressure buildup that would automatically occur after vasectomy. The presence of a sperm granuloma would result in a decreased risk of pain from pressure buildup and would make subsequent reversal of vasectomy much easier to perform.

Open-ended Vasectomy

I have recommended an approach to vasectomy that encourages the formation of a sperm granuloma while still preventing the complication of recanalization and failure. This is the so-called open-ended vasectomy. The major objection to open-ended vasectomy, and the reason it has not yet become widely popular, is fear of unjustified lawsuits. Now that some of the leading centers for vasectomy research are endorsing this approach, you probably will see it becoming the standard over the next five years. It is now the preferred technique for vasectomy in all of Australia, the major centers in Southern California, and in Ontario, Canada. Ten thousand such cases have been performed in Australia, over five thousand in California, and over five thousand in Ontario. The results keep coming back with overwhelming endorsement.

The technique is very simple, in fact simpler than both the standard close-ended cautery technique, and the old-fashioned "sloppy" approach (which often accomplished the same result in a hit-or-miss fashion). With open-ended vasectomy, after the vas is cut, the "testicular" end of the vas that would leak sperm is left alone and unsealed. The "ejaculatory" end, which leads toward the ejaculatory duct, however, is carefully sealed with the modern cautery technique. To prevent the subsequent sperm granuloma from resulting in a failure to achieve sterility, it is critical that the ejaculatory end of the vas be sealed for a long enough distance—from one-half to one inch. If this distance of vas is sealed on the ejaculatory side of the vasectomy, the chances of this open-ended vasectomy failing are very remote. Yet a sperm granuloma is allowed to form, and pressure buildup will be prevented.

If a shorter distance—for example, one-quarter inch—of vas on the ejaculatory side is sealed, then the risk of failure because of recanalization would be too high. Even doctors who had initially feared there would be too high an incidence of failure with this new technique are now endorsing it. They can protect their patients against recanalization failure simply by sealing a slightly longer length of vas on the ejaculatory side, and for an added precaution they will check the patient's sperm count until six months postoperatively.

This open-ended technique clearly reduces the incidence of post-operative pain and makes subsequent reversibility much easier. For those reasons it seems to be the optimal way to perform a vasectomy. Yet your vasectomy most probably will not be performed in this way unless you specifically ask about it. Your doctor may not even bring the subject up unless you take the initiative. The reason is that an unwanted pregnancy after vasectomy is the most popular cause for which urologists are sued. They can perform complicated operations for kidney or prostate cancer, take care of difficult kidney transplantations, do delicate bowel reconstructions to reroute urine, and never get sued. But let one woman have what should be the joy of pregnancy that she was not counting on, and the physician runs the risk of getting sued for the entire cost of raising that child.

Reversal of Vasectomy

As I have emphasized, vasectomy is one of the simplest methods of birth control and one of the most popular methods now used in the world. But it is generally best considered a last resort for those who have already tried more readily reversible methods of birth control, or who are sure they do not want any more children. Yet our lives and our families are held together by such thin threads that few of us can feel quite comfortable, at least while we are young, with the decision to be sterilized. Reversibility must be a high priority.

CHILD DEATH

The Lorens were a couple with two children and a "complete" family. The husband was forty-two, the wife was forty, and he had been vasectomized eight years ago. Six years after the vasectomy his son died in a car accident while he was playing in front of the house. Mr. Loren immediately went to have a vasectomy reversal, but the operation failed, and a year after that they came desperately to St. Louis. Despite being in their forties they still desperately wanted to have another child. They knew that a new child would not replace the little boy that they had lost, but that did not change their desire to have another child.

The MacIntoshes were younger, had two children, all they ever wanted, and he had a vasectomy right after the birth of the third child. They lived on a farm and were leading a beautiful life. Two months before they came to St. Louis for a vasectomy reversal, their little boy (by then two years of age) was kicked in the head by a horse no more than ten yards from his father and mother, who at that instant were not looking. He was dead instantly and never uttered a sound. For that reason, when they looked in his direction and saw him lying on the ground, they thought he was just sleeping. Only a few minutes later did they realize with horror what must have happened.

Mr. and Mrs. Johnson from a small Southern town had two healthy children, which was all they had wanted. When their youngest son was two-and-a-half years old he pushed the button to the garage door opener and then tried to run under it as he had done many times before. This time he was not fast enough and the garage door came down on him. Automatic garage door openers are supposed to have a safety mechanism that makes them go right back up again when they hit something, but on this particular day that safety mechanism was not working and the little boy was crushed to death.

Then there is the terribly sad case of the professor from England who was forty-four years old, had two children, a girl eighteen years old, and a boy who died at age fourteen in a train accident. He had an attempted reversal of the vasectomy in London right after the child died. The reversal was not successful and it was not until three years later that he came all the way to St. Louis for a reoperation. By then his wife (who was forty-three years old) had stopped ovulating properly, and despite a successful reoperation by me to reverse his vasectomy, it was too late for this couple to replace their loss. The wife was somewhat old from the fertility point of view when their child had died. If the husband had had an "open-ended" vasectomy, his original attempt at vasectomy reversal in London would have been easier to perform, and he might have gotten fertile early enough for his wife to have another child.

There are many patients who have had previous unsuccessful vasectomy reversals who were told they might as well give up, when actually in most of these cases fertility could be restored by a reoperation. One of my earliest patients was a very hardworking Mexican immigrant from California who was raising three beautiful children (two girls and a boy), holding several jobs, and saving up enough money to give them a home and the education he never had. Suddenly his boy came down with a rare and incurable illness that baffled his doctors and finally resulted in a deep coma and death. The man was beside himself with grief and decided shortly thereafter to go to one of the nation's leading medical centers nearby to try to reverse the vasectomy that had been performed three years earlier, when he thought his family was complete. The doctors at that medical center explored the patient's scrotum and found no vas deferens whatsoever. Apparently his vasectomy had been performed so radically that there was no vas at all left in the scrotal area. His doctor sadly closed the incision and when the patient woke up explained to him that there was no hope.

One year later the man chanced to read an article written by a former patient of mine in his local paper. He called the newspaper and talked to the reporter who suggested that the patient contact me. When I explained to him that the large amount of vas deferens removed should not make any difference in his prospects for recovering fertility, even though it would make for a much larger and more difficult operation, he seemed unable to believe me. He asked for several more opinions, all of which concurred with that of the medical center where he had his original surgery. He finally decided to come to our clinic anyway and have another attempt at surgery. As expected, we found that there was no vas deferens in the scrotum, and our incision had to be extended into the abdomen.

Every male is endowed with an excess length of vas deferens, more than he needs. Thus we were able to free this patient's vas up in the abdomen, bring it into the scrotum, and very accurately reconnect it under the microscope. The patient developed a normal sperm count postoperatively. He now has three more children, and he is working his head off to make enough money so they all can have an education.

SUCCESSFUL REVERSAL OF VASECTOMY WHEN PREVIOUS ATTEMPTS HAVE FAILED

There are countless other patients with similar stories who had given up simply because their first efforts at reversal of vasectomy had failed. In almost all these cases, the failure is caused by obstruction. Obstruction is either at the site of the vas reconnection (vasovasostomy), or in the epididymis from blowouts that have been caused by the pressure buildup after vasectomy. If the patient has obstruction at both sites, then reconnection of the vas deferens alone would not restore fertility, and doctors might be confused into thinking that the patient remains sterile for some obscure reason. But the reason never is obscure. It always is obstruction, and therefore reoperation always carries with it good hope for success if the microsurgical technique is sophisticated enough.

The length of vas removed at the time of vasectomy and the area of vas that was cut should have no effect on success rate. If a large segment of vas has been removed, the gap always can be bridged by making the incision larger and freeing up a large enough segment of vas. The success rate should not be any lower in cases where large portions of the vas have been removed. In the same fashion, the success rate should not be any lower where previous attempts to reverse the vasectomy have resulted in failure.

Sometimes patients may think they have had a successful vasectomy reversal operation because postoperatively there are some sperm in the ejaculate, but the sperm count may be very low and they are not really fertile. If an inadequate channel has been established and the site of reconnection is constricted, thus impeding sperm transport, this causes the sperm count to be too low. More importantly, this restricted channel results in continued pressure buildup, causing the sperm motility to be poor. Fertility is not likely with that sort of result, even though the operation may have been called successful. Failure to get one's wife pregnant in such a situation is caused by poor sperm quality as a consequence of blockage to sperm flow.

In patients undergoing vasectomy reversal with no damage in the epididymis, over 98 percent have adequate postoperative sperm counts, and 88 percent get their wives pregnant eventually. This is not significantly different from a normal population of couples trying to get pregnant. The results are certainly not this good when there is epididymal damage. Of patients who have had previous failures of vasectomy reversal coming to our clinic for reoperation, 81 percent have gotten their wives pregnant. Many of these patients get their wives pregnant with a moderately low sperm count, as I have discussed before. So how do we explain the fact that men with partial obstruction causing low sperm counts do not get their wives pregnant until they have a reoperation, whereas patients we operate on with meticulous microsurgical technique that have no partial obstruction but low sperm counts do get their wives pregnant?

David from California had a sperm count of consistently less than five million per cubic centimeter after we did his vasectomy reversal, but his motility (the percentage of sperm that were moving) was 50 percent, and the sperm looked healthy. He never expected to be able to get his wife pregnant because the doctors in California advised that his sperm count was too low. We knew, however, from quantitative studies of his testicle biopsy performed at the time of the surgery, that that was all of the sperm he was making, or ever did make. We know that before he had had his vasectomy his sperm count also had to be below five million per cubic centimeter, and he got his wife pregnant in those days with the same low sperm count that he now had after his vasectomy reversal.

After he and his wife got over the tension caused by the gloomy report their local doctors gave them, eventually she got pregnant several times. His low sperm count was not due to a failure of the vasectomy reversal, or partial obstruction, but because that was all the sperm he ever made. Men have sperm counts that range from 1 million to 120 million per cubic centimeter. Men come in different sizes, different shapes, and different sperm counts, and they are all normal. Low sperm count is a cause for infertility in people after vasectomy reversal only if it is dramatically lower than the amount of sperm the testicle is making, indicating that the cause of the low sperm count is partial blockage resulting in delayed sperm transport and increased epididymal pressure.

I saw a lovely couple who had a previous attempt at vasectomy reversal in Europe that had failed. Two and a half months after we reoperated, the wife got pregnant. The sperm quality was good (over 50 percent motile), but the sperm count was only three million per cubic centimeter. The testicle biopsy showed that was all the sperm the man was producing, and that was most likely what his sperm count was before he had his vasectomy.

The majority of men who have fewer than ten million sperm per cubic centimeter after vasectomy reversal are infertile, because in 90 percent of the cases it will have been caused by partial obstruction. They will have poor sperm motility as well as a poor sperm count. They are infertile not because the number of sperm is low but because the constricted reconnection is impeding sperm transport and thereby sperm quality. To reestablish fertility after vasectomy, the tiny, delicate duct must be microsurgically reconnected with extreme accuracy. The outer diameter of the vas deferens is about one-eighth inch, but the diameter of the inner canal that carries the sperm is about one-one-hundredths inch, or roughly the size of a pinpoint. This inner canal has a lining of mucosa about three cells thick. To achieve a nonobstructed reconnection, it is necessary to stitch this inner lining in a leakproof fashion using thread invisible to the naked eye (approximately one-one-thousandths inch in diameter). This must all be performed under a microscope with very high magnification using delicate instruments and suture (surgical thread) much of which I designed specifically for this surgery.

If there are epididymal blowouts causing blockage in the ductwork closer to the testicle, the operation becomes ten times more difficult (see Figure 7–4). The delicate wall of the epididymis is a thin, filmy membrane one-one-thousandths inch thick. The diameter is one-three-hundredths inch, or roughly one third the size of a pinpoint. If there is blockage in the epididymis caused by pressure-induced blowouts, the vas deferens must be microsurgically reconnected to this much more delicate epididymis, bypassing the blowouts. This means stitching together a tubule one-one-thousandth inch in wall thickness. Obviously a great deal of practice and skill are required for this kind of microsurgery. Of our patients who have undergone this kind of epididymal bypass, 80 percent develop adequate sperm counts, and about 65 percent produce a pregnancy. This is a considerably lower success rate than for those who had no blowouts and simply undergo vas reconnection, but it still is a very optimistic outlook for those who otherwise would have no chance for fertility if they simply had undergone reconnection of the vas.

How to Choose the Right Microsurgeon

This delicate surgery must not be undertaken lightly, and yet it is being performed by some doctors who are not very experienced. For example, Will had undergone a failed vasectomy reversal attempt by a very fine doctor who has had a reasonable success rate. Because this was a very difficult case that involved the epididymis, the doctor sent Will to our clinic in St. Louis for another attempt to restore fertility. Before sending the patient here, he called to say that he had gone into the operating room with several of the surgeons of his area, who were professing to be experts, to observe their technique with other patients. He told me that he was very disappointed to see that their technique was not at all what they claimed at professional meetings. He was

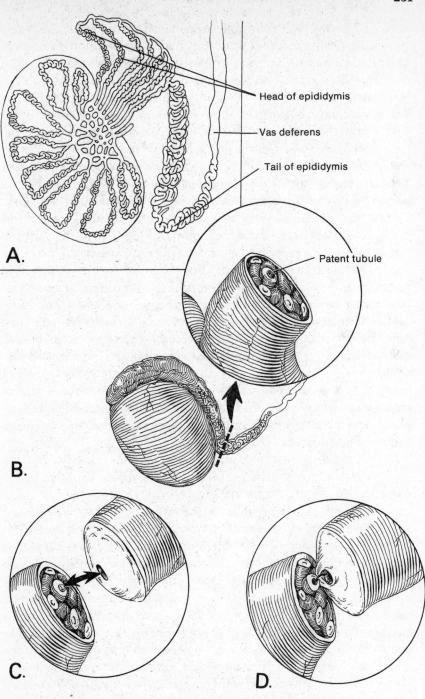

Head of epididymis

Vas deferens

Tail of epididymis

A.

Patent tubule

B.

C.

D.

FIGURE 7-4.

dismayed to find that there were many more doctors professing to be experienced microsurgeons who really had no more expertise than he, and yet they were attempting surgical procedures for which they had not had sufficient previous laboratory practice.

Another patient coming here for reoperation told me that the doctor who did his previous vasectomy reversal had told him he was going to use the microscope, but the patient, who had been pretending to be asleep, observed that the doctor had used no microscope or optical aid whatsoever. How could he have had very much chance of success? In fact, there has been a wave of popular interest in doing these delicate operations on an outpatient basis, supposedly to save the patient money. The savings is minimal. This kind of surgery requires good anesthesia and an overnight stay in the hospital. Anything short of that usually means that a very superficial approach is being taken to the surgery.

I have heard countless stories from patients who tell me they paid big surgical fees, went in as an outpatient, were sent home several hours later with a great deal of scrotal pain and swelling, received no communication with the doctor postoperatively, and elicited no interest from the doctor in the postoperative result. When I reoperate on this kind of patient I generally find that the scrotum is so filled with scar tissue from the previous surgery that it is as though cement were poured into it. It is true that this should not and does not affect the results of reoperation if the surgeon doing the reoperation is extremely experienced. But it makes for a more difficult procedure, a longer procedure, and much more postoperative pain.

It is important not only to choose a good microsurgeon for the vasectomy reversal, but also not to be confused about the postoperative course. One patient of mine had five previous children and wanted to have another child very badly, and he and his wife had seen several well-known doctors in their area. None of the doctors could give them any figures on results. These doctors knew nothing about epididymal complications and merely kept reiterating that they "knew how to do the surgery" and that the chances for success were "fifty–fifty." Whenever someone says, "fifty–fifty," that means that they are not quoting results based upon documented follow-up but rather are just pulling a number out of the air, trying to guess at what your chances might be. "Fifty–fifty" does not mean that your operation has a 50 percent chance for success. A 50 percent chance for success would mean that out of every thousand patients having the surgery, five hundred of them have a successful result. "Fifty-fifty" means that the doctor has not the foggiest idea what his or her success rate is.

Waiting for Pregnancy after Vasectomy Reversal

A patient of mine from the Seattle area who already had one child after we did a vasectomy reversal was anxious to have a second child. His postoperative sperm counts varied from thirty million to eighty-six million per cubic centimeter, and the sperm motility varied from 25 to 50 percent. When he and his wife decided to have a second child after the reversal operation, he had the sperm count repeated, and the local doctors told him it was only about two million per cubic centimeter, with 0 percent motility. They told him he had no chance at all ever to have another child. Yet two months later, his wife became pregnant. We discovered later that the sperm count on which the doctors were basing all this grim advice was in error.

If you have an adequate sperm count after vasectomy reversal, so long as you know the surgery was performed properly, you must have patience. If your sperm count is poor, you may need a second operation. Check with your doctor regularly. Many patients have to wait for several years before their wife becomes pregnant. The epididymis is so dilated by a long-term vasectomy that in many cases it can take as long as five years for it to recover and for sperm transport and motility to return to normal. Harold is a patient of mine who had a previous vasectomy reversal that had failed because the doctor had just tried to put the vas together without recognizing epididymal blockage. He came to St. Louis in 1980. When we operated we found that his vas had been put together properly but that he had complete epididymal blockage. We did a delicate microsurgical bypass of this epididymal blockage, but at four months postoperatively the patient still had no sperm. He seemed to give up at that point even though we had warned him that it might be a long wait and that we were sure we had made a good reconnection of the epididymis. We heard from him one year and ten months after surgery. He reported by phone that he had a sperm count of forty-nine million per cubic centimeter now, but zero motility. We encouraged him to be optimistic, but he found it difficult. Finally, three years after surgery, he sent us a sperm count report showing forty-three million per cubic centimeter, with 80 percent excellent-quality motility. Two months after that, his wife announced that she was pregnant. We knew that with the kind of difficult epididymal damage he had suffered, even after a perfect restoration of continuity of this delicate duct, it might take several years for sufficient epididymal function to return so that he would be able to get his wife pregnant. His patience paid off.

Other patients have fluctuating motility caused by the chronic epididymal damage, like Hal. Hal's sperm counts ranged from sixteen million to twenty-six million per cubic centimeter, and his motility varied from 0 to 20 percent. Hal figured that he could never get his wife pregnant because of his poor sperm motility. In his case, about three years postoperatively, his wife's doctor had become suspicious that she might have a problem and put her on Clomid to stimulate ovulation. That is when she got pregnant. Norman, on the other hand, had to wait five and a half years for his motility finally to come up to normal and for his wife to get pregnant. At one year postoperatively his sperm count had reached normal levels of about twenty million per cubic centimeter, but the motility was terrible. We encouraged him to be patient because there was no constriction or partial blockage causing this motility problem. His patience finally paid off, but it would have been impossible for him to be patient if he had not known that everything was anatomically and microsurgically normal, that no further treatment would help, and that only time was necessary for the epididymis to recover.

Sylvester was a different case. He had high sperm counts within the first three months after surgery, and yet it took four years for his wife finally to get pregnant. It was important for him to know that nothing needed to be done to improve his fertility, that his wife was completely normal, and that they were simply on the end of a bell-shaped random curve into which all couples trying to have children fit. As if to demonstrate how random this waiting period can be, their second pregnancy came within six months of the first child, for whom they had waited more than four years to conceive.

If there is no epididymal blockage and only the vas has to be reconnected, there should be sperm present by three months postoperatively, and the motility should be normal within three months to one year. However, when the epididymis is bypassed, there may be no sperm present at all for one year postoperatively, but some sperm should begin to appear by a year to a year and a half. It is in these epididymal cases that the motility of the sperm may not improve for several years. It is important to be reassured that the epididymal surgery was performed in the most meticulous and accurate microsurgical manner possible so that while waiting, you can feel comfortable that the epididymal duct is intact.

All these difficulties associated with epididymal bypass would disappear if the original vasectomy were routinely performed in an open-ended fashion. In that case, all that would be necessary to restore fertility is a microsurgically accurate vas reconnection, which is much easier than operating on the epididymis. This would go a long way toward minimizing the two major objections to vasectomy as a method of birth control: lingering pain and irreversibility. As you will see in the next chapter, if vasectomy is unappealing to you as a couple, we can also make sterilization readily reversible in the female, with an operation almost as simple and inexpensive as a vasectomy.

8

Tubal Ligation (Female Sterilization)

Tubal Ligation Can Be Reversible

Female sterilization is the most popular method of birth control today for married women in their mid-thirties who have had all the children they want. But it need not be considered a permanent procedure, and it is not always limited to women who have had all the children they want. In fact, sometimes it can be a saving grace for young women who have not been able to use other methods of birth control and desperately need some kind of immediate relief from what might otherwise inevitably turn into a tragic series of pelvic infections, pregnancies, abortions, unwanted children, and guilt. To make the sterilization easily reversible, however, it must be performed properly. Tubal ligation is immensely popular because in the past ten years it has become a simple one-day surgical procedure. But as women now become aware of its reversibility with microsurgery, it may become even more popular.

Ironically, some "reversible" methods of birth control may turn out to be more permanent than tubal sterilization. For example, the worst contraception for the young woman with more than one partner would be an IUD, because it is well known to allow infectious organisms an easier time getting up into the tubes and causing PID (pelvic inflammatory disease). This can damage the tubes in such a destructive fashion that the hope for pregnancy is poor even with delicate microsurgery. Ironically, sterilization may protect you from pelvic infections and thus preserve your fertility. With multiple sexual partners a young woman is very prone to catch one or more sexually transmitted diseases, but if she has been sterilized, these bacteria will not as easily be able to find their way up into the tubes.

Terri is a thirty-three-year-old professional woman who at age twenty-six found herself in a real bind. She came from a nice family. Her parents, however, had never taught her anything about sex, reproduction, or birth control. They just assumed she was a "nice" girl who would not have sex for "moral" reasons until she got married. What they did not realize is that everywhere around her (and around all of us), the movies, television, and magazines were sending clear messages that sex is fun, okay, and that there is no need to worry about birth control. All of these "beautiful people" on the screen have sex at the drop of a hat with new partners at a moment's attraction, and none of them ever seem to have trouble on the screen with venereal disease or pregnancy.

And so Terri by age twenty-one, unbeknownst to her parents, armed herself with birth control pills and got ready for some fun. Then she read some scary magazine articles about the pill. This, combined with the irresponsibility she had seen in screen heroes and television stars, helped her forget to take the pills. She then had several scares in which she was afraid she might have been pregnant. She thought that condoms and diaphragms were simply "kids' toys" and not used by the "beautiful people." How many times in a Hollywood love scene do you see a super-hero stop to put on a condom before engaging in an extremely explicit and graphic scene? At this point she made a rash decision that turned out to be, by a pure stroke of luck, the best decision she had ever made in her life.

Her choice boiled down to having an IUD inserted, or having a tubal sterilization. She did not think she would ever want to have children, as she was career-oriented. But she was only 75 percent sure of this, not 100 percent. Nonetheless, without any counseling she had no difficulty finding a resident at a university hospital who was quite willing to "tie her tubes." Ironically, this turned out to be absolutely the right decision for all of the wrong reasons. If she had had an IUD put in, the many cases of sexually transmitted diseases that she was to pick up in the next couple of years would have ascended through the vagina into her uterus, up into her tubes and pelvis, causing massive adhesions and doubtless destroying her tubes. This could have happened without the IUD, of course, but placing the IUD would have made it even easier. The IUD thus would probably have been an "irreversible" method of contraception. But because her tubes were "permanently" tied, they were saved from gonorrheal destruction.

When we reversed her tubal sterilization we discovered that her tubes would have been totally destroyed by infection were it not for the fact that the blockage of the tube prevented the infection from migrating any farther. It was a permanent protection against infecting organisms, and she did not have to worry about remembering to use condoms or a diaphragm every time she had sex. Ten years older and much wiser, Terri now was happily married, with a totally different view of life. She can have children because aside from the fact that her tubes had been tied, they were healthy and free of damage from infection. We successfully reversed her sterilization with delicate microsurgery.

Not so lucky was Linda who, in 1972, at age twenty, used an IUD for convenient, "reversible" contraception. She didn't have the patience or self-discipline to take the pill, use a diaphragm, or go "natural." She considered getting sterilized, but rejected this idea because she wanted to retain the option of having children at a later date. Now, fourteen years later, she wanted a child, but couldn't have one because at age twenty her IUD had caused massive infectious scarring of her tubes that was irreparable. If she had had a tubal sterilization, we could have easily restored her fertility with microsurgery.

But reversal of sterilization is easy only if the sterilization was performed properly. Janet was a nurse who had married very young because she did not know anything about birth control, became sexually active in her late teens, and figured she'd better get married to avoid having illegitimate children. Several years later she found herself not only unhappily married, but with two little children, a husband she did not love, and no time to pursue her career of nursing. Knowing nothing about birth control, she naturally opted for the "easy" route, sterilization. Five years later, she was happily remarried to a doctor, was an accomplished nurse, and in a sense had truly benefited from that interval in which she did not have to worry about getting pregnant. Now, naturally, she wanted more children, and had heard about our success with reversing tubal sterilizations.

But when we looked inside her abdomen, we were horrified to discover that the doctor who sterilized her had completely destroyed the fimbriated end of each Fallopian tube that is needed to pick up the egg from the surface of the ovary. At the time of ovulation the open end of the tube normally sweeps down around the ovary, coming to life like octopus tentacles, and literally grabs the egg off of the surface. Without this egg-collecting mechanism, the woman cannot possibly get pregnant. So Janet's decision in the heat of youth to have a sterilization turned out to be a poor choice, only because she chose the wrong doctor and was not well counseled.

Don't let this example dissuade you from recognizing the potential reversibility today of sterilization. If performed properly, tubal sterilization can be a safe, convenient, and potentially reversible birth control option. It should not be considered a routinely reversible birth control option, but for desperate young women, or for those who just hate to "burn their bridges," it can have a high degree of reversibility.

Who Gets Sterilized, and Why?

Voluntary female sterilization is the most widely used contraceptive method in the world, and its popularity is still rising. Over one hundred million women in the world have been sterilized. In the United States, Panama, China, and South Korea, over 25 percent of married women have been sterilized. When you include men who have had a vasectomy, sterilization is the birth control method of choice for almost two hundred million people around the world.

The reason for this increasing popularity of female sterilization is that it can be performed much more simply than twenty years ago. In the past it was a major operation that required several days to one week in the hospital. Although general anesthesia still is required in the vast majority of cases, surgery can be performed through a tiny incision with such minimal postoperative pain that often you can go home the same night. The failure rate of this contraceptive approach is only about two cases per thousand, or 0.2 percent. That makes it the most secure, and most convenient contraceptive method. What has kept it from being even more popular is that it still requires an operation, however simplified, and it has classically been viewed as a permanent, irreversible step.

In the United States alone, over 25 percent of married women use sterilization as a permanent method of birth control. Among married women ages thirty-five to forty-four, almost 40 percent rely on female sterilization. Oral contraceptives, by comparison, are used by only 14 percent. But the more amazing statistic is that prior to the new wave of popularity of sterilization beginning in the 1970s, almost 40 percent of American women eventually had a hysterectomy (complete removal of the uterus), supposedly for medical reasons. One has to speculate whether a side benefit of a hysterectomy might have been the more important unspoken reason of birth control. Since hysterectomy is a major procedure requiring up to one week in the hospital and fraught with possible complications, it is medically frowned upon as a method of sterilization. Hysterectomy clearly is becoming less popular as a method of sterilization, now that tying of the tubes has become so simple.

In China sixteen million female sterilizations and nine million male sterilizations are performed every year. In South Korea now, 25 percent of all married women have been sterilized, whereas in 1974 only 2 percent were sterilized. Even in Latin America, with its largely Catholic population, many countries have embraced this method of birth control. Panama, El Salvador, Costa Rica, the Dominican Republic, Barbados, Colombia, and Brazil have some of the highest rates of female sterilization in the world. This dramatic increase has resulted simply from the introduction of laparoscopy, whereby a little telescope can be placed through the belly button, to burn or block the tubes with great simplicity and very little pain. Only in Africa and the Middle East is sterilization rare or unusual.

Sterilization is most commonly chosen by women who are over thirty years of age, married, have several children, and don't want any more. Women who are sterilized under the age of thirty often come to regret it. Women who are sterilized over the age of thirty generally don't. Even women who have as many as three or four children before age thirty are very likely to want more. Furthermore, women who are unhappily married at the time of their sterilization are very likely to regret the procedure after they get divorced and remarried. Some women actually undergo sterilization hoping to cure their marriage problems, but this tactic almost inevitably fails.

In developed countries such as the United States, the most common reason women regret the operation is divorce, remarriage, and the desire to have children in a new marriage. Less commonly, the unexpected death of a child can prompt regret and the desire for more children. In poor, developing countries, child death is the major reason for regretting sterilization. Infant mortality rate in these countries is very high, and the chance of a child making it to young adulthood is low compared to the United States or Europe. These people are very likely to lose one or more children from infectious disease or malnutrition.

In the United States, child death is not that uncommon, either.

The most dangerous period in anyone's life is the first year, and particularly the first six months. Sudden infant death syndrome (SIDS) probably is more likely to claim your child's life than any other cause. Once your child has made it past his or her first year, it is relatively clear sailing from then on. In fact, the puzzling thing to me is why anyone should be at all confused or surprised about this terrible sudden infant death syndrome. Anyone who has ever listened to an infant breathe during the first three months of life while it is asleep has to wonder how such a fragile being could possibly survive.

Infants just don't breathe right. The infant pattern of breathing is based on oxygen deprivation. As we mature, normally the breathing center of the brain is regulated by the amount of carbon dioxide in our blood. This means that long before your oxygen levels get dangerously low, a buildup of carbon dioxide stimulates you to breathe more and thus constantly maintain an oxygen level very safely above the minimum required for survival. But this carbon dioxide breathing center in the brain is not well developed in infants. Their breathing is stimulated purely by oxygen deprivation. As they sleep, when their oxygen levels go too low, this stimulates them to start breathing again. After they have gotten their oxygen level back up again to adequate levels, they just stop breathing until the oxygen levels go down again. It is absolutely amazing that more infants do not die of sudden infant death syndrome.

So how can a woman who is sterilized immediately after delivering her baby possibly feel assured that one year from now her baby still will be alive? Although population planners do not emphasize this issue in the United States (or, for that matter, in the developing world), infant death still is a major reason why women may later regret having had a "permanent" sterilization.

For example, Cynthia had her second baby in 1977. It was born with multiple birth defects, including congenital heart disease. Yet she had a tubal ligation performed right at the time of the Caesarean section for the clearly logical reason that all she ever wanted was two children, and she figured that raising a child with all of these birth defects was going to be very expensive. She assumed that sterilization was permanent and wanted it that way. Even when the little infant died six weeks later, the emotional ordeal of having a child with birth defects was so overwhelming that she still was quite satisfied with her decision to be sterilized, and she did not want to have any more children. Yet five years later she came to our office begging to have microsurgery to reverse her sterilization so she could once again try for a second child.

Decisions made during the emotional strain of birth and delivery rarely hold up later.

Nancy had two children who were both quite healthy, but she and her husband were schoolteachers with a limited income and wanted to provide the best they could for those two children. So she had her tubes tied right after delivery, an approach frequently used because tubes are so accessible immediately after childbirth, when the enlarged uterus is pushing them up toward the abdominal wall. With this sort of timing the woman never has to worry about birth control after going home from the hospital. The problem is that her child died two months later of SIDS, and three months later she was in our office hoping we could tell her that her sterilization could be reversed.

Thus clearly the women most likely to regret being sterilized are those who have the procedure performed under the age of thirty, who are now in an unhappy marriage, or who have the procedure performed within one year of having their last child. At present sterilization is not commonly performed on single, young women or teenagers with a history of sexual promiscuity and who may already have had one or more abortions. This is because most doctors are quite rightly concerned that ten years later these women will be likely to regret their decision and want to have children. Nonetheless, a significant minority of women do get sterilized under these circumstances because they are just so desperate. These women may regret their decision later. But as will unfold in the rest of this chapter, these are not necessarily women to whom a sterilization should be denied. Certainly they would be better off developing a sense of sexual responsibility so they don't ruin their lives. But if they have difficulty achieving this, sterilization may very well be their best move, as long as it is performed in a way that can be easily reversed.

Comparison of Tubal Sterilization in the Female to Vasectomy in the Male

The Fallopian tube in the female works quite differently from the vas deferens in the male. The entire ductal system that transports sperm out of the testicle is a closed one, and therefore blocking it by vasectomy causes pressure buildup. In the female tube, the system is an open one. The Fallopian tube drains freely through the fimbria into the abdominal cavity. There is no pressure buildup caused by tubal ligation. Therefore, the duration of time that has passed since the tubal ligation is not of any consequence for the restoration of fertility with tubal reversal. No effort need be made to leave one end of the tube open after the ligation, because the tube is open at the end anyway.

However, the length of the Fallopian tube which has been damaged or removed by the sterilization procedure, unlike with vasectomy, has a tremendous effect on the reversibility. No matter how much tube has been removed, a good microsurgical technique can reconnect it. The problem is that if so much tube has been destroyed that this results in too short a tube, the fimbriated end will not be able to reach the surface of the ovary to pick up the egg. Furthermore, because the tube nourishes the egg during the first two days of the embryo's life, if the wrong area of the tube is removed, subsequent fertility would be unlikely despite a good reconnection.

The failure rate for tubal sterilization in the female should be about the same as for vasectomy (about two per every thousand cases). But failures with female sterilization are less predictable and more dangerous than failures with male sterilizations. At least 50 percent of accidental pregnancies that occur following tubal sterilization are ectopic. That means that although the sperm were able to get through the attempted blockade and reach the egg, the blockade did successfully prevent the egg from being transferred into the uterus to grow. Thus the pregnancy developed in the tube, creating a surgical emergency. The embryo cannot possibly survive in the tube, and in fact surgery very similar to an appendectomy is necessary to remove the ectopic pregnancy before the tube ruptures and the mother hemorrhages. Failure of sterilization after a vasectomy, however, simply results in a normal pregnancy.

Failure after tubal sterilization also is less predictable than failure after vasectomy. With vasectomy, a man's semen can be checked at regular intervals after the operation to see whether sperm are present. If sperm continue to be present, he knows the operation has failed, and he knows to use other birth control methods. With the female there is no easy way to check to see whether the operation was successful. Furthermore, when a vasectomy fails, it almost always occurs within six months. In the female, the tube can recanalize two or three years later, when she least suspects it. Thus a woman won't know that her tubal sterilization has failed until she becomes pregnant, and half of the time it is a potentially dangerous pregnancy that requires surgery. With the vasectomized male who has been properly counseled, such an unpredictable pregnancy would be very rare.

When are you safe from getting pregnant after vasectomy or after tubal sterilization? With vasectomy it can be a long wait, from six weeks to six months. During that time you are advised to use other birth control methods. In the female, if the sterilization operation has been successfully performed, you should be "safe" immediately.

Women are generally less likely to regret their sterilization, change their minds, and come back later for a reversal. Whether it is fair or unfair, in our society women have the bigger role to play in childrearing and do the most work. For men, childrearing often is a very casual and brief effort, and they may be very unrealistic about the amount of work involved in having more children. Women have a much truer perception of what having another child involves because generally they have done all of the work. Furthermore, women become biologically incapable of reproducing at a younger age than men. As evidenced by octogenarian Senator Strom Thurmond, who had a baby at age eighty-one, men virtually never lose their fertility simply by aging. But women become increasingly infertile over the age of thirty-five, and by age forty-two or forty-three are very infertile. By age forty-five or forty-eight it is almost impossible, despite great effort, for a woman to conceive. Thus a woman who has her sterilization at age thirty-three is pretty much near the end of her reproductive career and usually has no designs on reversing this decision. Men at age thirty-three have about fifty more years of reproductive viability ahead of them, and if they should get remarried, particularly to a young woman, they are more likely to request a reversal of their sterilization.

Sterilization in a man is simpler, safer, and easier to perform than in a woman. Vasectomy can be performed under local anesthesia in a doctor's office in less than twenty minutes. There is no major risk to health. Tubal sterilization, even with the modern techniques we will describe shortly, still involves penetrating the abdomen, risking damage to vital organs or blood vessels, and requires a general anesthetic in most cases. Even on an outpatient basis, female sterilization must be performed in a hospital setting, and this involves sophisticated instrumentation and ancillary personnel. The total cost of a tubal sterilization is about $2,000 ($1,000 doctor's fee and $1,000 for the hospital and anesthesia), whereas a vasectomy costs between $250 and $500.

In the past there was concern that tubal sterilization might affect a woman's menstrual periods, but many subsequent studies have shown that this is not true. Sterilization has no other effect on her reproductive organs. In the man, however, there are occasionally aggravating side effects on his reproductive system. The pressure buildup from the vasectomy can occasionally cause mild discomfort in the scrotum that every now and then may be aggravating enough to prompt him to have the operation reversed, despite its efficacy and lack of any overall negative effect on his health. Because the female tube is an open system with no pressure buildup, there is no such effect on the woman's reproductive system.

So who should get sterilized, the husband or the wife? It is clear that just as I recommended in the chapter on vasectomy, the person who should step forward is the person who wants it more. Comparing advantages and disadvantages of vasectomy to tubal sterilization really is a wash. The spouse who wants birth control more is the one who should be sterilized. If neither is willing to go through this step, then one spouse should not pressure the other, but other forms of birth control should be considered.

How Do the Fallopian Tubes Work?

First let's quickly review the anatomy from the first chapter. The uterus, or womb, is a pear-shaped, hollow structure into which the vagina leads. Two Fallopian tubes, one on each side, extend from the corners of the uterus and hang freely in the abdomen. The first part of the tube, called the isthmus, is about one inch long with a tiny inner canal and a thick, muscular, outer wall. The second portion of the tube is about three inches long. It is narrow at the isthmus and widens into a section called the ampulla, which has a trumpet-shaped opening at the end called the fimbria. The ovary sits freely in the abdomen, hanging from the uterus by a stalk called the ovarian ligament.

The ovary is not connected to the tube. When you ovulate, the egg does not simply fall out of the ovary into the tube. Rather, the tube seems to come to life as the muscles in its wall, and the wall of its ligaments, contract rhythmically, causing the tube to sweep over the surface of the ovary. The fimbriated end literally grabs the egg from the surface of the ovary and draws it into the interior of the tube. Millions of microscopic, hairlike projections called cilia constantly beat in the direction of the interior of the tube twelve hundred times per minute. These cilia function like a powerful, microscopic conveyor belt to pull the egg inside.

If the cilia are not functioning because the tubal lining has been damaged by infection, or if the tube has been dramatically shortened so it cannot reach the surface of the ovary, then pregnancy cannot result. If the ampulla is destroyed, pregnancy cannot possibly take place because that is where the embryo has to be fertilized and nourished for the first few days of life. However, if the isthmus is completely destroyed, the ampulla can be reconnected to the little opening coming out of the uterus (the cornu), and pregnancy can still easily occur. Thus the isthmus is not necessary for pregnancy, but the ampulla is.

How the Tube Is Approached Surgically

The only thing that makes tubal sterilization more difficult than vasectomy is that the tubes are inside the abdomen. There are three ways to reach the tubes. The old-fashioned method was through a major incision in the abdomen. This resulted in a great deal of postoperative pain, and all the potential complications of any major surgery. That is why sterilization of the female was so unpopular before the 1970s.

Today there are two very simple approaches to the tubes. One is minilaparotomy (minilap), which is the method used in most of the developing world. The second is laparoscopy, which is the most popular method in the United States, Europe, and the rest of the developed world. The minilap is a small surgical incision in the lower part of the abdomen about an inch to an inch and a half long. It can be performed extremely safely without sophisticated equipment in a very simple operating room. But the minilap is somewhat uncomfortable postoperatively and cannot be performed in obese women. It is perfect for thin women in developing countries.

Minilap can be performed under local anesthesia, but the patient will be more comfortable with general anesthesia. An incision is made just above the pubic hairline about an inch to an inch and a half long. At the same time a manipulator is placed into the cervix to move the uterus right up to the abdominal wall so that each Fallopian tube can be maneuvered into the area just under the small abdominal incision. A part of the tube is pulled out of the abdomen and occluded. The small incision in the abdomen is then closed, and the woman can leave the same day. Minilap is very difficult (and probably impossible) when the woman is obese. If it is mistakenly attempted on an obese woman the "small" incision frequently has to be lengthened quite a bit so it now becomes a big operation instead of a little one. In an appropriately thin patient, under local anesthesia, with an experienced surgeon, minilap may be the safest type of female sterilization. But under local anesthesia it does hurt, and for that reason most American physicians performing this method of sterilization put the patient to sleep.

The truly popular method of female sterilization in the United States, however, is laparoscopy (Figure 8–1 and Figure 8–2). The laparoscope is a narrow, stainless-steel telescope that is placed into the abdominal cavity through a tiny half-inch incision in the belly button (see Figure 8–3). Through this telescope most of the abdominal cavity can be visualized, and the Fallopian tubes can easily be grasped and either burned with an electrical current or occluded with a plastic ring or clip (Figure 8–4). The reason that this approach is so popular is that there is virtually no incision other than a puncture site in the belly button. This makes the procedure relatively painless postoperatively, and it can be used in all women, even those who are fairly obese, without any difficulty. But it does require sophisticated equipment, and it can be dangerous if not performed properly.

Although some family planners in the developing world are suggesting that this procedure be routinely performed under local anesthesia, the motivation for this is quite simply the lack of available, properly qualified general anesthesia personnel and facilities. I have seen experts perform this type of sterilization under local anesthesia, and I am convinced that it is not painless. In fact, it would be excruciatingly painful except that many of the women in developing countries on whom laparoscopy has been performed with only local anesthesia are very stoic people who can tolerate pain much more easily than Westernized patients in the United States and Europe. Therefore, in this country almost everyone undergoing laparoscopic tubal sterilization does so under general anesthesia.

Because the incision is so tiny, when the procedure is over there is virtually no pain. The reason that anesthesia is required is that for the laparoscope to be put in the abdomen with a clear view of the abdominal structures, the abdomen has to be inflated with about four to five pints of carbon dioxide gas. This inflation of the abdomen with gas allows the procedure to be performed safely and easily but precludes trying to do it while the patient is awake.

Laparoscopic Tubal Sterilization

Here is a step-by-step description of how sterilization is performed using the laparoscope. After the patient is asleep, a small, extremely

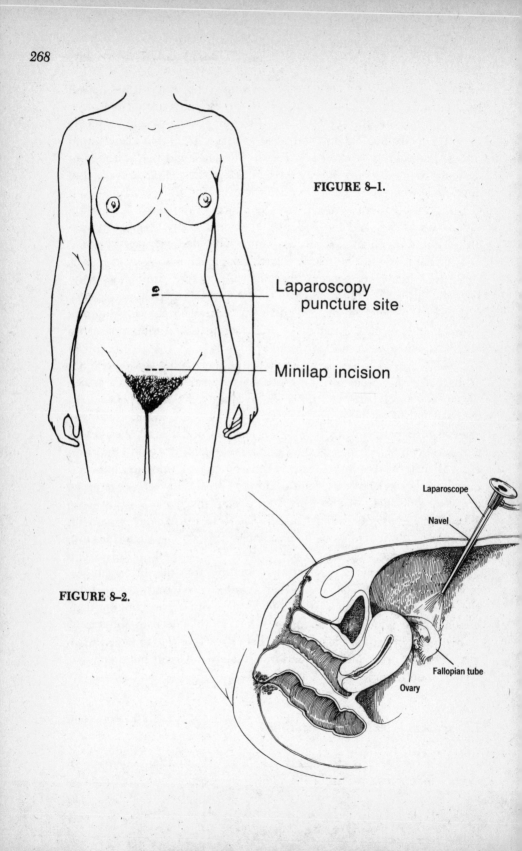

FIGURE 8–1.

Laparoscopy
puncture site

Minilap incision

FIGURE 8–2.

Laparoscope

Navel

Fallopian tube

Ovary

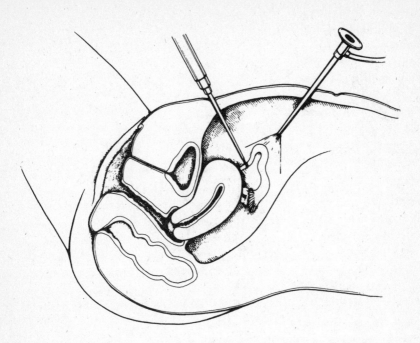

FIGURE 8–3.

safe needle is inserted into the abdominal cavity through the belly button. This needle is truly ingeniously designed. What makes it so safe is that it has a blunt outer edge that is spring-loaded, so that when you push against the abdominal wall the blunt edge is retracted and the sharp inside edge allows you to puncture the abdomen. The very instant that the needle goes through the abdominal wall, the decrease in resistance causes the blunt edge to spring back and protect the bowel from being punctured. Even if the bowel were accidentally punctured (which is virtually impossible with this needle), it would do no significant damage because such a small hole would heal on its own.

The needle is then connected to a flexible tube coming from a carbon dioxide inflation machine. An extremely safe system of backup valves ensures that the carbon dioxide does not come out of this inflator too rapidly. Even if these valves were to fail, the tiny hole in the needle through which carbon dioxide is transported puts an absolute limit on the amount of gas that can be transferred into the abdomen in a given

Tubal ligation

Healed tubal ligation

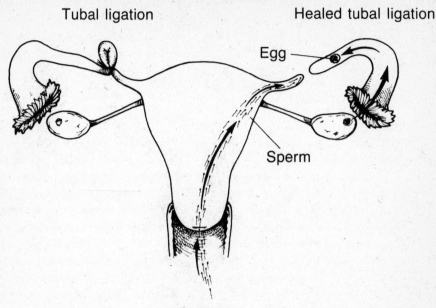

Egg

Sperm

FIGURE 8–4.

period of time. As the abdomen fills with this carbon dioxide gas, the physician can monitor the inflation of the abdominal wall and easily determine when to turn off the gas. Thus the abdominal wall is lifted far away from any important vital structures.

Next, a small half-inch incision is made in the skin of the belly button, and the outer sheath of the telescope is inserted, using a sharp inside "trocar" to puncture the belly button. The sharp trocar then is removed from the sheath, and the telescope is placed through the sheath into the abdominal cavity.

There are three major elements going through the telescope. The first is a fiberoptic light source, which travels via a flexible cable leading down a fiberoptic light pathway to the tip of the scope. The second is a carbon dioxide line that is used to maintain a constant flow of carbon dioxide gas to make up for the small amount that continues to leak out. Thus the abdomen remains inflated during the procedure. The third element of the telescope is the actual lens through which the operator looks to view the inside of the abdomen.

Once the abdomen is examined and the tubes are located, a tiny second puncture is made lower in the abdomen, just above the hairline. This puncture is no more than one-eighth inch in diameter, and through it, under direct vision, a narrow manipulating probe is inserted. This manipulating probe has on its end either a forceps that carries an electrocoagulating current to burn the tubes, or a silastic ring or clip to occlude the tubes mechanically. Once the tubes have been blocked, the manipulating probe is withdrawn, and carbon dioxide is completely removed from the abdomen by opening up a valve in the laparoscope. The laparoscope then is pulled out. A few little stitches are used to close the puncture site in the skin. The only dressing necessary is a Band-Aid. That is why this is so frequently referred to as the Band-Aid operation.

At least half a million of these laparoscopic tubal sterilizations are performed in the United States every year, safely, painlessly, and efficiently. I've explained the details of the operation so graphically in order to give you an appreciation of the potential for disastrous complications if the operator is not extremely proficient and well trained. In fact, proficiency is not as important as a carefully disciplined mentality that refuses to rush through, skipping the steps so as to imperil the safety of the patient. I will give you an example of the potential horror that can result from choosing the wrong surgeon.

Maxine went to the hospital to have a "simple little sterilization operation." She and her husband had two children and decided they did not want to have any more children because they wanted to give everything they could to the two they already had. Because of the fear of the side effects and dangers of reversible methods of contraception, they decided to take the safe, permanent step. The wife's obstetrician was a good-looking, fast-talking, fast-operating surgeon who had good manual dexterity in the operating room but always was in a hurry. Nobody ever was moving fast enough for him. A year or so earlier he had come to the conclusion that he was so good at laparoscopy that he could insert the trocar in a *deflated* abdomen without having to wait the time required to insert a needle and inflate the abdomen with carbon dioxide.

He was even in a bigger hurry this morning because he had a "lot of patients to do," and even had to attend to one or two pregnant women in labor. He inserted the trocar through the belly button almost effortlessly in this thin young woman, and when he looked inside through the laparoscope to burn her tubes, all he could see was red, nothing but red. This lady's husband did not go home that evening with a wife. He went home only with memories of what had been a happy marriage. His wife was dead. The doctor had stuck the trocar right into her vena cava, the central vein in the body.

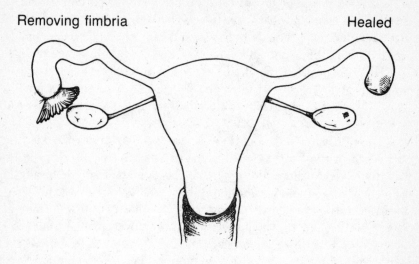

Removing fimbria   Healed

FIGURE 8–5.

Methods of Blocking the Tubes

Whether by minilap or by laparoscopy, there are four basic methods for occluding the tube. The classic method is to use a piece of surgical thread to ligate the tubes. This approach can be used only through the minilap—that is, when the abdomen is actually opened with a surgical incision. It cannot be used through the laparoscope. A variation of this classical tubal ligation is fimbriectomy, in which the entire fimbriated end of the tube is ligated with a tie and then removed (Figure 8–5), but this is an outdated method of sterilization that nobody should be using anymore because it not only makes the sterilization irreversible but also ironically leads to the highest failure rate of all the methods. I shall explain later how to make sterilization reliably reversible in the female by destroying only a minimum length of tube.

There are three methods for occluding the tube through the laparoscope. The most common method is simply to "burn" the tubes with an electrocoagulating current transmitted through a special forceps. There are two types of electrocoagulation current, bipolar and unipolar. Bipolar, the safer option, is much newer and limits the burn just to the tissue between the two tongs of the forceps. The electricity flows down one tong and across the tips to the other tong. There is no spread of the electrocoagulation effect.

Unipolar electrocoagulation is more dangerous. With this method, the current goes down both sides of the tongs of the forceps at once and then disperses from that point throughout the body, where it is picked up again by a grounding electrode, usually taped to the thigh or the back. With unipolar cautery, the patient is essentially a capacitor between two electrodes: a small electrode with an intense concentration of current where the tube is being burned, and a huge, flat, grounding electrode on the thigh that has a very minimum concentration of current. Actually unipolar electrocautery is much safer than it sounds, because the electric coagulating current becomes weak before it spreads out from the forceps. Nonetheless, there is some risk of damage to distant structures, and certainly a large area of tube usually is destroyed with this technique.

It used to be thought that sterilization with this unipolar cautery was irreversible because of so much tubal destruction. But my colleagues and I have been able to reverse even these difficult cases successfully for the following reasons: The current always tends to spread along the tube toward the uterus, the largest structure in its vicinity (which acts as a ground). Thus when the tube is grasped in the midpoint and burned extensively, usually it is burned only in the direction of the uterus, and the other side of the tube is spared. To reverse such a sterilization requires an extraordinarily delicate microsurgical reconnection of the tube to the tiny opening coming out of the uterus, and for that reason unipolar cautery is not recommended for making a tubal sterilization easily reversible. But because the electrical current burns toward the uterus rather than the end of the tube, even these cases can be reversed successfully.

The remaining two methods involve physical occlusion of the tube rather than cautery. The Hulka Clip (named after the gynecologist who invented it) reliably occludes the tube, and damages only the tiniest portion. The Fallope Ring is a small silastic rubber band with a special applicator that cinches around a doubled-up loop of the midportion of the tube. The Fallope Ring also damages only a small portion of the tube, is easy to apply, and probably is the most commonly used of the easily reversible methods of tubal occlusion (Figure 8–6).

The methods of tubal occlusion that are most easily reversible are

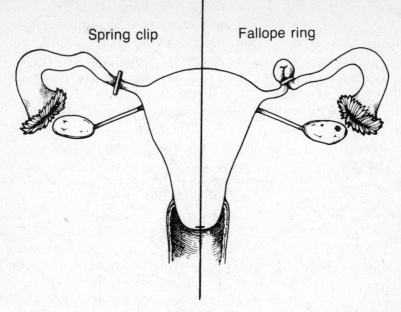

Spring clip   Fallope ring

FIGURE 8–6.

"bipolar" cautery, the silastic ring, and the clip. These three methods damage only a very small area of tube, leaving a small space in between. It would be unreliable simply to put a piece of thread around the tube and tie it down, hoping that this would prevent the egg and sperm from meeting. Such an approach would inevitably lead to a recanalization and pregnancy. Every method of occlusion must destroy some small segment of tube, which then scars down. This will be important to understand when I explain how the sterilization can be performed to make it more reversible and yet prevent failure.

Failure of the Sterilization to Work

Averaging together all of the millions of tubal sterilizations that have been reported, the failure rate of this method of contraception is about two pregnancies per thousand women. This extremely low failure rate makes it one of the securest methods of birth control. In fact, the failure rate may be much lower than two per thousand because many of those pregnancies occurred during the same cycle as the sterilization, and it has to be assumed that many of these women, unknown to the doctor, were already pregnant at the time they were sterilized. This is not truly a failure of sterilization, but rather a failure to get sterilized soon enough. Nonetheless, there are a small number of true failures of sterilization, and half of such pregnancies are very dangerous to the mother.

The reasons for failure of the sterilization to work are:

1. The woman already is pregnant at the time of the operation.
2. Surgical error is made, and another structure, such as the round ligament, is mistaken for the Fallopian tube and is cauterized instead.
3. The ends of the Fallopian tube actually grow back together again, creating a new connection, very similar to recanalization after vasectomy.
4. Surgical error is made in which the tube is properly identified, but is either not cauterized completely or the ring or clip is improperly applied.

The likelihood of failure is directly related to how inexperienced the surgeon is. The more experienced and disciplined the surgeon, the less likelihood there is for failure.

Recanalization means that the tube was completely occluded, but over the course of time the two ends have grown back together again and reestablished a connection. How does this occur? It virtually never occurs if the tube is occluded in the narrow isthmus region. Almost all spontaneous recanalizations occur when the sterilization occlusion was performed in the wide ampullary region. The large diameter of the ampullary region of the tube, combined with the lush inner lining with all of its many folds and projections, make it very easy for a small imperfection in the scarred ends to open up, allowing the lush lining mucosa to then spread across the gap, reestablishing the connection. This is a disaster because the pregnancy that results is usually ectopic and never gets into the uterus, thus requiring emergency surgery.

Also in the ampulla, an incomplete burn or an improper application of the Fallope Ring or Hulka Clip is more likely to occur. In the narrow isthmic region of the tube, it is easier completely to burn and coagulate the entire circumference of the narrow tube with cautery. It is similarly easier completely to occlude the narrow isthmic portion of the tube with an application of a clip or elastic band. For all these reasons, the only sensible region of the tube to occlude when doing a sterilization is the narrow isthmus.

Does making the tubal sterilization more reversible increase the risk of failure? There are many reasons for making the sterilization reversible. Three percent of women who were carefully counseled to consider sterilization as permanent, request a reversal later. Various studies have shown convincingly that even more patients would undergo sterilization if they thought it were reliably reversible. There have been many erroneous ideas about how to make the sterilization more reversible, and I will get into this in more detail later in the chapter. There is no question and no controversy that the sterilization technique that damages the minimal amount of tube is the easiest to reverse. Yet there has been fear that damaging only a small amount of tube will increase the chances for failure. We now know that this fear is erroneous. Failure of sterilization is related to incorrectly identifying the tube (thereby occluding the wrong structure), improperly occluding the tube (which almost always occurs in the ampulla, not in the isthmus), or properly occluding the tube but choosing to do it in the ampullary region (where recanalization is possible) rather than in the isthmus. Simple, minimally destructive occlusion of the narrow isthmus region of the tube makes the sterilization eminently reversible and at the same time gives you the lowest possible risk of failure of the sterilization.

Jennie was a twenty-seven-year-old housewife with a boy age three and a girl age six. She had her tubal ligation performed laparoscopically after the boy was about six months old, and she was relatively sure that he was healthy and growing normally. The doctor doing the sterilization wanted to make sure there was no unwanted pregnancy because this couple did not think they could afford any more children. So he burned the tubes with unipolar cautery all the way down to the uterus. Luckily, no matter how severely he tried to burn the tubes, he was not fully aware of that law of physics I explained earlier whereby the unipolar current tends to spread toward the largest surface, namely the uterus, and not in the opposite direction toward the end of the tube. So despite all of his destructive efforts there still was some tube left, although there was nothing on the uterine end to connect it to.

Three years later the little boy who was riding with his father on a tractor on a calm, beautiful Sunday afternoon, unexpectedly jumped off, and the big wheel ran right over him. He was dead instantly, and Jennie longed to have another child but was told that her tubes were just too badly burned to be repaired. Fortunately for her, we were able to reconnect the tubes to the microscopic openings coming out of the uterus. She has had two more children since then and has no intention of ever being sterilized again. But if she had had a more conservative tubal sterilization in which only a minimal amount of tube in the narrow isthmic region had been cauterized, she could have been just as safely protected against a sterilization failure and yet had a much easier time with reversibility.

When to Do the Sterilization, and on Whom?

Probably the most convenient time to perform the tubal sterilization is the worst time to do it, immediately after the delivery of the last child. The uterus is enlarged, and the tubes therefore are pushed up toward the abdominal wall. So the procedure is very easy. At this moment, when the mother is burdened with the discomfort of the delivery, the thought of the tremendous amount of work ahead of her in raising that child, and a touch of postpartum depression, it is the easiest conceivable time to convince her to have a sterilization. For that reason so-called postpartum sterilizations have been extraordinarily common, and for the same reasons, in most cases they should be condemned.

In the developing world, postpartum sterilization offers the advantage that for many women, childbirth is their major contact with health services and thus their best opportunity to obtain a sterilization. After delivery they go back to a village where they have no access to health personnel. After delivery these women also are highly motivated to avoid having more children because of the pain, the hospitalization, and the years of hard work ahead. The procedure can be performed extraordinarily easily through a minilaparotomy, which is the most common and easiest method of sterilization in the developing world in that it does not require the complex instrumentation of laparoscopy.

I knew a patient who had a postpartum sterilization because she wanted to know when she left the hospital that she would never have to worry about getting pregnant again. The child she had just carried was an "accident," and although she was dedicated to loving it, she was dreading the work ahead of her. Several days after the postpartum sterilization, however, the child developed unexpected respiratory stress syndrome and in less than one week was dead. Despite what the mother thought was a clear desire not to have more than two children, her present two children still turned out not to be enough. Several years later she came for a sterilization reversal. The first few months of life with a newborn are the most fragile we ever face, and it is the worst time for a couple to be making a permanent birth control decision.

Another popular time for performing a sterilization is at the time of, or shortly after, having an abortion. A World Health Organization committee found that up to 10 percent of women sterilized at the time of an abortion subsequently changed their minds about the sterilization. On the other hand, of women who ask for sterilization at the time of the abortion but for whom plans are not made to have the sterilization until three or four months later, 4 percent of them became pregnant before they could come in for the subsequent sterilization and then wound up having another abortion. So although it seems that when a woman is having an abortion is not the best time psychologically to make a permanent decision about future childbearing, there is a high risk that without sterilization, before too long these women will be coming back for another abortion.

For example, at age twenty-one Judy became pregnant and had an abortion. She felt extreme guilt and remorse about doing this and felt for sure that this "mistake" would not happen again. But she obviously had unresolved problems stemming from a conflict between wanting to have sexual relations and yet feeling too guilty about it to frankly and openly go on birth control pills. Her hit-or-miss approach of contraception failed once more, and then she had her second abortion. At this point she knew she was in trouble. Almost beside herself, she requested that sterilization be performed at the same time as the abortion. The clinic sensed this might be an error and told her to come back in six months after the abortion and rediscuss the issue then. When she came back in six months she was pregnant once more, had a third abortion, and this time did succeed in talking them into tying her tubes. Eight years later Judy was not just a flighty little girl who could not control her own life, but a very pleasant young woman happily married, doing volunteer work at the church, and who wanted more than anything else to have her sterilization reversed. Apparently she had been following the work at our clinic over the previous five years and told me in a letter before coming to visit us in St. Louis, "Although we have never met, just knowing that you exist has meant a lot to me over the last five years."

I finally did operate on Judy, and now she has several children whom she is doing a beautiful job of raising. Thus, while it is clear that a woman who is about to undergo an abortion is likely to regret her sterilization later, the mere fact that she has rejected a multitude of birth control methods or at least not been successful with them, means that she is very likely to become pregnant again if something isn't done.

So is sterilization the right answer for young women who just can't seem to stick to less permanent methods of birth control that require a little more effort and a little more discipline? Or is tubal ligation best intended strictly for the mature woman, happily married, who already has had all the children she ever wants? To help answer that question, let's look at Tammy, Jo Anne, and Eileen.

Tammy was a thirty-three-year-old nurse who had been on birth control pills before age twenty-one. She read an article that scared her because it suggested that birth control pills might cause fibrocystic disease of the breast. The ridiculous thing about the article is that studies have shown that birth control pills actually prevent fibrocystic disease of the breast. But because of the scare that was created, she decided she would not take birth control pills and decided to rely on the diaphragm. She said she just didn't understand why, but she was apparently just "irresponsible" about using the diaphragm and became pregnant. She had an abortion, and even now, nine years later, she tells me that she still grieves for this. Since the birth control pills were "too dangerous" and the diaphragm required too much discipline, she felt her choice was basically between an IUD or sterilization. She decided quite correctly that the IUD would not be safe for her. So she had a sterilization, knowing only full well that she was only partially sure that she wanted no children. She figured that she had no choice.

When the sterilization was performed, the doctors told her that her tubes were already badly inflamed from venereal disease, which she did not doubt, since at that stage of her life she had had quite a few sexual partners. When we performed her microsurgical sterilization reversal nine years later, she was expecting that we would find pretty terribly diseased tubes that would never allow her to get pregnant, and so she was rather despondent about it. What she had not realized is that the sterilization process itself, by blocking most of the tube off from the pathway of infectious organisms coming up from the uterus, protected the tube from any further infection or inflammation. Thus what we found nine years later was a beautifully preserved tube despite the fact that she had had numerous infections in the past. Now she was in a stable, happy, monogamous marriage with no threat of developing any more sexually transmitted diseases; wanted to have a happy, stable family; and was indeed able to do so *because of* rather than *in spite of* her tubal ligation nine years earlier.

Eileen was not so fortunate. She was very disciplined and faithfully went on birth control pills, preventing herself from having any pregnancies while she was sowing her wild oats. She never had a tubal ligation, and when she came to our clinic after three years of trying to get pregnant, we found tubes that had been badly damaged by pelvic inflammatory disease caused by sexually transmitted infection. Fortunately, the birth control pills offer some measure of protection against ascending venereal infections, because they make the cervical mucus sticky, creating a relative barrier to bacterial invasion. Otherwise, Eileen, too, would have been hopelessly sterile beyond surgical correction. As it is, there is only about a 40 percent chance that she will get pregnant after the intricate surgery we performed, whereas if she had had a reversible sterilization years ago, her chances of getting pregnant would have been normal.

Jo Anne had a relatively unpromiscuous life, did not believe in multiple relationships throughout her teens, twenties, and early thirties, and had only had a few serious sexual encounters before getting married in her late thirties. After several years of marriage and trying to get pregnant unsuccessfully, she came to us for evaluation, and naturally we suspected that due to her increasing age, she probably had some ovulatory inadequacy, but we certainly didn't expect pelvic inflammatory disease. When we looked inside with the laparoscope, we were surprised to find tubes that were no less damaged than Eileen's by pelvic inflammatory disease. Jo Anne, who had very few boyfriends in her life, who was totally faithful, who never dreamed she had ever contracted a sexually transmitted disease, had suffered tubal damage far less reversible than sterilization, damage from which either a sterilization, condoms, or a diaphragm could have protected her.

These tragic stories are not meant to sell the notion that every young woman with frequent sexual exposure or multiple partners should have a tubal sterilizaton. She is far better off insisting on condoms, or using a diaphragm without fail, or possibly even taking birth control pills because of the moderate level of protection they give from infectious disease. But when all else fails, either because the woman may be too young and undisciplined to remember to take the pill, insist on her boyfriend using a condom every time, or remember to go to her purse and put in her diaphragm before fully engaging in the throes of passion, or who may have already had one or more abortions, sterilization may well be the rest from worry that she needs. An IUD in such a woman would be very convenient but surely would court the disaster of pelvic inflammatory disease. As serious a step as it might seem, having a sterilization despite youth and no children might be exactly the right ticket so long as the tubes are spared enough to make the sterilization easily reversible.

Of course, the obvious candidate for a tubal sterilization is a happily married woman over thirty-five years of age who has at least two children and doesn't want any more. But many married women who have all the children they want are not so happily married. Yet they get a sterilization performed with absolute confidence that it is the best thing for them, thinking it may even save the marriage. Such women usually get divorced several years later and find themselves remarried, often in a much better relationship.

Many happily married women over the age of thirty with all of the children they want, who have no doubt in their mind that sterilization is the easiest, best birth control for them, suffer from heavy menstrual periods, severe menstrual cramps, or premenstrual syndrome (PMS). These symptoms, which are so common in women over age thirty-five, will not in any way be improved by having a tubal ligation. In fact, the best treatment for these conditions may very well be the new low-dose, triphasic birth control pills. These could reduce their periods dramatically and in many cases help alleviate the PMS symptoms. Of course, I am not advocating birth control pills for women over thirty-five in preference to tubal sterilization. I just want to warn women with severe menstrual symptoms that would best be managed by the new, safer, low-dose birth control pills, or even by hysterectomy, that they should consider carefully before thinking that tubal sterilization is the answer to all their worries.

Reversal of Sterilization

The major worry of the doctor performing your sterilization is that you will get pregnant when you don't want to. For this they can get sued. Generally they are not worried about how to make the operation reversible. In fact, if you ask them to make it reversible, they may be afraid to perform the operation in the first place for fear you will sue them for sterilizing someone who should not be sterilized. They also worry that if they damage the least amount of tube, perhaps there is a very, very outside risk that the operation will fail, the tubes will grow back together again, you will have an unwanted pregnancy, and then you will sue them. There have been several lawsuits where women have sued the doctor on behalf of their child for "wrongful life." If you can believe it, the contention of such suits is that the child had a right not to exist because his mother had chosen sterilization. The failure of the sterilization resulted in the birth of a child whose right not to exist was denied.

Well, fortunately the courts have decided that such a lawsuit is absurd. But the courts have a funny way of compromise. As I mentioned earlier, if a "wrongful birth" occurs and the child is handicapped, then the doctor may be found liable for the entire cost of raising the child for the rest of his or her life over and above what it would cost to raise a normal child. Once again the chaotic court system has clouded up the issues, but fortunately there are doctors who will discuss and consider your individual case according to your particular needs and do what is right regardless of the fear of an irrational lawsuit. But you can certainly see why they may lean heavily away from a reversible approach to sterilization. As we have discussed before, for the sterilization to be maximally reversible and yet not fail, the tube must be blocked or destroyed in the isthmus region and preferably only a small segment damaged.

If the tubal sterilization destroys the fimbria, or damages too huge a segment of ampulla, then despite perfect microsurgery, the woman is unlikely to get pregnant. We do not feel that there is any case of tubal obstruction too technically difficult to reconnect. The tubal sterilization procedure can often create a very difficult microsurgical problem for correcting obstruction, but we feel virtually all of these problems can be solved and the tube reopened. But then pregnancy depends on whether the reconstructed tube has an adequate fimbria, and enough length to reach and pick up the egg, as well as enough ampulla to nourish it.

REVERSING THE IMPOSSIBLE

Jan had three children, a happy marriage, and had decided to have a sterilization three years earlier. Two years after the sterilization, Jan and her husband, Roger, knew they wanted a larger family and could afford more children. They had done such a good job of raising the three they already had that I felt quite sure there was room for more children if they wanted them. Yet, when their local gynecologist, a well-known fertility expert, looked at her tubes through the laparo-

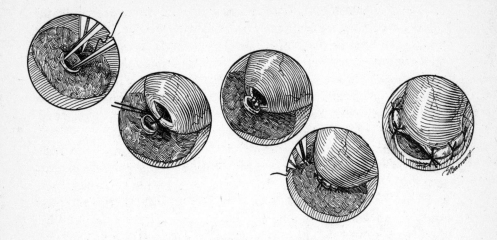

FIGURE 8–7.

scope to decide whether a reversal procedure could be performed, he sadly concluded that nothing could be done. The tubes had been "too badly damaged" by the original sterilization procedure. When we looked at his report we realized that the fimbria was not damaged, and although the ampulla was short, it certainly was long enough to nourish the egg. What had concerned her gynecologist was what looked like a technically very difficult operation because of a unipolar cautery sterilization that had burned all the way down to the uterus. The opening to the uterus is so tiny that such an operation requires a great deal of microsurgical skill (see Figure 8–7). But still, virtually all such cases can be reconnected, and I knew there was enough healthy tubal length for pregnancy to occur. So Jan came to St. Louis so we could operate. Jan and Roger now have two more children.

Katie had a tubal sterilization performed in 1979, and a relatively inexperienced surgeon attempted a reversal three years later. The operation was poorly performed, and she wound up with total blockage on the right and partial blockage on the left. Two and a half years later, she got pregnant on this left side. The sperm were able to find their way through the partial blockage to the egg, but unfortunately the egg was not able to move into the uterus two days later. This resulted in an ectopic pregnancy, which required emergency surgery. Thus when I saw her in 1985 she only had one tube remaining, and never dreamed that it still would be technically possible to make her fertile. But when we operated we found a long, healthy tube that just needed to be reconnected properly, this time to the cornu, the tiny little opening coming out of the uterus. Her case was the same as that of countless others emphasizing the same point. She had an adequate length of normal tube, but it required a technically difficult operation to restore continuity. As long as there is enough tubal length even on just one side, a technically difficult operation is not a problem. Katie is also now fertile.

We have seen many patients who had a poor attempt at sterilization reversal, failed to get pregnant, and then went through *in vitro* fertilization attempts. *In vitro* fertilization is an exciting new treatment designed for cases where the tube is totally destroyed. In this case, the ovary is stimulated with hormones to make many follicles. These follicles then are removed through a laparoscope and fertilized in a laboratory dish with the husband's sperm after they have been suitably washed. Then conception takes place in that dish. The fertilized embryo then is placed into the womb, and the hope is that a pregnancy will result. Unfortunately, the pregnancy rate even in the very best clinic is very poor, with only about 8 percent of such women coming home with a baby.

It is no surprise that most of these women who went through the *in vitro* fertilization treatment after sterilization reversal failed did not get pregnant with that approach either. In each one of these cases we have seen, there was enough healthy tube for pregnancy to occur, but the restoration of tubal continuity required a very technically involved operation. In all these cases we were able to reestablish fertility, and these women achieved pregnancy. But it would have been better if the original sterilization procedure were performed cautiously enough to make the reversal operation easier.

How the Type of Sterilization Affects the Technique for Reversal

Unipolar cauterization (burning) through the laparoscope has been the most common method of sterilization over the past ten years. This usually results in destruction of a fairly large segment of tube. Fortunately, the burn always seems to spread from the grasping forceps to the uterus, sparing the end of the tube leading toward the fimbria. It burns all of the isthmus right down to the uterus, and some of the ampulla. Thus it is technically the most difficult type of sterilization to reverse. But because tubal length often is quite adequate, we still have an extremely high success rate with reversing this type of sterilization. But the technical difficulty of such a procedure usually overwhelms the doctor who is not extremely experienced in microsurgery. For that reason unipolar cautery is not an easily reversible sterilization.

The type of reconnection required after unipolar cautery is called ampullary-cornual, meaning that the large-diameter ampulla has to be reconnected to the tiny cornual opening of the uterus. To perform such an operation requires either making a tiny opening in the scarred ampulla so that openings of the same microscopic size can be connected, or else cutting out the scar and tailoring this enlarged opening down to the tiny one-seventieth-inch diameter that will allow it to match up with the tiny one-seventieth-inch opening of the cornual end (see Figure 8–8). Any tubal reconnection requires a microsurgical technique, but this operation requires the most delicate microsurgical technique possible. Therefore, unipolar cautery through the laparoscope cannot be considered an easily reversible method of sterilization, even though in very technically skilled hands this sterilization can be reversed most of the time.

There are four approaches to obstructing the tube that usually do very little damage and make the sterilization an *easily reversible one*. Bipolar cauterization (also performed through the laparoscope) allows the current to go down one tong of the forceps across the tissue to the other tong and never spreads anywhere but between those two points. Thus the tube is burned wherever it happens to be grasped, and the burn does not spread in either direction. This type of cautery will damage very little tube, and if the tube is grasped in the narrow isthmus region, should result in the blocked ends of the tube being of relatively equal size and not very difficult to reconnect with microsurgery (see Figure 8–9). The only catch here is that many doctors are so afraid that this bipolar cautery does not burn the tube adequately that they may burn the tube in several different places. This does not mean the sterilization is irreversible, but once again means that more complex surgical techniques are required for the reversal.

The classic technique for occluding the tubes from years ago is the original tubal ligation. This is where the tube is actually tied off with surgical suture. This cannot be performed through the laparoscope but is the most common method of blocking the tube through a minilap. This type of sterilization is technically easier to reconnect than unipolar

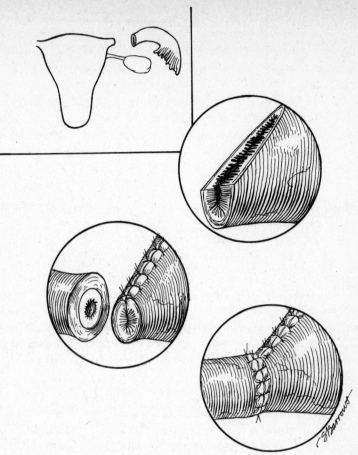

FIGURE 8–8.

cautery or bipolar cautery done in multiple areas of the tube. But still it destroys an inch to an inch and a half of tube and results in some scar tissue that has to be freed. Thus although within the grasp of most microsurgeons to reverse, tubal ligation still is not as favorable for easy reversibility as either the Fallope Ring or the Hulka Clip.

The Fallope Ring is a tiny, silastic band that looks like a very thick, round rubber band with an internal diameter of about one-eighth inch. It comes loaded on a device which through the laparoscope, or minilap, grasps the Fallopian tube and then pulls a loop of it up through the ring. Because the ring is so tight, the loop of Fallopian tube loses its bloody supply and disappears into scar tissue over the course of several weeks. Usually it destroys no more than one-half inch to at most an inch of tube and virtually always leaves enough tubal length for subsequent reversibility. Like the bipolar cautery, it virtually never dam-

1.

2.

3.

4.

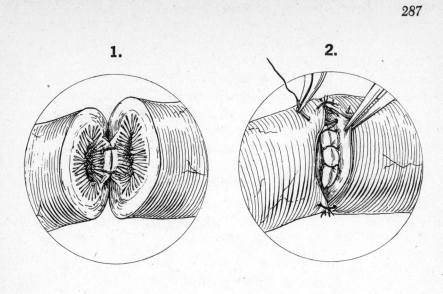

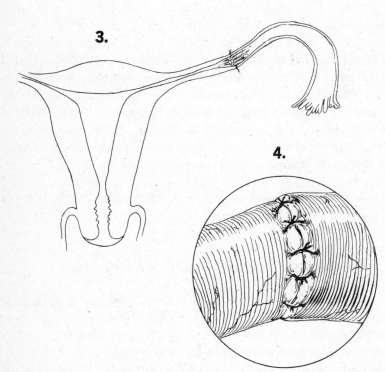

FIGURE 8–9.

ages the tube all the way down to the uterus, and thus a difficult cornual reconnection never is required. The only technical problem sometimes created by the Fallope Ring and the classic tubal ligation is that often an area of isthmus and ampulla, rather than just isthmus alone, is destroyed. This means that to reconnect the tube means surgically uniting the relatively large diameter of the ampulla to the somewhat smaller diameter of the isthmus. This is not a terribly difficult surgical problem and does not compare to the difficulty of reconnecting the ampulla to the cornu coming out of the uterus.

The easiest surgical reconnection is with lumens of the same diameter, and that is where the Hulka Clip comes in. The Hulka Clip never damages more than one-quarter inch of tube. So if it is applied to the isthmus region, the reversal operation simply would involve reconnecting isthmus to isthmus, lumens of the same diameter.

To summarize, the Hulka Clip, if applied to the narrow isthmus, damages the least amount of tube and is the easiest technically to reverse. Bipolar cauterization, as opposed to unipolar, should damage almost as little tissue as the Hulka Clip, but many doctors are so fearful that they haven't really burned the tube adequately with the bipolar that they may burn it in several different locations. The Fallope Ring, in my view, is just as reversible as the Hulka Clip, and I advise patients that using the Fallope Ring is virtually a completely reversible sterilization procedure. But because it may damage slightly more tube than the Hulka Clip and may damage both ampulla and isthmus, the Fallope Ring may present slight technical difficulties for less experienced microsurgeons. Unipolar cautery, which is now becoming less popular, damages the most tube and creates a technical need for the most difficult reconnection procedure.

What Factors Affect Successful Sterilization Reversal?

If we look at the success rates in various groups of patients on whom we performed a sterilization reversal, we get a clear picture of what factors affect reversibility. Virtually all our reversal patients have had a good connection with open tubes postoperatively. But despite near-perfect surgical results, not all our patients got pregnant after reversal of tubal sterilization. Looking at the various categories of these patients helps to tell us what makes the sterilization reversible and not reversible after a proper microsurgical reconnection.

When we first began doing microsurgical sterilization reversals for women in 1977, we decided that we would start with no preconceptions and offer the operation to absolutely any woman who requested it. At that time there were many prejudicial misconceptions about what type of sterilization and what type of patient would be most easily reversed, who could get pregnant, and who couldn't. We knew that none of these preconceptions was based on genuine observations of women undergoing truly meticulous, careful microsurgical technique for reversal. Many doctors just assumed, for example, that reversal of a laparoscopic unipolar cautery sterilization was impossible to perform. Many assumed that if a woman had had a previous attempt at reversal that failed, there would be too much scarring ever to allow a subsequent reattempt at reversal to succeed. Many felt that women over thirty-five, or women whose sterilization was performed over five years earlier, would have no chance for success, and these women were turned down. Of the hundreds of women coming to us for sterilization reversal, we turned no one down based on any preconception, but kept accurate, meticulous records of every aspect of their situation to see which patients were mostly likely to get pregnant.

The observations recorded for each patient were the age of the husband; the age of the wife; the sperm count of the husband; the number of previous children (if any); the duration of time since the sterilization was originally performed; the type of sterilization procedure performed (whether through laparoscopy, laparotomy, or minilaparotomy); whether unipolar or bipolar cautery, Fallope Ring, Hulka Clip, or ligation was used; the area of the tube that was destroyed; the areas of the tube that had to be reconnected; and finally the total length of tube remaining after the reconnection was achieved. Furthermore, we observed the character of the anatomic appearance of the ovaries, the quality of the menstrual cycle before and after the reversal surgery, and the amount of general scarring (adhesions) in the pelvis.

Thus we hoped to find the answer to three specific questions that would help us advise women who were getting sterilized as to how it could be made more easily reversible. The first two questions were: What type of sterilization procedure is easiest to reconnect surgically? Are there any types of sterilization procedures that are impossible to reconnect surgically? The third question was: Assuming a good reconnection is achieved, would anything else about the way the sterilization was originally performed stand in the way of getting pregnant now that the tubes are properly reconnected?

What we found is that the only thing affecting whether these women got pregnant after sterilization reversal surgery is the *length of tube on the longer side*. None of the other myriads of factors we carefully and assiduously studied made any difference. As long as there was a fimbria left to pick up the egg, there was nothing else about the sterilization procedure that prevented pregnancy other than the length of tube that was left after the reconnection. If there was very little tube left, so that only about an inch of tube remained after the reconnection, the pregnancy rate was a very low, only 18 percent (despite a perfect reconnection of the tube). If there were an inch and a half of tube left, the pregnancy rate went up to 55 percent. If there were over two inches of tube left after the reconnection, on either side, every woman in this category got pregnant. The duration of time since the sterilization made no difference. The age of the woman, as long as she was under forty, made no difference. The type of sterilization, whether through a laparoscope or a minilap, made no difference. Whether the tube was blocked by unipolar cautery, bipolar cautery, Fallope Ring, Hulka Clip, or ligation, made no difference. Nothing made any difference except the total length of the tube, and if the tube was over two inches long when the procedure was completed, every patient in the original study got pregnant.

Now, of course, to retract slightly, no woman can ever be guaranteed a pregnancy. For example, in a normal population of women, about 15 percent are going to be relatively infertile. So a 100 percent pregnancy rate actually makes no sense except for the fact that these were women who, before they had the sterilization, were extremely fertile and got pregnant rather easily. Thus after the sterilization they also are by and large more fertile than a random population of women, 15 percent of whom would have difficulty getting pregnant. If by any chance some other illness would cause such a woman to develop infertility later on in life, then she may not be expected to get pregnant as easily as she did before the sterilization. In addition, if she has a new husband he might not be as fertile, and this could affect her chances of getting pregnant. Therefore, we cannot guarantee fertility to women who have more than two inches of tube left after the sterilization reversal. But we can assure them that the sterilization procedure itself most likely has had no effect on their fertility, and after the reversal they should be just as fertile as they would have been at this stage in their life had they never had sterilization.

A good example of this is Dena. Dena came from the West Coast to have her sterilization reversal performed at our clinic. Because her original sterilization, performed with unipolar cautery, burned the tube right down to the uterus, she required an ampullary-cornual reconnection. Postoperative X rays confirmed that we had achieved a beautiful microscopic reconnection of the tube, and her tubal length was over two inches. Thus we could assure her that pregnancy was extremely likely, and certainly could assure her that she was just as fertile now as she would have been had she never undergone a sterilization procedure years ago. Yet after several years she did not get pregnant, and another X ray, performed in her hometown, demonstrated once again perfectly normal tubal anatomy. What was not expected is that she had ovulatory dysfunction, with multiple little cysts in her ovaries. She required fertility drugs to get her pregnant. This kind of problem could have intervened in any woman of any age at any time. Indeed, it is commonly found in almost 15 percent of the population who have trouble getting pregnant without being treated for infertility. Therefore, having a successful sterilization reversal operation with adequate-length tubes does not guarantee pregnancy, but it does assure you that you have the same chance of getting pregnant that you would have had if you had never had the sterilization years before. Depending on the random size of the number of patients a given surgeon has operated upon, and assuming the woman is not already in her late thirties, the pregnancy rate is about 90 percent. But if too much tube has been destroyed, the pregnancy rate can be as low as 18 percent.

Unusual Cases of Sterilization Reversal

We have seen many requests for reversal of sterilization by women whose husbands also need vasectomy reversal. If we weren't so certain about the return to normal fertility of women who have two inches or more of tube left, we would have difficulty suggesting that both the husband and the wife undergo surgery to try to have children. Because it is clear that any such woman not in her late thirties with two inches or more of tube has a 90 to 100 percent chance of pregnancy (assuming her husband has sperm) we can easily recommend to such patients that both have a reversal operation.

Wanda and Bert were the first such couple I had seen. Each had several children from previous marriages. They were now blissfully married to each other in a happy, stable relationship, and both they and their present children wanted them to have more kids. Wanda was told there was no hope for reversing her sterilization because it had been performed with unipolar cauterization with too much tubal destruction. As in all cases of female sterilization reversal, only two issues mattered: Could we technically accomplish a surgical reconnection? Was there enough tubal length? As we have stated before, despite the fact that the tube was burned all the way to the uterus, we were able to establish a beautiful ampullary-cornual reconnection and had no doubt we would be able to do this. Her tubal length was only about one inch on each side, and thus her fertility rate would have been extremely low after reconnection. Therefore we transplanted a portion of her tube from one side to the other side so that instead of having two short tubes, which would have a difficult time picking the egg up from the ovary, she had one two-inch long tube that had no difficulty picking up the egg.

With confidence we then suggested that Bert also go through vasectomy reversal surgery. Three months later, despite the dire predictions given by her regular doctors, Wanda became pregnant. In most of the cases we have seen where both the husband and the wife had previously been sterilized in an earlier marriage, reversing the sterilization on both of them resulted in pregnancy.

Some doctors have a negative view about women who change their minds and decide they want to have a sterilization reversed. This merely reflects a chauvinistic male attitude that does not admit to the vicissitudes of unpredictable problems that life presents. If your doctor takes that attitude when you ask about sterilization reversal, you might want to consider another doctor.

Sterilization Is "Natural" Birth Control

A final point that should emerge from this chapter is that sterilization is, in a sense, a very "natural" method of birth control. It causes no hormonal changes, and really no changes in the body's functioning whatsoever. It doesn't make you liable to develop infections or heavy bleeding, such as the IUD. It does not suppress ovulation or in any way change the chemistry of your body, like the birth control pills. It does not rely on remembering to use it just before sex while in the heat of passion, as the condom, the diaphragm, and foam often unrealistically require. If performed with minimal damage to the tube, sterilization is potentially reversible, very convenient, and ultimately "natural" method of birth control. The only reservations are that it requires a surgical operation, however simple; and to reverse it requires a surgical operation that is not so simple, and the results cannot be guaranteed.

When I visited a very busy birth control research clinic and talked with knowledgeable nurses who were guiding hundreds of women through difficult decisionmaking, I met one nurse who put it all in simple perspective. Her life's work was to carry out procedures and counseling for brilliant doctors who were trying to develop safer, totally convenient, reliable, and yet totally reversible new approaches to birth control for women. With all the many avenues available, I wanted to know which of the new approaches she thought would be the best. She just looked at me and said, "Doc, I would just forget all these complicated new approaches and have my tubes tied."

9

Newer Methods

Injectable Contraception Once Every Three Months

For women who would like all of the benefits of the birth control pill but simply can't remember to adhere to a rigid, daily, pill-taking routine, injectable contraception may be the answer. Just one shot of Depo-provera (the brand name for a progesterone hormone made by the Upjohn Company) every three months gives you incredibly safe protection from pregnancy (less than 0.5 percent per year). This makes it every bit as effective as the birth control pill in preventing pregnancy and provides all the progesterone-related beneficial effects of the pill, such as decreasing the risk of cancer of the uterus, cancer of the ovary, benign breast tumors, and pelvic inflammatory disease. It has been used for over twenty-five years in over a hundred countries with no evidence of any serious risk to health. But if you live in the United States, you can't have it. Before you start packing your bags again to plan another trip to Canada or another foreign country to obtain an effective, convenient contraceptive that is available everywhere else in the world but the United States, you should realize that this time the problem isn't litigation-hungry lawyers with dollar signs in their eyes but rather timid government bureaucrats.

The injectable contraceptive we are talking about is Depo-provera. It has been used since the mid-1950s as a long-acting progesterone that provides a remarkable cure for endometriosis, as well as advanced cancer of the uterus that has spread to all parts of the body that would be uniformly fatal except for the remarkable ability of long-acting progesterone in humans to cause endometrial tissue that lines the uterus to soften and eventually shrivel away. In 1963 this long-acting progesterone began to be used as an injectable contraceptive that would provide the same remarkable protection against pregnancy as the birth control pill but without the need of daily pill-taking. The reason you can't have it is that the very cancer that Depo-provera prevents (and can cause to go away if you are unfortunate to have it already) is feared by some congressmen to be caused by it. If this sounds strange to you, you are not alone. Despite assurances from one scientific committee after another that Depo-provera is safe and does not cause cancer in humans, the bureaucrats are undaunted in their refusal to approve it for use as a contraceptive.

Actually, Depo-provera is available in the United States, but not for use as a contraceptive. The U.S. Food and Drug Administration has approved its use to prevent and treat the very cancers it is supposed to cause. Are you puzzled? Well, so are many scientists and physicians who have yet to figure out how to get around this bureaucratic no-win barrier. But the good news is that because the drug is approved for treating and preventing cancer, it is available to American doctors to prescribe for you. Furthermore, the law is such that a doctor can give it to you for injectable contraception quite legally as long as he or she informs you that in his or her judgment it is safe but that the U.S. Food and Drug Administration has not approved it for this use.

For all practical purposes no private doctor is going to administer this safe contraceptive to you under those circumstances, because if you develop any illness whatsoever, whether related to the contraceptive or not, he or she will be a sitting duck for your lawyer. However, if you go to a physician who is relatively immune from being sued (such as a full-time university salaried physician), you may very well be able to go on this contraceptive without having to travel to Canada or another foreign country every three months.

Like all contraceptives, injectable Depo-provera is not a panacea without any problems. You will remember that the birth control pill involves three weeks of taking an estrogen and progesterone pill followed by one week of no hormones at all, during which you menstruate. A three-month injection of Depo-provera does not in anyway mimic this monthly cycle. It just means that a continuing high level of progesterone throughout the entire month for three consecutive months inhibits ovulation and prevents the cervical mucus from ever becoming receptive to sperm invasion. You do not build up the lining of your uterus every three weeks followed by a one-week interval when you menstruate. Rather you have a continual, nonfluctuating level of hormone that interferes with rather than mimics the natural cycle. Therefore most women on Depo-provera experience a disruption of their menstrual cycle.

The changes in your cycle are unpredictable and are basically that of a nonovulating woman. You will have irregular spotting and staining without any predictability or regularity. Your total amount of menstrual bleeding will be less than in a normal cycle because the progesterone causes dramatic thinning of the endometrial lining of the uterus. Eventually you stop menstruating. Once you reach this stage, the Depo-provera becomes much more acceptable, because you no longer have to worry about when you are going to have your menstrual bleeding, because you just won't have any. You should not worry about the fact that the menstruation has ceased, because whenever you decide to have children and stop taking the Depo-provera injections, your menstruation eventually will return to normal, generally after six months or a year.

Other disadvantages in anywhere from 1 to 17 percent of women include a possible two- to ten-pound weight gain related to increased appetite, and progesterone-induced headaches. So injectable progesterone contraception every three months, despite its great convenience and superior effectiveness, may not be your choice because of some of these harmless but potentially aggravating side effects. But most physicians feel that this decision should be made by you as an informed choice rather than by a government bureaucrat with no scientific training.

In 1967 Upjohn applied to the U.S. Food and Drug Administration to study the use of Depo-provera as a contraceptive. In 1974, after seven years of extensive testing in this country, the Obstetrics and Gynecology Advisory Committee of the Food and Drug Administration issued a notice to doctors that they had reviewed this drug favorably and were going to approve it for use in women who had difficulty with other, more conventional contraceptive methods. Doctors were very enthusiastic about the availability of this contraceptive because of the growing awareness that the estrogen component of the birth control pill is what caused nausea, vomiting, and blood clots, and that the progestin in the pill is what provided most of the protection the pill affords against various diseases already discussed. The Food and Drug Administration officially announced its intent to approve Depo-provera for this use in September 1974.

Shortly thereafter, a U.S. congressman questioned whether Depo-provera might increase the risk of cervical cancer. Thousands of studies had indicated that it did not, but the Food and Drug Administration, responding to this ignorant but powerful political pressure, suspended its intended approval. One year later, after more study by more scientific advisory committees, it was proven conclusively, without a shadow of a doubt, that Depo-provera did not increase the risk of cervical cancer, and the FDA committee once more recommended approval of Depo-provera. Three years later, again responding to tremendous pressure from Congress and the scare tactics of certain special-interest groups, the FDA formally denied approval of the drug for the following reasons:

1. Studies in beagle dogs indicating the development of breast nodules when they were given Depo-provera.
2. Potential risk of birth defects if the woman should get pregnant while on Depo-provera.
3. Estrogens might be needed to control irregular menstrual bleeding and then the benefit of a no-estrogen contraceptive would be diminished.
4. A significant need for Depo-provera in the United States had not been demonstrated.

The last three objections can be dismissed very simply. There has been no report at all showing any injectable contraceptive such as Depo-provera to cause birth defects, but it is true that some progestins already approved and available in birth control pill preparations can cause a more masculine appearance of the external genitalia of female babies when taken sometime between the ninth and twelfth weeks of pregnancy. These cases are very rare, not very difficult to treat surgically, and have been known to occur only in association with the progestins already approved for use in the birth control pill.

Progestins that have been approved for use in the birth control pill are quite different from Depo-provera in that they are derived chemically from the male hormone testosterone. Therefore you can understand how, if birth control pills were given between the ninth and the twelfth weeks of pregnancy, when the external genitalia are developing, there might indeed be some risk of masculinization. It is well demonstrated that taking birth control pills during the first several weeks of pregnancy does not produce this or any other fetal abnormality (see Chapter 4). Yet it is because of this rare risk of masculinization of the female genitalia caused by a contraceptive preparation already fully approved by the FDA, that the FDA decided not to approve Depo-provera, which, in fact, has not ever been shown to cause masculinization of the fetus and would not rationally be expected to because, unlike the already approved contraceptives, it is not derived from the male hormone testosterone.

The case against the FDA's concerns is even stronger when you realize that pregnancy would not occur after discontinuation of Depo-provera until the hormone levels of Depo-provera dropped to almost undetectable levels. It is true that if Depo-provera injections were given sometime in the middle of the cycle, it would most likely not prevent a pregnancy from occurring, and in that case the fetus would be exposed to three to five months of the hormone. That is a very legitimate reason to study the issue carefully. But if you make sure to give the injection within the first five days of the beginning of the menstrual period only, you can be virtually certain that the woman is not pregnant, and the chances of becoming pregnant are incredibly low because it is such a reliable contraceptive. Over four million women around the world are using Depo-provera for contraception, it has been available for over twenty-five years, and yet there have been no reports of increased risk of birth defects in the human. To put this concern in perspective, it has also groundlessly been alleged that rhythm birth control, the diaphragm, and contraceptive vaginal spermicides all might cause fetal abnormalities.

The concern of the FDA that estrogens might be needed to control irregular menstrual bleeding and thereby reduce the benefit of the progestin-only injection is answered simply by the fact that no physician today recommends using estrogen in combination with Depo-provera. If a woman is bothered by the irregular menstrual bleeding of Depo-provera and is not willing to wait until she stops spotting, then she simply should not take Depo-provera. It is as simple as that.

The argument that there is no significant need for such a contraceptive in the United States is so frivolous and irresponsible as to be unbecoming to any properly constituted governmental regulatory agency. That brings us to the major controversy—the issue of whether Depo-provera causes cancer.

DOES DEPO-PROVERA CAUSE CANCER?

No evidence to date links the use of any progestin to cancer in humans. In fact, it is clear that progestins retard the growth of cancer in reproductive organs and certainly help prevent development of cancer of the uterus. But there are two animal studies that have created great concern for the Food and Drug Administration. One study demonstrates the development of breast cancer in beagle dogs injected with Depo-provera, and the other study demonstrates development of endometrial cancer of the uterus in monkeys receiving the drug. As I explain what these studies showed, you need to keep in mind one basic fact from Chapter 1 of this book, "How You Get Pregnant." The human female is hormonally unlike any other animal on the face of the earth, including monkeys, in that she menstruates. Menstruation is peculiarly human, and the effect of hormones on female sexual behavior as well as on her reproductive tract is also peculiarly human. If you keep this fact in mind you may be able to understand better the confusion caused by studies performed in dogs and monkeys.

Dogs have a peculiar reaction to progesterone, behaving quite differently from humans and many other species. The dog is the only species in which progesterone or other progestins are known to increase breast tissue growth. This abnormal growth of breast tissue caused by progesterone occurs in no other species. In humans, breast growth is stimulated by estrogen rather than progesterone, and long-term estrogen unopposed by progesterone certainly will cause benign breast enlargement and conceivably could lead to cancer. Exactly the opposite is true with progesterone in humans.

Another peculiarity about dogs is that they normally have reservoirs of microscopic tumors in the breast. These tumors, normally present in beagle dogs in particular, then grow and develop in response to progesterone or any other progestin. Thus the fact that Depo-provera caused beagle dogs to develop benign and malignant breast tumors should be no surprise. Similarly, the fact that Depo-provera has not been shown to cause benign breast enlargement, or breast malignancy in humans despite over twenty-five years of use involving four million people a year, should not be surprising either. No other government licensing authority in the world requires that progestins be tested on beagle dogs.

Another study demonstrated that there was endometrial cancer of the uterus in two of twelve monkeys that received fifty times the equivalent human dose of Depo-provera. Again, the monkey uterus's response to progestin is expectedly quite different from that of humans. Remember, only humans menstruate. In all other species, including monkeys, the production of progesterone in the second half of the cycle does not just soften up the uterine lining so that if the animal does not get pregnant the lining then sloughs in what we call menstruation. In all other animals, both estrogen and progestin stimulate the uterine lining, and when the hormone levels go down after "heat," the uterine lining thins down because it is no longer stimulated. Naturally, therefore, you can understand how when beagle dogs are given a progestin, it stimulates the endometrial lining of the uterus so much that a severe plethora of tissue grows within the uterus, which can get infected, become cancerous, and even kill the animal.

For this particular reason the FDA for years has advocated that all other hormonal experiments performed on female dogs should wait until the dog first has a hysterectomy. So all these studies on dogs that were supposed to demonstrate whether Depo-provera would be safe in humans were performed on dogs who had first undergone a hysterectomy because everyone knew that they would otherwise run a high risk of uterine complications from progestin intake. In the human, on the other hand, progesterone causes the endometrium to become soft and then slough despite continued progesterone stimulation. That is why we shouldn't be surprised that giving Depo-provera to monkeys (who were not hysterectomized) caused them to develop many tumors in the uterus, the very tumors that in humans Depo-provera would prevent.

Countless studies in hundreds of thousands of humans around the world since the 1960s in women of all ages have demonstrated that progestin causes no increased risk of cancer of the uterus or cancer of the breast. The use of progestins like Depo-provera to treat and indeed prevent the development of cancer of the uterus is accepted throughout the world. Studies on oral contraceptives that contain progestins that were clearly proven to cause breast nodules and breast cancers in beagles have been shown not to increase the risk of breast cancer in humans at all and to decrease significantly the risk of the development of benign breast disease. Thus most doctors and scientists view the U.S. government's failure to approve Depo-provera for this purpose as another example of how politics and bureaucracy are interfering in the United States with your receiving the best possible health care.

HOW DOES DEPO-PROVERA WORK?

If you can talk your doctor into giving you Depo-provera for contraception, or if you are going on a trip to Canada or another foreign country, you will want to know a little bit more about how Depo-provera works. A 150-milligram dose is given by shot once every three months. The initial shot must be given within five days of the beginning of menstruation, so your doctor can be sure you're not already pregnant. If you wait until eight or nine days after the beginning of menstruation and you have had intercourse, it is very possible for you still to get pregnant that first month. In the future it may be possible to lower the dose to only 100 milligrams every three months, as some early studies now are showing that that lower dosage may be just as effective in preventing conception. Provera can be given as a long-acting injection, or taken as a short-acting pill. In the Depo-provera form, it is given as a shot that has a very slow release over a prolonged period of time. That is why a single injection provides safe contraception for a full three months. By the end of three months there is still enough Depo-provera in the system to provide contraception, but by five months most of the hormone is gone from the system. Nonetheless, small, traceable amounts still can be detected as long as six or seven months later. The decision, therefore, to have the injection every three months makes you quite secure that the contraceptive effect will not have worn off before you get your next injection.

Depo-provera provides its contraceptive effect by reducing the pituitary secretion of both FSH and LH. In this way the constant presence of this progestin agent prevents follicle development and subsequent ovulation. In addition, the constant progestational effect dries up the cervical mucus and makes it impermeable to sperm invasion. Finally, the endometrial lining of the uterus becomes thinned out so that it would never support a pregnancy anyway. After cessation of the drug, this thinned-out endometrial lining comes right back up to normal, and the pituitary starts secreting FSH and LH again.

Within one week of injection of 150 milligrams of Depo-provera, blood levels of the drug begin to peak, remain elevated for two to three months, and then begin to decline steadily. Depo-provera may be undetectable in the blood as early as seventy-three days after injection, or may continue in the bloodstream in tiny amounts until seven months after injection. Regardless of this variation in disappearance rate, blood levels do not accumulate with long-term use of Depo-provera in these doses. Nonetheless, a more even, constant level of hormone in the blood can be achieved with a more modern type of injectable contraceptive using implantable plastic rods or capsules underneath the skin. This approach will be discussed in the next section.

The most troublesome side effect of this extremely simple and extraordinarily reliable method of birth control is menstrual disturbances. Fifty percent of the patients do not mind these menstrual disturbances too badly, and if they stick with it long enough, after one year they are not menstruating at all. If they can get through this difficult first year until they reach the stage of no menstruation, most of these patients feel like they are in nirvana. Imagine not having to worry about getting pregnant, not having to remember to take a pill every day, not having to put on a condom or diaphragm every time you want to make love, no dangerous side effects to worry about, and on top of that you don't even have to menstruate.

But don't take too lightly the aggravation associated with that irregular bleeding during the first year and the 50 percent possibility that after a year you still may have irregular bleeding. In one birth control clinic I visited, the nurse who gives the Depo-provera injections and instructs the patients in many of these new birth control devices introduced me to a typical patient who had had a lot of irregular bleeding during the first year, necessitating many trips to the clinic to be reassured that everything was working fine. This patient had stuck it out for a year, was still having occasional spotting, but was looking forward to the day soon when she figured she wouldn't be menstruating anymore. I congratulated the nurse on being so supportive to the patient and helping her get through this difficult time. The nurse then surprised me by confiding that if it were she, she simply would have had her tubes tied long ago.

It is possible to get a variety of other aggravating side effects from Depo-provera, and if these side effects are so troublesome that you decide against this method of contraception, you are going to have to wait three months or longer to get rid of them. This is not the case with a birth control pill that you simply can stop taking, or an IUD that you can have removed, or even an implantable progesterone rod (see the next section) that you can have removed if the symptoms of constant progestin release disturb you. These symptoms in some women can include headache, weight gain caused by increased appetite, abdominal bloating, and even mood changes. These are symptoms typically associated occasionally with women with premenstrual syndrome related to variations in progesterone level just prior to menstruation. Anytime you give a progestin-type drug, it is possible to get symptoms. But women are variable, and most women report no such problems. In fact 20 to 40 percent of women note weight loss rather than weight gain, which quite pleases them.

How long does it take for fertility to return after discontinuing Depo-provera? Although the 150-milligram injection of Depo-provera is not considered to provide contraceptive protection for more than ninety days, in most women it prevents pregnancy for several months longer. On the average, it takes a month and a half to three months longer for women to conceive after discontinuing Depo-provera than after discontinuing birth control pills. On the average, it takes about five and a half months from the time the next injection would have been given for Depo-provera users to get pregnant. There is no evidence to show that any injectable progestin permanently impairs fertility. More than 50 percent of women are menstruating by six months after stopping Depo-provera, and 85 percent by one year. However, note that 15 percent do not resume menstruation until after one year. Only 60 percent of the women seeking to become pregnant do so within one year after stopping Depo-provera, which represents a significant retardation in recovery of fertility. However, two years after discontinuing the drug, over 90 percent have gotten pregnant. Furthermore, long-term users of Depo-provera conceive, on an average, just as rapidly as women who have had only a few injections for half a year, proving that there is no long-term, cumulative effect of taking the drug.

There will always be a certain small percentage of women who fail to resume menstruation after any hormonal contraceptive. In this respect, Depo-provera is no different from the birth control pill. But keep in mind that progestin-only contraception such as Depo-provera is much less likely to have this permanent inhibitory effect on the hypothalamus. In most such women, just as for all nonovulaters, treatment with clomiphene citrate should be able to stimulate the suppressed hypothalamus to start working again. The pregnancy rate in treating women with postpill amenorrhea and, in like fashion, amenorrhea subsequent to Depo-provera usually is quite high.

Norplant—Birth Control Under the Skin

Major objections to Depo-provera are, first, that if it gives you side effects you don't like, you have to wait five months, on an average, before all these side effects go away, and you can use another method. A second problem is that you do have to remember to get the injection every three months, which may be a more formidable task than it seems. By the time three months are up, you may have gotten so used to the convenience of not having to worry about it that you may very well forget. The third objection is that right after the injection your levels of Depo-provera go up fairly high, and then slowly diminish over the next several months.

The Population Council of the United Nations, working in cooperation with a company in Finland, has developed a new long-term progesterone implant that solves all these objections. The implant consists of a silastic rod or capsule that is designed to release slowly a progestin called levonorgestrel in doses far lower than present birth control pill formulations. The level of levonorgestrel in the blood is thus at the same constant level all the time for up to a full five years without the need of any other injection or treatment. Unlike with Depo-provera, the method is instantly reversible simply by removing the silastic implant.

In the early clinical trials, over four thousand women used this method of contraception, and about 80 percent stick with it despite the menstrual irregularities at the end of one year. At the end of five years, 50 percent of the women remain happy with the Norplant implant. The pregnancy rate is very low—less than 0.2 percent per year. This approach to long-term, injectable contraception is very advantageous in women who wish an extended period of "thoughtless" protection from getting pregnant but who wish to have the freedom to be able to discontinue the method anytime they like by having the implant removed. Norplant will probably be available in the United States in the next year or so unless government officials block this also.

The Norplant progestin-only implants are inserted underneath the skin of a woman's arm using a local anesthetic, in an operation that requires only about five or ten minutes in a doctor's office. The system consists of one to six flexible capsules or rods, about as long as a popsicle stick, containing levonorgestrel, a potent progestin that has been in oral contraceptives for twenty years. Removing the implant is just as easily done under local anesthesia in a matter of minutes in the doctor's office. The effect on the menstrual cycle is virtually identical to that of Depo-provera and the potential side effects are identical. The total amount of progestin released into the body is very small, half the dose of progestin that is absorbed in the usual low-dose oral contraceptives. The implants are not painful, and are fairly unobtrusive.

There is a major tactical advantage that Norplant has over Depo-provera in getting the approval of the U.S. Food and Drug Administration. The drug Depo-provera has never been tested or officially approved for use as part of a contraceptive program. However, the drug levonorgestrel, despite being more potent and needing a more critical review than Depo-provera, already has been approved by the FDA years ago for use as an oral contraceptive. Thus in the inscrutable ways of bureaucratic licensing, Norplant has gotten a friendlier reception thus far than the equally safe Depo-provera did.

The strongest advantage of Norplant over Depo-provera is that Norplant yields a constant, even delivery of progestin, provides protection for many years without the need of reinjection, and is very rapidly reversible the instant the rod is removed. Unlike with Depo-provera, where only about 60 percent of women get pregnant in the first year after discontinuation, with Norplant 84 percent of women get pregnant within the first year after discontinuation. This is absolutely no different from a normal population of women trying to get pregnant. As soon as the Norplant is removed from under the skin of the arm, hormone levels go down precipitously, and the woman rapidly returns to her precontraception condition, unlike with Depo-provera, where a prolonged wait sometimes is necessary before all the hormone leaves the system and she once again becomes fertile.

GNRH—Birth Control Nosedrops

The birth control nosedrops, which you may have read about a couple of years ago, have not panned out as well as was hoped. You need to understand how they work, because if they ever are perfected, you will be rushing to get them. You may recall from the first chapter that the pituitary gland would not secrete its stimulating hormones, FSH and LH, unless there were a continual episodic release from the brain of a substance called GNRH (gonadotropin-releasing hormone). The primitive region of the brain called the hypothalamus releases a short one-minute pulse of this hormone every ninety minutes directly into the pituitary gland, which sits right under the brain. This area of the brain also is the seat of many of our emotions and the location of our thirst and appetite center. If this part of the brain is turned off, as occurs when you take birth control pills, or when you are given a Depo-provera injection, the pituitary gland will no longer make FSH and LH, and consequently the ovaries and the testicles will not function.

What is absolutely amazing is that if GNRH were to be *released continually*, it would shut off the pituitary gland. There would be a very transient increase in FSH and LH production by the pituitary, but within a matter of a few days a process called down regulation would exhaust the pituitary's receptors and make it unreactive to the GNRH. This discovery has led to an explosion of interest in finding a way to regulate reproductive function simply by changing the "pulse frequency" of GNRH in the circulation.

One simple way to do this is to give a drug that behaves exactly like GNRH except that it stays in the system for a prolonged period of time. When your brain normally releases GNRH to your pituitary, it is chemically changed within a matter of minutes into an inactive compound that has no effect on the pituitary. But if GNRH were to be altered slightly so that it would not disappear within a matter of minutes but stay around for hours or days, it would completely turn off the pituitary's production of FSH and LH.

We now have drugs that do exactly that, and they are called GNRH agonists. In fact, they have been already approved for turning off the testicles' production of testosterone in patients with prostate cancer, and to halt temporarily the production of hormones from the ovary or the testicles in children with precocious puberty. Men with prostate cancer that has spread throughout the body usually have to have their testicles surgically removed to stop the testosterone production which stimulates that cancer's continued growth. By using this GNRH agonist instead, these men can accomplish the same thing without having to be castrated. More impressive than that, children who are going through premature puberty at age seven or eight used to represent a tragic scene in which modern medicine could do nothing. They would have stunted growth, never reach full height, and undergo all the changes of puberty long before they had the emotional maturity to deal with it. With GNRH agonists we can simply turn off their ovaries or their testicles until the appropriate time for them to have puberty along with their peers. When the GNRH agonist is no longer given, the pituitary immediately starts making FSH and LH again, and the children then go through a normal puberty as though they never had a problem.

Because these GNRH agonists are so easily destroyed by your stomach juices, they must be given either by injection in an oil base, or via a nasal spray. Most people interested in contraception would rather squirt a few drops of GNRH in their nose once or twice a day than give themselves a daily injection. But the form of GNRH agonist that is now approved can be given by injection only, and it has only been officially approved for the treatment of prostate cancer and precocious puberty.

There are some serious problems associated with trying to use this new wonder drug as a contraceptive. First, if you give a woman a high enough dose to suppress the ovary completely, you create artificial menopause with hot flashes and potential long-term problems associated with lack of estrogen in the system, such as weak bones and a dry, painful vagina. So clearly you do not want to give a dose so large that the ovary is completely turned off. However, if you decrease the dose gradually to the level where the ovary still can make estrogen but not ovulate, what you wind up with is a so-called unopposed estrogen effect, which we have talked about many times in this book because it leads to cancer of the uterus. The human uterus simply must have a periodic production of progesterone to soften up the hard lining created by the estrogen in order to prepare it for sloughing. Production of estrogen alone will result in a heaped-up uterine lining that eventually leads to cancer. So it doesn't appear that this new wonder drug is going to be advisable, as yet, for contraception in the female.

In the male, you get exactly the opposite of what you would hope for. You would hope to be able to reduce the sperm production to zero but have minimal effect on testosterone production. But in truth the opposite occurs. You reduce the testosterone production of the testicle to literally castrate levels, but you just can't seem to get the sperm count down to zero. As has been shown on numerous occasions, even a very low sperm count can result in pregnancy. Newer more potent GNRH drugs in the future may be able to push the sperm count down to zero, but then there will still be the problem that the testicle won't make testosterone either. Thus the GNRH agonist is great for cancer of the prostate and represents a miracle for children with otherwise tragic precocious puberty, but for the moment these miracle nosedrops won't quite do as a contraceptive.

The Male Pill

Why should there be a "pill" for women only? Men have barrier methods available to them (the condom) and sterilization (vasectomy), but with all we know today, why can't there be a pill for the male as simple as the female birth control pill that would provide men with easily reversible protection from fertility? Well, the answer is there is a male "pill"—in fact, several varieties of male pill. But a lot of bugs need to be worked out, which will require the same amount of financing and commitment that the women's movement lent in the 1950s toward efforts to develop a female "pill." Perhaps the slowness in progress is related to the fact that most of the researchers in this field are male. But a more important stumbling block is the conviction of drug companies that the majority of women will not feel comfortable trusting a man to remember to take his pill every day. They fear that after the infusion of huge amounts of capital into such a venture, it would wind up being a commercial fizzle.

Studies coming from China, where one quarter of the world's population lives, indicate that the drug companies may be wrong. There are two types of approaches to the "male pill": (1) drugs that directly interfere with the testicle's production of sperm without affecting the production of testosterone, and (2) male hormones that (as with the female pill) suppress the pituitary's release of FSH and LH.

The first type of pill is already widely available in China. It is called Gossypol, and its story is fascinating. Gossypol is a yellowish compound found in the seeds, leaves, and roots of the cotton plant. Chemists knew about it as far back as 1899, and by 1958 it could be commercially synthesized. But no one was aware of its remarkable future as a male birth control pill until 1971, when Dr. Qian from the Nanjing Institute in China came across an obscure report from the 1930s prepared by a Dr. Liu, who had studied a strange "curse" that had hit the village of Wang Cun in Jiangsu Province in the 1920s.

For fifteen years, between the 1920s and the early 1930s in this small village, a strange, inexplicable phenomenon had occurred: During that time not a single child was born. The village was panic-stricken. They tried praying to Buddha, and moving their ancestors' tombs to "luckier" sites, as their fortune-tellers had directed. Some villagers married widows from other villages who earlier had given birth to children, but these fertile women strangely enough became barren after coming to Wang Cun village. Then suddenly in the mid-1930s the "curse" was lifted, and women began to get pregnant again.

It was later realized that during those no-baby years, villagers who previously had lived on soybean oil switched to a crude cottonseed oil for their daily cooking. In the mid-1930s, when the price of soybean oil again went down, the villagers switched back to it and no longer used cottonseed oil. Cottonseed oil does not necessarily cause infertility. If the oil has been prepared by first heating the cottonseed and then pressing the oil out of it, the Gossypol is inactivated. But if the oil is prepared by a process of pressing it out without preheating, what is left is a very excellent antifertility agent.

In 1978 the Chinese first presented their exciting research on Gossypol, and in 1980 they reported their results in over ten thousand men using Gossypol as a family's sole method of birth control. Gossypol does not affect sperm production in any hormonal way at all. It is not even distantly or remotely similar to the female pill. It simply has a direct effect on the testicle, which stops its sperm production but has no effect on the production of testosterone. Therefore there is no difficulty with impotence or hormone deprivation. Gossypol does not even affect the early stages of sperm production, which are so important to maintaining the testicle's ability to restore sperm production after the drug is discontinued. It affects only the later stage of sperm production. The problem with Gossypol as it is now available in China is that it is not always reversible, and there are some side effects that preclude its approval in the Western world until these kinks are smoothed out.

Here are the specific details of how the Chinese use this birth control method: A twenty-milligram pill is given to the men every day for thirty-five days. By the fourth week, most of the men have very low sperm counts but aren't definitely protected yet from getting their wives pregnant. By the sixth week, 99.1 percent of the men have no sperm and are quite safe contraceptively. In the second and third phase after the first thirty-five days, the dose is reduced to a single seventy-five- or one-hundred-milligram pill every two weeks. Although the drug was remarkably effective (99.1 percent successful), unfortunately five to 10 percent remained sterile even three years after discontinuing the Gossypol. In some subgroups an even greater percentage remained permanently sterile.

Certain men could be identified who were more likely to suffer this complication. Older men, men with smaller-size testicles, and men with poor dietary nutrition were most likely to fail to regain fertility after discontinuing the pill. Furthermore, men who took the pill for only a brief interval for birth control were less likely to suffer permanent sterility than men who took it for a prolonged period of time. Thus the young man who is well nourished and who has large, or at least normal-size testicles and who takes the drug for a limited period of time may avoid this terrible complication.

Gossypol has some other side effects as well. The main one is the drop in the body's potassium level, which results in muscle weakness and the risk of heart damage. This occurred in 4.7 percent of the ten thousand men but was strictly limited to those with a very deficient amount of potassium in their diet. By incorporating a potassium supplement in the pill, the Chinese have solved this problem. But they haven't yet solved the problem of irreversibility, and until they do, Gossypol will not be available in the West.

The other type of "male pill" is not really a pill but a shot. In fact, it is not really a drug in the strict sense of the word but simply the natural male hormone testosterone. As you have already learned, the pituitary makes two hormones, FSH and LH, which stimulate the ovary in the female to make estrogen from its follicle, ovulate, and then make progesterone from the ovulated follicle. These same two hormones stimulate the testicle in the male to make the hormone testosterone, and sperm. By interfering with the pituitary's release of FSH and LH, we should be able to provide effective birth control to men in exactly the same manner that we do in women with the birth control pill. The reason we can't just give female birth control pills to men (although there is no doubt whatsoever that it would work) is that the estrogen component would create the undesirable side effects of breast enlargement and female body contour, and the drop in testosterone would result in impotence and loss of libido. So all we need for men is a hormone that would suppress FSH and LH, just as the female pill, but would not have the side effects of the female hormones.

To understand this simple concept, however, you have to realize that when you give the female birth control pills to women, the very hormones you are giving to suppress ovulation are an absolute requirement for the female's health and well-being. As soon as you stop the ovary's production of hormone by suppressing FSH and LH from the pituitary, you are depriving the woman of hormones she needs for multiple body functions. She needs estrogens for maintaining bone strength; a healthy, pliant vagina; breast size; and feminine characteristics. If you were simply to give her a GNRH agonist (discussed in the previous section) so that the ovaries simply stopped releasing eggs and stopped making hormones, she would suffer from all the symptoms of menopause, including hot flashes, weak bones, and a dried-up vagina. Therefore, the very estrogen and progesterone in the pill, which are inhibiting her FSH and LH, are necessary to replace the hormone that the pill is preventing her ovaries from making.

The same principle must apply for any hormonal male birth control pill. When you turn off sperm production by suppressing the pituitary gland's release of FSH and LH, you also turn off testosterone production. But if testosterone is the drug you are giving to suppress the pituitary's production of FSH and LH, you won't have a problem. When the newfangled studies attempting to use GNRH to turn off the pituitary gland produced a great wave of excitement, sophisticated researchers who have been working on this for the past ten years simply shook their heads. GNRH was an exciting new toy that could turn off the pituitary gland, but in so doing, turned off the testicles as well, without providing a replacement for the testosterone that the testicles would otherwise be making. So men who were given a shot of GNRH agonist every day had a dramatic reduction in sperm count, but they also had all of the symptoms of castration, including hot flashes, decreased libido, and impotence. Adding insult to injury, most of them still had some sperm production, albeit reduced in amount, so that although they were impotent, they weren't sterile (which is the only reason they went on the GNRH agonist in the first place).

The obvious solution to this problem, which currently is being worked on, is to combine the administration of testosterone replacement with the GNRH agonist. In that way you could turn off the pituitary's production of FSH and LH, but not suffer symptoms of impotence and hot flashes caused by the cessation of testosterone production. If all of this sounds complicated, you will be relieved to hear that there is a simpler approach, which dates back to the mid-1970s, before the fancy new GNRH agonists were available. As you might have expected, much of the confusion generated over the past ten years is related to the commercial undesirability of producing a male birth control method that doesn't make anybody any money.

The pure male hormone testosterone is a very inexpensive drug. The profit margin is very low, because virtually anyone can make it. Many researchers contend that the male system simply is so vigorous that it is impossible to turn off sperm production completely with testosterone. No birth control method for males can be considered reliable unless absolute zero sperm counts are achieved. Many fear that the system in the male is so vigorous that it just cannot be completely turned off as in the female, using normal hormonal feedback mechanisms.

Most efforts to suppress sperm production to zero using testosterone have failed, but one researcher, Dr. Emil Steinberger, considered to be the father of modern male reproductive endocrinology, contends that the difficulty has frequently been in not administering the right dose at the right time. Dr. Steinberger administered testosterone in a very scientific fashion with a dosage regime designed to mimic the body's normal, natural levels of testosterone completely. This was quite different from anybody else's approach. After testing many different dosage schedules, he determined the dose that made the most physiological sense in keeping the testosterone level normal. Using this method, he was able to reduce sperm production to zero in the vast majority of men tested, and to less than one hundred thousand per cubic centimeter in the few remaining. It seemed in the mid-1970s that with his wonderful results we were on the brink of having available a simple, reversible method male birth control. Yet his approach never caught on, probably because everyone who used testosterone before and since then used dosage schedules that were simpler to administer but that anyone should have predicted were bound to fail.

Dr. Steinberger's patients were given a shot of two hundred milligrams of testosterone twice a week for two weeks as an initial induction phase, which reduced the sperm count to zero in virtually all patients who adhered to that schedule. This was a higher dose than anyone else had ever used, and it resulted in a higher than normal level of testosterone for a brief interval. This was necessary initially to turn off sperm production. Thereafter, however, sperm production would remain turned off if that same dose of testosterone were given just once every ten days instead of twice a week. This "maintenance phase" resulted in a normal testosterone level in all the patients, and therefore no hormonal side effects whatsoever, and yet still prevented the testicle from making sperm. When discontinued, all patients recovered normal sperm production and fertility.

Dr. Steinberger also discovered how vigorous the male system is when he tried giving the maintenance dose of testosterone at more convenient intervals of once every fourteen days instead of once every ten days. With just this slight change in schedule, the pituitary began to release LH, and these men developed "breakthrough" sperm production. The reason for this peculiar importance of having a tightly observed ten-day injection schedule really is quite simple. The form of testosterone that is commercially available (and has been available for decades) when given to men who were born with no testicles, maintains normal levels on average for about ten to eleven days. Most such patients who require testosterone injections are placed either on a weekly, nightly, or monthly schedule of testosterone injections. But this schedule is simply for weekly convenience and has nothing to do with the kinetics of how long this hormone lasts in the body after a single injection. Most of such patients notice between about ten and fourteen days after the initial injection that they develop symptoms of hormone deprivation, such as decreased libido, irritability, and even hot flashes.

Therefore, it only makes sense that if you are using this same exact hormone in normal men to suppress sperm production, you should expect its contraceptive effect to be diminished after ten days following the previous injection.

When you examine most of the studies which show that the male system simply is too vigorous to be suppressed completely by testosterone alone, you realize that all of their injections were given at intervals of two weeks and four weeks, or did not have an initial induction phase. Many investigators then began to add female hormones (progestins) to the testosterone in hopes that the two acting together could do a better job of stopping sperm production and yet not create the bad side effect that administering female hormones alone to men would cause. But none of these approaches worked either, because they were all designed to meet a convenient monthly calendar schedule rather than to meet the realities of the schedule required by the particular form of testosterone that is presently available.

Furthermore, what drug company is going to give money to researchers to study a male contraceptive that is so cheaply and readily available that there would be no commercial value in it? The answer to that question finally is at hand, and it gives me great hope that in the next five years there may be a very simple solution to this problem. Few people are going to want to give themselves a shot twice a week for two weeks, and then every ten days thereafter. Even if the schedule were every two weeks, it would be easier to deal with than every ten days. A ten-day schedule of anything simply does not conform to the modern lunar or solar calendar. But now a technology is available that not only will solve this problem but also is likely to make a lot of money for the people who developed it, so these people are going to pour money into research.

This involves silastic microcapsules just like those being used by the manufacturers of Norplant (see previous discussion in this chapter), or by an injection of so-called microspheres. Any hormone can be put either into a silastic capsule for implantation under the skin, or can be injected in microspheres that ensure a constant, steady delivery of the hormone over a prolonged period of time. The problem with silastic capsules is that the hormone must be very potent, as in Norplant, because only a small amount can be delivered at any time from the surface area of the silastic. This, however, is not a problem with microspheres, and therefore virtually any hormone in its natural form can be delivered with this system. This delivery system is quite reliable and has already been shown to provide effective hormonal replacement for female hormones. It is only a matter of time before the companies who developed this technology get approval for human studies utilizing the male hormone. When this occurs, the inconvenience of the Steinberger dosage schedule of testosterone injections will be obviated. In that event, hormonal birth control for the male could conceivably become far and away more popular than for the woman. Here is the reason.

The major difficulty with modern low-dose birth control pills in the woman (which by now you should know are very safe) is the adherence to a daily pill-taking routine. The main problem with a long-term injectable female contraceptive (which is certainly available today in the form of Depo-provera or Norplant) is the menstrual irregularities caused by it. Normally, women have a changing amount of estrogen and progesterone production, resulting in regular, predictable monthly menstruation. When you take away that monthly cycle and give a woman an even, continual level of hormone throughout the month and throughout the year, even though it is quite safe, she is going to have menstrual irregularities.

But in men, the normal mode of hormone production is constant. There is no monthly cycle of hormone production in men, and therefore hormonal contraception is ideally suited for men rather than women. If women can have a simple injection of Depo-provera every three months, or a simple implant of Norplant once every five years that will reduce their risk of pregnancy to 0.2 percent, a similar approach now can be made available for men. Contrary to the negative expression of male researchers who feel that the male system is just too vigorous to suppress, this method of contraception is perfectly suited for men but never was ideally suited for women.

A New Morning-After Pill: RU 486

You may soon be hearing about a controversial new pill that will be a blessing for rape victims, but a source of agonizing debate for those embroiled in the politics of abortion. The pill has a terrible name that no commercially savvy American businessperson would have ever dreamed up: RU 486!

This drug, developed recently by the French, supported by the World Health Organization, is an excellent oral contraceptive but also can be used to cause a relatively symptom-free early abortion. As a backup method of birth control, it can be used if a condom breaks or a diaphragm becomes dislodged. A single use prevents pregnancy by blocking the uterine lining from absorbing progesterone. Thus it renders the uterus unreceptive to sperm or egg, and causes a prompt menstruation. Early studies show it to be relatively symptom-free and reliable for preventing conception and promptly ending the cycle.

RU 486 has been tested in France on one hundred women who were already less than ten days pregnant. That means they had only noticed a missed period for ten days or less, but pregnancy was suspected because of rape or some contraceptive foul-up such as a dislodged diaphragm. Early pregnancy was proven by a super-sensitive blood hormone assay for HCG (see Chapter One). Eighty-five of these one hundred women simply menstruated promptly after taking the pill, and never carried their pregnancy. The drug is expected to get prompt approval in France and Sweden. However, in the United States there is bound to be a storm of controversy. Those concerned about the 50 percent of New York teenagers who get pregnant will demand the availability of RU 486, and those who oppose abortion will be horrified. Ironically, abortion clinics may worry over the loss of business (because RU 486 is certainly safer than a surgical abortion), and it may only be non-profit groups such as Planned Parenthood that push for its approval. This is unfortunate because what's non-controversial is that the drug would be a relief for victims of rape or incest who could take this pill right after the incident occurs.

It may be years before this drug becomes available, and even then it may run into problems of government approval because it can also be used for up to a month after pregnancy to cause an intentional miscarriage. This contraceptive is bound to become the center of a heated debate, if anyone can remember its ungainly name.

Index

Birth control pill (*continued*)
of, 113–114, 122; and reduced bleeding, 131–133; side effects of, 2, 9, 16,
50, 52, 99, 106, 107–122, 131; triphasics, 52, 111, 122, 127, 128–129; use
after childbirth, 137–138
Birth defects, 261; and Depo-provera, 297–
298; and diaphragm use, 179–180, 197;
and failed vasectomy, 235. *See also* Fetal abnormalities
Bottle feeding, health hazards of, 94–95,
112
Breakthrough bleeding, 134–136
Breast cancer, 179; and birth control pill,
111–113; and Depo-provera, 299, 300
Breast disease, 112, 140; birth control pill
prevention of, 2, 16, 98, 114, 122; and
Depo-provera, 299, 300
Breast-feeding, 8–9, 87; advantages of, 94–
96; animal vs. human, 91–92; and
birth control pill, 93, 137–138; and
IUD, 138
Breast-feeding as birth control, 18–19, 90–
96, 137; reliability of, 91, 95
Bulbous urethra, 41

Calendar method of rhythm birth control,
49, 58–61, 65, 73, 83; failure rate, 85
Cancer: and birth control pills, 111–116,
122, 141, 300; and Depo-provera, 294–
295, 297, 298–300. *See also* Breast
cancer; Cervical cancer; Ovarian cancer; Uteran cancer
Capacitation, 45
Cardiovascular disease, and birth control
pill, 116–122, 137
Career vs. childrearing, 17–18
Catholicism, and birth control, 49, 54, 61,
73, 201, 260
Cats, ovulation in, 29–30, 55
Cautery: in tubal sterilization, 272–274,
275, 276, 283, 284–289, 291, 292; in
vasectomy, 221, 236, 239, 241
Cervical cancer, 15, 173, 175; and birth
control pill, 115–116; condom and diaphragm protection against, 171, 176,
189; and Depo-provera controversy,
297
Cervical cap, 181, 194–195
Cervical mucus, 26, 28, 31; birth control
pill effect on, 101, 106; cyclic changes
in production of, 43–44, 56–57, 75–
82; Depo-provera effect on, 295, 301;
sperm invasion of, 43–45, 76, 81
Cervical mucus (Billings) method, 75–83;
failure rate, 85–86
Cervix, 25, 26, 28, 31, 41; definition of, 21;
and IUD insertion, 155–157, 162;
monthly changes in, 56–57, 75–82;
sperm invasion of, 43–45
Chancroid, 173
Child death, 260; crib death, 210, 260–261;
and sterilization, 245–247, 260–262
Child spacing, breast-feeding as aid in, 90–
96

Chinese IUDs, 166–167
Chinese male pill, 308–309
Chlamydia, 15, 106, 174, 175, 189
Choice of birth control, 16–17
Cigarette smoking, and birth control pill,
116, 120–121, 138, 140
Cilia, 32, 265
Clomid, 10, 103, 123, 141, 243
Coil spring rim diaphragm, 185
Coitus interruptus, 199, 201
Combined temperature and cervical mucus
method (symptothermal), 82–83
Condoms, 2, 14, 16, 84, 170–172, 197–201,
280; defective, 200; disadvantages of,
172, 179–180, 200; as disease protection, 15–16, 115, 170–171, 176, 179,
189, 197, 200; failure rate, 124, 144,
172, 182–183, 191, 199; history of,
197–198; Japanese, 172, 198; popularity of, 170, 171–172, 198, 199–200;
purchase of, 171, 177; spermicide, 196;
types of, 200
Congenital abnormalities, 136, 139, 152,
179–180, 235. *See also* Fetal abnormalities
Contraceptive spermicides, 2, 4, 16, 136,
195–197; and birth defects, 179–180,
197; as disease protection, 196; failure
rate, 124, 196; foam, 2, 4, 196; risks
of, 179–180, 196–197; use with diaphragm, 181–184, 185, 188, 189, 196
Copper IUDs, 146–151, 159–160, 165,
168–169; Copper 7, 7, 53, 147–150,
153, 165, 169
Corpus luteum, 28, 31, 48, 82, 100
Cumulus oophorus, 46

Dalkon Shield IUD, 5–6, 143, 146, 148,
159, 163, 167–169
Demulen, 128, 129
Depo-provera, 294–303; and cancer controversy, 294–295, 297, 298–300; disadvantages, 295–298, 302, 303; failure
rate, 294, 301; FDA approval denied,
294–298, 300; fertility reestablished
after, 303; how it works, 300–303;
menstrual cycle disrupted by, 295–
296, 298, 301, 302, 303; vs. Norplant,
304–305
Diabetes, 140
Diaphragm(s), 2, 16, 105, 115, 170, 181–
189, 280; as disease protection, 170–
171, 176, 179, 189; dislodged, 188–
189; failure rate, 124, 144, 172, 191,
193; and fetal abnormalities, 179–180,
197; history of, 181–182, 194; how it
works, 183–184; insertion of, 185–188;
risks of, 179–180, 197; spermicide
used with, 181–184, 185, 189, 196; and
toxic shock syndrome, 193–194; types
and fitting of, 184–186
Diarrheal infections, in infants, 94–95
Divorce, 14
Dogs, hormonal tests on, 299–300
Douching, 82, 184